Management of the Breast and Axilla in the Neoadjuvant Setting

Atilla Soran • Faina Nakhlis
Editors

Management of the Breast and Axilla in the Neoadjuvant Setting

Springer

Editors
Atilla Soran
Breast Surgery
University of Pittsburgh Medical Center
Pittsburgh, PA, USA

Faina Nakhlis
Dana-Farber Harvard Cancer Centar
Brigham and Women's Hospital
Boston, MA, USA

ISBN 978-3-030-88019-4 ISBN 978-3-030-88020-0 (eBook)
https://doi.org/10.1007/978-3-030-88020-0

This Springer imprint is published by the registered company Springer Nature Switzerland AG
The registered company address is: Gewerbestrasse 11, 6330 Cham, Switzerland

Preface

Over the last several decades, breast cancer management has made great strides in the improvement of oncologic treatment outcomes, particularly so in patients with early stage disease. While widespread access to screening resulting in early detection is undoubtedly to be credited for this trend, at the same time, the management of breast cancer has evolved to be an intricate multidisciplinary collaboration between breast imagers, surgeons, medical oncologists, and radiation oncologist. As a result, with better mutual understanding of multidisciplinary goals and challenges, the treatment strategies have become more individualized, with a great emphasis being placed on the intrinsic disease biology. Furthermore, the indications for neoadjuvant systemic therapy have significantly broadened, with a substantial number of patients with early stage breast cancer being able to take advantage of this strategy to decrease the extent of breast surgery they would undergo at its completion. As such, the management of the axilla in these patients has presented new challenges as well as new opportunities to de-escalate the extent of local therapy and, consequently, its toxicity.

This text is designed to present a comprehensive and state-of-the-art approach to contemporary multidisciplinary management of the axilla in early stage breast cancer patients treated with neoadjuvant systemic therapy. Parts will address issues faced by breast imagers, medical oncologists, surgeons, and radiation oncologists involved in the care of these patients. Written by experts in the respective fields, each of these parts will address characterization of the extent of axillary disease at presentation, appropriate selection of neoadjuvant systemic therapy to maximally downstage the axilla, and refinement of subsequent axillary surgery and radiation to maximize patient safety and minimize toxicity. A thorough review of the existing literature addressing the particular topic will be included in each part, enriched with extensive illustrations.

Editors and authors believe that this book, with its comprehensive summary of contemporary data on the management of the axilla in patients receiving neoadjuvant systemic therapy, will serve as a valuable guide in daily clinical practice.

Pittsburgh, PA, USA — Atilla Soran
Boston, MA, USA — Faina Nakhlis

Contents

Contributors

Gabrielle M. Baker Department of Pathology, Beth Israel Deaconess Medical Center, Boston, MA, USA

Department of Pathology, Harvard Medical School, Boston, MA, USA

Jose G. Bazan Department of Radiation Oncology, The Ohio State University Comprehensive Cancer Center – Arthur G. James Cancer Hospital and Solove Research Institute, Stefanie Spielman Comprehensive Breast Center, Columbus, OH, USA

Kristie Bobolis Department of Medicine, Sutter Roseville Medical Center, Roseville, CA, USA

Adam M. Brufsky University of Pittsburgh Physicians, Pittsburgh, PA, USA

UPMC Hillman Cancer Center, Magee Women's Hospital, Pittsburgh, PA, USA

Allyson L. Chesebro Breast Imaging Division, Department of Radiology, Brigham and Women's Hospital, Dana-Farber Cancer Institute, Boston, MA, USA

Stephanie Chung Division of Breast Imaging, Department of Radiology, Brigham and Women's Hospital, Boston, MA, USA

Beth Z. Clark UPMC Magee-Women's Hospital, Pittsburgh, PA, USA

Eva C. Gombos Breast Imaging Division, Department of Radiology, Brigham and Women's Hospital, Dana-Farber Cancer Institute, Boston, MA, USA

Vikram Gorantla Department of Pathology, University of Pittsburgh School of Medicine, Pittsburgh, PA, USA

John W. Hall IV UPMC Department of Radiology, Pittsburgh, PA, USA

Tara Hyder University of Pittsburgh Physicians, Pittsburgh, PA, USA

Ronald R. Johnson Breast Surgical Oncology, University of Pittsburgh, Pittsburgh, PA, USA

Olga Kantor Division of Breast Surgery, Department of Surgery, Brigham and Women's Hospital, Boston, MA, USA

Breast Oncology Program, Dana-Farber/Brigham and Women's Cancer Center, Boston, MA, USA

Joanna S. Lee Breast Surgical Oncology, University of Pittsburgh, Pittsburgh, PA, USA

Mina Makary Department of Hematology/Oncology, Geisinger Health System, Danville, PA, USA

Juan Luis Gomez Marti Department of Pathology, University of Pittsburgh School of Medicine, Pittsburgh, PA, USA

Priscilla F. McAuliffe Breast Surgical Oncology, University of Pittsburgh, Pittsburgh, PA, USA

Azadeh Nasrazadani University of Pittsburgh Physicians, Pittsburgh, PA, USA

UPMC Hillman Cancer Center, Magee Women's Hospital, Pittsburgh, PA, USA

Beth Overmoyer Susan F. Smith Center for Women's Cancer, Dana Farber Cancer Institute, Boston, MA, USA

Leah H. Portnow Breast Imaging Division, Department of Radiology, Brigham and Women's Hospital, Dana-Farber Cancer Institute, Boston, MA, USA

Sughra Raza Division of Breast Imaging, Department of Radiology, Brigham and Women's Hospital, Boston, MA, USA

William M. Sikov Breast Health Center, Program in Women's Oncology, Women and Infants Hospital of Rhode Island and Warren Alpert Medical School of Brown University, Providence, RI, USA

Victor G. Vogel Department of Hematology/Oncology, Geisinger Health System, Danville, PA, USA

Uzma Waheed Breast Imaging Division, Department of Radiology, Stanford University, Palo Alto, CA, USA

Adrienne Waks Department of Medical Oncology, Breast Oncology Program, Dana-Farber Cancer Institute, Boston, MA, USA

Anna Weiss Division of Breast Surgery, Department of Surgery, Brigham and Women's Hospital, Boston, MA, USA

Breast Oncology Program, Dana-Farber/Brigham and Women's Cancer Center, Boston, MA, USA

Julia R. White Department of Radiation Oncology, The Ohio State University Comprehensive Cancer Center – Arthur G. James Cancer Hospital and Solove Research Institute, Stefanie Spielman Comprehensive Breast Center, Columbus, OH, USA

Margarita Zuley Breast Imaging Division, Department of Radiology, University of Pittsburgh Medical Center, Pittsburgh, PA, USA

Part I
History of Neoadjuvant Systemic Therapy in Breast Cancer

Chapter 1
Neoadjuvant Therapy for Breast Cancer

Mina Makary and Victor G. Vogel

Evolution of the Indications for Neoadjuvant Therapy

Neoadjuvant therapy, initially used only for locally advanced breast cancer, has become more common for patients with operable disease. This allows more individuals to undergo breast-conserving procedures and enables observation of response to treatment. Long-term treatment outcome correlates significantly with both clinical and pathologic tumor response rates. In 2008, Rastogi and her colleagues provided an update of extended outcomes for two preoperative chemotherapy trials of the National Surgical Adjuvant Breast and Bowel Project (NSABP), Protocols B-18 and B-27 [1]. NSABP Protocol B-18 was designed to determine whether four cycles of doxorubicin and cyclophosphamide (AC) administered preoperatively improved breast cancer disease-free survival (DFS) and overall survival (OS) compared with AC administered postoperatively [2–4]. Protocol B-27 was designed to determine the effect of adding docetaxel (T) to preoperative AC on tumor response rates, DFS, and OS [5, 6].

Eligible patients for B-18 had operable, palpable breast cancer (T1–3, N0–1, M0) diagnosed by core needle biopsy or fine-needle aspirate (FNA). NSABP Protocol B-27 was opened to accrual in December 1995 and closed in December 2000 after 2411 patients had been randomly assigned. Patient characteristics for B-27 are listed in Table 1.1. Women who had primary operable breast cancer (T1c–3, N0–1, M0 or T1–3, N1, M0) diagnosed by core biopsy or FNA were eligible. The stratification variables for both studies were age, clinical tumor size, and clinical nodal status. Because FNA results could be used to establish eligibility, hormone receptor status was not available at random assignment for these patients, so it was not used as a stratification variable.

M. Makary · V. G. Vogel (✉)
Department of Hematology/Oncology, Geisinger Health System, Danville, PA, USA
e-mail: mmmakary@geisinger.edu; vgvogel@geisinger.edu

A. Soran, F. Nakhlis (eds.), *Management of the Breast and Axilla in the Neoadjuvant Setting*, https://doi.org/10.1007/978-3-030-88020-0_1

Table 1.1 Chemo-immunotherapy regimens for neoadjuvant therapy [9]

Breast cancer phenotype	Regimens
HER2-positive	Docetaxel, carboplatin, trastuzumab, and pertuzumab (TCHP) Docetaxel, carboplatin, and trastuzumab (TCH) Paclitaxel and trastuzumab Doxorubicin and cyclophosphamide followed by paclitaxel and trastuzumab (higher incidence of declines in left ventricular ejection fraction), with or without pertuzumab
Estrogen receptor-positive	Dose-dense doxorubicin/cyclophosphamide followed by weekly paclitaxel (or paclitaxel every 2 weeks) Docetaxel and cyclophosphamide Epirubicin and cyclophosphamide Cyclophosphamide, methotrexate, and 5-fluorouracil; anthracycline is contraindicated
Triple-negative	Weekly paclitaxel with carboplatin and pembrolizumab in weeks 1, 4, 7, and 10 followed by dose-dense doxorubicin and cyclophosphamide with pembrolizumab every 3 weeks

In Protocol B-18, patients were randomly assigned to either surgery (lumpectomy and axillary lymph node dissection or modified radical mastectomy) followed by four cycles of AC chemotherapy (doxorubicin 60 mg/m^2 and cyclophosphamide 600 mg/m^2) every 21 days or the same chemotherapy followed by surgery. Before random assignment, surgeons were required to disclose the intended surgical procedure (lumpectomy or mastectomy) without considering possible downstaging by chemotherapy. Patients ≥50 years of age received tamoxifen 10 mg orally twice a day for 5 years, starting after chemotherapy, regardless of hormone receptor status, whereas women less than 50 years of age did not receive hormonal therapy. Patients undergoing lumpectomy received whole-breast irradiation [2–4].

In Protocol B-27, all patients were assigned to receive four cycles of AC every 21 days before surgery. Patients in groups 1 and 3 did not receive further preoperative chemotherapy, whereas patients in group 2 were assigned to receive four cycles of T preoperatively at 100 mg/m^2 every 21 days. After the completion of AC in groups 1 and 3 or AC followed by T in group 2, patients underwent surgery (either lumpectomy plus axillary node dissection or modified radical mastectomy). Patients in group 3 received four cycles of postoperative T (100 mg/m^2). In all study patients, tamoxifen (20 mg/d for 5 years) was to be initiated on the first day of chemotherapy regardless of age or hormone receptor status [5, 6].

In Protocol B-18, 751 patients were assigned to receive preoperative AC, and 742 patients were assigned to receive postoperative AC. In B-27, 784 patients were assigned to receive preoperative AC followed by surgery, 783 patients were assigned to AC followed by T and surgery, and 777 patients were assigned to AC followed by surgery and then T.

Results from Protocol B-18 showed no statistically significant differences in DFS and OS between the two groups. However, there were trends in favor of neoadjuvant chemotherapy for DFS and OS in women less than 50 years old (hazard ratio [HR] = 0.85, $P = 0.09$ for DFS; HR = 0.81, $P = 0.06$ for OS). DFS that was conditional on being event-free for 5 years also demonstrated a strong trend in favor of the preoperative treatment (HR = 0.81, $P = 0.053$).

Protocol B-27 demonstrated that the addition of T to AC did not significantly impact DFS or OS. Preoperative T added to AC did, nevertheless, significantly increase the proportion of patients having pathological complete responses (pCRs) compared with preoperative AC alone (26% vs. 13%, respectively; $P = 0.0001$). In both studies, patients who achieved a pCR continued to have superior DFS and OS outcomes compared with patients who did not achieve a complete response. The B-18 and B-27 trials concluded that preoperative therapy is equivalent to adjuvant therapy. B-27 showed that the addition of preoperative taxanes to AC improves response. These trials and others set the stage for the development of current preoperative therapy for operable breast cancer.

Current Evolution and Application of Preoperative Treatment Strategies

The extent of invasive breast disease and its biologic aggressiveness are the principal determinants of the outcome of chemotherapy for breast cancer. Clinical and pathologic staging help in assessing the extent of disease, but each is imprecise. Tumor grade, hormone receptor assays, HER2 oncogene amplification, and genomic assays have prognostic value and are key to determining systemic therapy. Controversy has surrounded the choice of primary therapy of stage I, II, and III breast carcinoma. Neoadjuvant therapy has become popular given its three potential advantages: (1) the neoadjuvant approach initiates systemic therapy early and avoids delays imposed by a primary surgical procedure; (2) primary chemo- and/or immunotherapy can decrease the size of the primary tumor and convert a mastectomy to a lumpectomy; and (3) preoperative therapy constitutes an in vivo sensitivity assay allowing an assessment of treatment response. In addition, in some cases of either triple-negative or HER2-amplified breast cancer, the response to neoadjuvant therapy determines the need and type of postoperative, or adjuvant, systemic therapy.

Patients with hormone receptor-negative, triple-negative, or HER2-positive breast cancers are more likely to have a (pCR) (meaning no residual invasive cancer in either breast or lymph nodes at the time of surgery) in response to neoadjuvant chemotherapy than those with hormone receptor-positive breast cancer [7]. A pCR at the time of surgery, especially in hormone receptor-negative tumors, is associated with improvement in event-free and overall survival.

Survival after neoadjuvant chemotherapy is like that seen with postoperative adjuvant chemotherapy [8, 9]; that is, no improvements in disease-free or overall survival have yet been demonstrated with preoperative systemic therapy. Randomized trials have demonstrated equivalent mortality for pre- or postoperative delivery of similar systemic therapy [4, 10–21]. A meta-analysis conducted by the Early Breast Cancer Trialists' Collaborative Group based upon data from 4756 women in ten trials that were initiated between 1983 and 2002 [22] showed there were no significant differences between neoadjuvant chemotherapy and adjuvant chemotherapy in the risk of distant recurrence (15-year rate of 38% in both arms) or breast cancer mortality (34% in both arms). The use of neoadjuvant chemotherapy was associated, nevertheless, with an increased frequency of breast-conserving therapy (65% vs. 49%). Importantly, it was also associated with an increased risk of local recurrence (15-year local recurrence rate, 21.4% vs. 15.9%; rate ratio 1.37, 95% CI 1.17–1.61). This increased risk of recurrence may not be seen, however, with current therapies.

Candidates for Neoadjuvant Therapy

Candidates for neoadjuvant therapy for breast cancer are listed in Fig. 1.1. Discussions among the surgical oncologist, radiation oncologist, and medical oncologist are important in determining the goals and potential benefits of neoadjuvant therapy for a given patient.

1. Locally Advanced Breast Cancer
Patients with locally advanced breast cancer (stage III disease, T3, or T4 lesions), no matter the subtype, are recommended to receive neoadjuvant therapy because their cancers, due to their locally advanced nature, are not amenable to a negative margin resection or breast conservation (the latter is not applicable to patients with inflammatory breast cancer, who require a modified radical mastectomy upon completion of neoadjuvant chemotherapy) and because their risk of distant recurrence warrants prompt initiation of systemic treatment. Many patients with tumors larger than 5 cm (T3), even if potentially operable, are considered to have locally advanced disease and have been included in neoadjuvant therapy clinical trials.

2. Selected Cases of Early-Stage Breast Cancer
Patients with early-stage breast cancer (stage I or II) are appropriate candidates for neoadjuvant therapy if breast-conserving surgery is not possible due to a high tumor-to-breast size ratio or if their anticipated cosmetic outcome would be

Fig. 1.1 Candidates for neoadjuvant systemic therapy

- Locally advanced breast cancer
- Early-stage breast cancer
  With a large tumor-to-breast size ratio
  Large tumors (>4 cm)
- Node-positive breast cancer
  Bulky or matted nodes
  N3 nodal disease
- T4 tumors
- Patients who have temporary contraindication(s) to surgery

suboptimal due to tumor location [23]. Additionally, patients with smaller (T1c) triple-negative breast cancers or HER2-positive cancers may be offered neoadjuvant therapy, particularly if they might benefit from additional treatments in the adjuvant, postsurgical setting if residual disease is identified.

The role of neoadjuvant therapy in patients with early-stage hormone receptor-positive, HER2-negative breast cancers is less clear. Neoadjuvant treatment can induce tumor shrinkage that may allow breast conservation in a patient who otherwise would have required mastectomy. Whether such patients should be offered neoadjuvant chemotherapy or neoadjuvant endocrine therapy depends on many factors, including patient age, comorbidities, and clinical stage. Tumor characteristics including grade and intensity of hormone receptor expression may help differentiate between patients more or less likely to respond to chemotherapy versus endocrine therapy. Proliferation indices or gene expression assays such as Oncotype Dx may help oncologists select between these treatment options [7].

3. Limited Clinically Node-Positive Disease
Neoadjuvant chemotherapy may be used to downstage the axillary nodes in patients with limited clinically node-positive disease (cN1). Neoadjuvant chemotherapy can convert cN1 patients to pN0, especially in patients with more aggressive breast cancer subtypes. Results of recent studies suggest that many of these patients can be managed effectively with sentinel lymph node biopsy with much lower rates of lymphedema and other complications [24].

Patients with Temporary Contraindications for Surgery

NST is a treatment option for patients who have medical contraindications to undergoing surgery at diagnosis but in whom surgery is anticipated at a later date, such as women with breast cancer diagnosed during pregnancy or patients requiring short-term anticoagulation such as those with recent pulmonary embolism, deep-vein thrombosis, or placement of drug-eluding coronary stents. It is also a possible strategy for the elderly with significant comorbidities.

Regimens for Neoadjuvant Therapy (Table 1.1)

1. HER2-Positive Breast Cancer
Standard neoadjuvant therapy for patients with HER2-positive disease consists of chemotherapy and HER2-directed therapy, specifically trastuzumab, with or without pertuzumab. Results from trials using these regimens will be reviewed below.

Chemotherapy

The phase III TRAIN-2 trial of 438 patients with stage II–III HER2-positive breast cancer was randomly assigned to anthracycline-containing chemotherapy (three cycles of 5-fluorouracil, epirubicin, and cyclophosphamide followed by six cycles of paclitaxel and carboplatin) versus non-anthracycline-based chemotherapy (nine cycles paclitaxel and carboplatin), with trastuzumab and pertuzumab administered every 3 weeks with all chemotherapy cycles [25]. The rates of pCR did not differ between the arms (67% vs. 68%). Updated results from this study demonstrated equivalent 3-year event-free (94% vs. 93%) and overall (98% vs. 98%) survival for the anthracycline-free versus the anthracycline-containing regimens, respectively [26]. No patient subgroup could be identified whose long-term outcomes benefited from inclusion of the anthracycline, and patients who received the anthracycline experienced higher rates of febrile neutropenia (10% vs. 1%) and significant decline in left ventricular ejection fraction (36% vs. 22%).

Targeted (Biologic) Therapy

Dual anti-HER2 blockade associated with trastuzumab plus lapatinib or with trastuzumab plus pertuzumab has shown significant improvements in the pCR rate when compared with chemotherapy associated with one anti-HER2 agent in the neoadjuvant setting [27].

The NeoALTTO trial enrolled women with HER2-positive early breast cancer and randomly assigned them to receive oral lapatinib and trastuzumab or lapatinib plus trastuzumab in combination for 6 weeks, followed by an additional 12 weeks of the assigned anti-HER2 therapy in combination with weekly paclitaxel [28]. Surgery was done 4 weeks after the last dose of paclitaxel. After surgery, women received three cycles of FEC (fluorouracil 500 mg/m^2 plus epirubicin 100 mg/m^2 plus cyclophosphamide 500 mg/m^2) given intravenously every 3 weeks followed by 34 weeks of the same assigned neoadjuvant anti-HER2 therapy. Analyses showed that the 3-year event-free survival was improved significantly for women who achieved pathological complete response compared with those who did not (HR 0.38, 95% CI 0.22–0.63, $P = 0.0003$), as was 3-year overall survival (0.35, 0.15–0.70, $P = 0.005$).

Trastuzumab

In the phase II NOAH trial ($n = 235$), the addition of every-3-week trastuzumab to neoadjuvant anthracycline- and taxane-based chemotherapy was associated with a pCR rate of 38% compared with 19% with chemotherapy alone; patients assigned to trastuzumab resumed this treatment after surgery to complete a full year of treatment [28, 29]. Long-term follow-up (5.4 years) revealed improved event-free survival (EFS) with the addition of trastuzumab (43% vs. 58%; HR 0.64, 95% CI 0.544–0.930) [21]. Among patients who achieved a pCR, those treated with trastuzumab had significantly better EFS than those who did not (HR 0.29, 0.11–0.78), demonstrating the superiority of the neoadjuvant chemotherapy plus HER2-targeted therapy combination at eradicating occult metastatic disease even among patients with an excellent locoregional response [29, 30].

Pertuzumab

Pertuzumab is a monoclonal antibody that binds to a different epitope on HER2 than trastuzumab, blocking the formation of HER2/HER3 heterodimers, which is believed to be an important mechanism of resistance to trastuzumab. The NeoSphere study, a randomized multicenter, open-label, phase 2 trial, showed that patients given pertuzumab and trastuzumab plus docetaxel had a significantly improved pCR rate compared with those given trastuzumab plus docetaxel, without substantial differences in tolerability [31]. Treatment-naive women with HER2-positive breast cancer were stratified by operable, locally advanced, and inflammatory breast cancer and by hormone receptor expression to receive four neoadjuvant cycles of trastuzumab (8 mg/kg loading dose, followed by 6 mg/kg every 3 weeks) plus docetaxel (75 mg/m(2), escalating, if tolerated, to 100 mg/m(2) every 3 weeks; group A) or pertuzumab (loading dose 840 mg, followed by 420 mg every 3 weeks) and trastuzumab plus docetaxel (group B) or pertuzumab and trastuzumab (group C) or pertuzumab plus docetaxel (group D). Patients given pertuzumab and trastuzumab plus docetaxel (group B) had a significantly improved pathological complete response rate (45.8% [95% CI 36.1–55.7]) compared with those given trastuzumab plus docetaxel (group A; 29.0% [20.6–38.5]; $P = 0.0141$). Twenty-four percent (24.0% [15.8–33.7]) of women given pertuzumab plus docetaxel (group D) had a pathological complete response, as did 16.8% [10.3–25.3] given pertuzumab and trastuzumab (group C).

The TRYPHAENA trial assessed long-term efficacy and cardiac safety outcomes in patients with HER2-positive early breast cancer treated with neoadjuvant pertuzumab plus trastuzumab with anthracycline-containing or anthracycline-free chemotherapy. During post-treatment follow-up, only 2–5% of patients had any grade of left ventricular systolic dysfunction; 11–16% of patients experienced left ventricular ejection fraction declines ≥10% from baseline to <50%. Long-term disease-free and progression-free survivals were similar between groups. Patients who achieved a pCR had improved disease-free survival [32].

2. Hormone Receptor-Positive, HER2-Negative Breast Cancer

Patients with hormone receptor-positive breast cancer have a lower chance of achieving a pathological complete response with neoadjuvant therapy than those patients with triple-negative or HER2-positive breast cancers. Studies indicate similar response rates with neoadjuvant endocrine therapy compared to neoadjuvant chemotherapy. Typically, responses are not appreciated unless 4–6 or more months of hormonal therapy are given. Outside a clinical trial setting, the use of neoadjuvant hormonal therapy is generally restricted to postmenopausal patients who are unable or unwilling to tolerate chemotherapy [9]. According to the NCCN, neoadjuvant endocrine therapy alone may be offered to those with strongly hormone receptor-positive tumors. The endocrine therapy options include an aromatase inhibitor (with ovarian suppression for premenopausal women) or tamoxifen. The preferred endocrine therapy option for postmenopausal women is an aromatase inhibitor.

3. Triple-Negative Breast Cancer

Neoadjuvant chemotherapy leads to pathological complete response in up 50% or more of patients with triple-negative breast cancer [33]. Patients who achieve a pathological complete response seem to have a similar prognosis to other breast cancer subtypes with pathological complete response [9].

A randomized phase 2 trial (GeparSixto) was aimed to assess the efficacy of the addition of carboplatin to neoadjuvant therapy for triple-negative and HER2-positive breast cancer [34]. Patients were treated for 18 weeks with paclitaxel (80 mg/m^2 once a week) and non-pegylated liposomal doxorubicin (20 mg/m^2 once a week). Patients with triple-negative breast cancer received simultaneous bevacizumab (15 mg/kg intravenously every 3 weeks). Patients with HER2-positive disease received simultaneous trastuzumab (8 mg/kg initial dose with subsequent doses of 6 mg/kg intravenously every 3 weeks) and lapatinib (750 mg daily); 296 patients were randomly assigned to receive carboplatin and 299 to no additional carboplatin, of whom 295 and 293 started treatment, respectively. In this final analysis, 43.7% (95% CI 38.1–49.4) in the carboplatin group achieved a pathological complete response, compared with 36.9% (31.3–42.4) without carboplatin (odds ratio 1.33, 95% CI 0.96–1.85; $P = 0.107$). Of the patients with triple-negative breast cancer, 53.2% achieved a pCR with carboplatin, compared with 36.9% without ($P = 0.005$). The addition of neoadjuvant carboplatin to a regimen of a taxane, an anthracycline, and targeted therapy significantly increases the proportion of patients achieving a pathological complete response. This regimen seems to increase responses in patients with triple-negative breast cancer, but not in those with HER2-positive breast cancers. CALGB 40603 [35] and ADAPT [36] triple-negative trials showed improved pCR rates with platinum-based neoadjuvant therapy.

Pembrolizumab

In a phase 3 trial, patients with previously untreated stage II or stage III triple-negative breast cancer were randomly assigned to receive neoadjuvant therapy with four cycles of pembrolizumab (at a dose of 200 mg) every 3 weeks plus paclitaxel and carboplatin or placebo every 3 weeks plus paclitaxel and carboplatin [37]. The two groups then received an additional four cycles of pembrolizumab or placebo, and both groups received doxorubicin-cyclophosphamide or epirubicin-cyclophosphamide. After definitive surgery, the patients received adjuvant pembrolizumab or placebo every 3 weeks for up to nine cycles. The primary end points were pCR at the time of definitive surgery and event-free survival in the intention-to-treat population.

At the first interim analysis, 64.8% of women in the pembrolizumab-chemotherapy group achieved pCR, compared with only 51.2% (95% CI, 44.1–58.3) in the placebo-chemotherapy group. After a median follow-up of 15.5 months, 7.4% of patients in the pembrolizumab-chemotherapy group and 11.8% of patients in the placebo-chemotherapy group had disease progression that precluded definitive surgery, had local or distant recurrence or a second primary tumor, or died from any cause (hazard ratio, 0.63; 95% CI, 0.43–0.93). Across all treatment phases, the incidence of treatment-related adverse events of grade 3 or higher was 78.0% in the pembrolizumab-chemotherapy group and 73.0% in the placebo-chemotherapy group, including death in 0.4% (three patients) and 0.3% (one patient), respectively.

Incorporation of some immunotherapy in the neoadjuvant management of TNBCs remains investigational in the USA [38]. Atezolizumab plus neoadjuvant chemotherapy for triple-negative breast cancer was assessed in the IMpassion031 trial. Among over 300 patients with treatment-naïve stage II–III TNBC, the addition of the PD-L1-targeted monoclonal antibody atezolizumab to neoadjuvant chemotherapy improved pathological complete response rates (58% vs. 41%). Additional studies are needed to assess fully the role of atezolizumab in the neoadjuvant treatment setting.

Achieving a Pathological Complete Response

Pathological complete response (pCR) to systemic therapy is associated with an extremely favorable disease-free and overall survival, particularly in situations in which all treatment is given preoperatively. The correlation between pathological response and long-term outcomes is strongest for TNBC, somewhat less so for HER2-positive disease and least for ER-positive disease. Staging following neoadjuvant therapy is designated with "yc" or "yp" prefix to the T and N classification. There is no anatomical stage group assigned if there is a pCR to neoadjuvant therapy, for example, ypT0ypN0M0. The cellular fibrous reaction to invasive tumor cells is generally included in the measurement of a tumor prior to treatment; however, the dense fibrosis observed following neoadjuvant treatment is generally not included in the pathological measurement because its extent may overestimate the residual tumor volume [27].

Evaluation of tumor response at surgery and its association with long-term outcome, as well as the definition of pCR and its prognostic impact on survival in intrinsic breast cancer subtypes, has been reported [39]. Among 6377 patients with primary breast cancer receiving neoadjuvant anthracycline-taxane-based chemotherapy in seven randomized trials, pCR was defined as no invasive and no in situ residuals in breast or lymph nodes. In this way, pCR can discriminate between patients with either favorable or unfavorable outcomes. Patients with noninvasive or focally invasive residual disease or with involved lymph nodes should not be considered as having achieved pCR. Additionally, pCR is a suitable surrogate end point for patients with luminal B/HER2-negative, HER2-positive (non-luminal), and triple-negative disease, but not for those with luminal B/HER2-positive or luminal A tumors.

Investigators have compared responses to neoadjuvant chemotherapy and survival between patients with TNBC and non-TNBC [40]. Clinical and pathologic parameters, pCR, survival measurements, and organ-specific relapse rates were compared between patients with TNBC and non-TNBC. Two hundred fifty-five patients (23%) had TNBC. Patients with TNBC compared with non-TNBC had significantly higher pCR rates (22% vs. 11%; $P = 0.034$) but decreased 3-year progression-free survival rates ($P < 0.0001$) and 3-year overall survival rates ($P < 0.0001$). TNBC was associated with increased risk for visceral metastases ($P = 0.0005$), lower risk for bone recurrence ($P = 0.027$), and shorter post-recurrence survival ($P < 0.0001$). Recurrence and death rates were higher for TNBC only in the first 3 years. If pCR was achieved, patients with TNBC and non-TNBC had similar survival ($P = 0.24$). In contrast, patients with residual disease had worse overall survival if they had TNBC compared with non-TNBC ($P < 0.0001$). The study concluded that patients with TNBC have increased pCR rates compared with non-TNBC, and those with pCR have excellent survival. However, patients with residual disease after neoadjuvant chemotherapy have significantly worse survival if they have TNBC compared with non-TNBC, particularly in the first 3 years.

The CTNeoBC trial pooled data obtained from 12 international trials that enrolled nearly 12,000 patients [41]. Eradication of tumor from both breast and lymph nodes (ypT0 ypN0 or ypT0/is ypN0) was associated with both improved event-free survival (ypT0 ypN0: hazard ratio [HR] 0.44, 95% CI 0.39–0.51) and overall survival (0.36, 0.30–0.44; 0.36, 0.31–0.42) than was tumor eradication from the breast alone (ypT0/is; event free survival HR = 0.60, 95% CI 0.55–0.66; overall survival HR = 0.51, 0.45–0.58). The association between pCR and long-term outcomes was strongest in patients with triple-negative breast and in those with HER2-positive, hormone receptor-negative tumors who received trastuzumab. In the trial analysis, there was little association between increases in frequency of pCR and event-free survival. The study concluded that patients who attain pCR defined as ypT0 ypN0 or ypT0/is ypN0 have improved survival, and the prognostic value was greatest in aggressive tumor subtypes. The pooled analysis could not validate pCR as a surrogate end point for either improved event-free or overall survival.

Treatment of Residual Disease in Either Breast or Lymph Nodes

Patients with residual tumor in either breast of axillary lymph nodes benefit from additional treatment following neoadjuvant chemotherapy or immunotherapy (Table 1.2). The specific postoperative treatment is dependent upon the phenotype of the initial breast cancer diagnosis.

1. Patients with HER2-Positive Residual Disease

The phase 3, open-label KATHERINE trial enrolled patients with HER2-positive early breast cancer who were found to have residual invasive disease in the breast or axilla at surgery after receiving neoadjuvant therapy containing a taxane (with or without anthracycline) and trastuzumab [42]. Patients were randomly assigned to receive adjuvant T-DM1 (ado-trastuzumab emtansine) or trastuzumab for 14 cycles. Among 1486 randomly assigned patients, invasive disease or death occurred in 12.2% of patients in the T-DM1 group and 22.2% of patients in the trastuzumab

Table 1.2 Treatment after neoadjuvant chemo-immunotherapy and surgery

Breast cancer type	Complete pathological response	Residual disease in breast and/or axillary lymph nodes
Estrogen receptor-positive (hormonal suppression for premenopausal women)	Hormonal therapy with an aromatase inhibitor	Hormonal therapy with an aromatase inhibitor
HER2-positive	Herceptin for a total of 17 pre- and postoperative cycles	Ado-trastuzumab emtansine every 21 days for 14 cycles
Triple-negative	No further therapy	Capecitabine BID for 6 months

group. The estimated percentage of patients who were free of invasive disease at 3 years was 88.3% in the T-DM1 group and 77.0% in the trastuzumab group. Invasive disease-free survival was significantly higher in the T-DM1 group than in the trastuzumab group (hazard ratio for invasive disease or death, 0.50; 95% confidence interval, 0.39–0.64; $P < 0.001$). Distant recurrence as the first invasive disease event occurred in 10.5% of patients in the T-DM1 group and 15.9% of those in the trastuzumab group. The study concluded that among patients with HER2-positive early breast cancer who had residual invasive disease after completion of neoadjuvant therapy, the risk of recurrence of invasive breast cancer or death was 50% lower with adjuvant T-DM1 than with trastuzumab alone.

2. Hormone Receptor-Positive, HER2-Negative Breast Cancer
The CALOR study was a pragmatic, open-label, randomized trial that accrued patients with histologically proven and completely excised isolated locoregional recurrence of breast cancer after unilateral breast cancer who had undergone a mastectomy or lumpectomy with clear surgical margins [43]. Eligible patients were randomized to chemotherapy or no chemotherapy and stratified by previous chemotherapy, estrogen-receptor and progesterone-receptor status, and location of the recurrence. Patients with estrogen-receptor-positive local recurrence received adjuvant endocrine therapy, radiation therapy was mandated for patients with microscopically involved surgical margins, and anti-HER2 therapy was optional. Eighty-five patients were randomly assigned to receive chemotherapy and 77 were assigned to no chemotherapy.

At a median follow-up of 4.9 years, 28% of patients had disease-free survival events in the chemotherapy group compared with 44% in the no chemotherapy group. Five-year disease-free survival was 69% (95% CI 56–79) with chemotherapy versus 57% (44–67) without chemotherapy (hazard ratio 0.59 [95% CI 0.35–0.99]; $P = 0.046$). Adjuvant chemotherapy was significantly more effective for women with estrogen-receptor-negative local recurrence, but analyses of disease-free survival according to the estrogen-receptor status of the primary tumor were not statistically significant. Based on these results, adjuvant chemotherapy should be recommended for patients with completely resected isolated local recurrence, of breast cancer, especially if the recurrence is estrogen-receptor negative. Current recommendations for the treatment of residual ER-positive disease after NCT are currently in evolution, but additional chemotherapy is not recommended routinely [7].

3. Triple-Negative Breast Cancer
The CREATE-X clinical trial randomly assigned patients with HER2-negative residual invasive breast cancer after neoadjuvant chemotherapy (containing anthracycline, taxane, or both) to receive standard postsurgical treatment either with capecitabine or without [44]. The primary end point was disease-free survival. Secondary end points included overall survival. Disease-free survival was longer in the capecitabine group than in the control group (74.1% vs. 67.6% of the patients were alive and free from recurrence or second cancer at 5 years; hazard ratio for recurrence, second cancer, or death, 0.70; 95% confidence interval [CI], 0.53–0.92; $P = 0.01$). Overall survival was longer in the capecitabine group than in the control group (89.2% vs. 83.6% of the patients were alive at 5 years; hazard ratio for death, 0.59; 95% CI, 0.39–0.90; $P = 0.01$). Among patients with triple-negative disease, the rate of disease-free survival was 69.8% in the capecitabine group versus 56.1% in the control group (hazard ratio for recurrence, second cancer, or death, 0.58; 95% CI, 0.39–0.87), and the overall survival rate was 78.8% versus 70.3% (hazard ratio for death, 0.52; 95% CI, 0.30–0.90). Therefore, after standard neoadjuvant chemotherapy containing anthracycline, taxane, or both, the addition of adjuvant capecitabine therapy is safe and effective in prolonging disease-free survival and overall survival among patients with HER2-negative breast cancer who had residual invasive disease on pathological testing.

Summary

Radiographic monitoring during neoadjuvant chemotherapy to predict pCR is notoriously inaccurate [45] and should not be done routinely. Imaging can be done during treatment if there are clinical signs of disease progression and should be done at the completion of NCT to assist in surgical decision-making. Although those patients with a poor initial response have a worse prognosis, modification of chemotherapy after an observed poor response has not resulted in clinically meaningful improvements in outcome. As noted above, multiple studies have demonstrated that the burden of pathologically detected residual disease after neoadjuvant chemotherapy is associated with long-term prognosis. There has been little agreement, however, regarding the precise definition of pathological complete response. Patients with triple-negative breast cancer are much more likely to have a pathological complete response, and those who achieve a pCR have a much better outcome [46]. Neoadjuvant chemotherapy and immunotherapy should be offered to appropriate surgical candidates based on the clinical parameters of newly diagnosed invasive breast cancer.

References

1. Rastogi P, Anderson SJ, Bear HD, Geyer CE, Kahlenberg MS, Robidoux A, et al. Preoperative chemotherapy: updates of National Surgical Adjuvant Breast and Bowel Project Protocols B-18 and B-27. J Clin Oncol. 2008;26:778–85.
2. Fisher B, Brown A, Mamounas E, et al. Effect of preoperative chemotherapy on local-regional disease in women with operable breast cancer: Findings from National Surgical Adjuvant Breast and Bowel Project B-18. J Clin Oncol. 1997;15:2483–93.
3. Fisher B, Bryant J, Wolmark N, et al. Effect of preoperative chemotherapy on the outcome of women with operable breast cancer. J Clin Oncol. 1998;16:2672–85.
4. Wolmark N, Wang J, Mamounas E, et al. Preoperative chemotherapy in patients with operable breast cancer: nine-year results from National Surgical Adjuvant Breast and Bowel Project B-18. J Natl Cancer Inst Monogr. 2001;(30):96–102.
5. Bear HD, Anderson S, Brown A, et al. The effect on tumor response of adding sequential preoperative docetaxel to preoperative doxorubicin and cyclophosphamide: preliminary results from National Surgical Adjuvant Breast and Bowel Project Protocol B-27. J Clin Oncol. 2003;21:4165–74.
6. Bear HD, Anderson S, Smith RE, et al. Sequential preoperative or postoperative docetaxel added to preoperative doxorubicin plus cyclophosphamide for operable breast cancer: National Surgical Adjuvant Breast and Bowel Project Protocol B-27. J Clin Oncol. 2006;24:2019–27.
7. Caparica R, Lambertini M, Pondé N, Fumagalli D, de Azambuja E, Piccart M. Post-neoadjuvant treatment and the management of residual disease in breast cancer: state of the art and perspectives. Ther Adv Med Oncol. 2019;11:1–23.
8. Gralow JR, Burstein HJ, Wood W, et al. Preoperative therapy in invasive breast cancer: pathologic assessment and systemic therapy issues in operable disease. J Clin Oncol. 2008;26:814–9.
9. Giuliano AE, Hurvitz SA. Carcinoma of the female breast. In: Current medial diagnosis and treatment. Appleton & Lange; 2021.
10. Schwartz GF, Hortobagyi GN. Proceedings of the consensus conference on neoadjuvant chemotherapy in carcinoma of the breast, April 26-28, 2003, Philadelphia, Pennsylvania. Cancer. 2004;100:2512.
11. Kaufmann M, Hortobagyi GN, Goldhirsch A, et al. Recommendations from an international expert panel on the use of neoadjuvant (primary) systemic treatment of operable breast cancer: an update. J Clin Oncol. 2006;24:1940.
12. Scholl SM, Fourquet A, Asselain B, et al. Neoadjuvant versus adjuvant chemotherapy in premenopausal patients with tumours considered too large for breast conserving surgery: preliminary results of a randomised trial: S6. Eur J Cancer. 1994;30A:645.
13. van der Hage JA, van de Velde CJ, Julien JP, et al. Preoperative chemotherapy in primary operable breast cancer: results from the European Organization for Research and Treatment of Cancer trial 10902. J Clin Oncol. 2001;19:4224.
14. Davidson NE, Morrow M. Sometimes a great notion--an assessment of neoadjuvant systemic therapy for breast cancer. J Natl Cancer Inst. 2005;97:159.
15. Gianni L, Baselga J, Eiermann W, et al. Feasibility and tolerability of sequential doxorubicin/paclitaxel followed by cyclophosphamide, methotrexate, and fluorouracil and its effects on tumor response as preoperative therapy. Clin Cancer Res. 2005;11:8715.
16. Mauri D, Pavlidis N, Ioannidis JP. Neoadjuvant versus adjuvant systemic treatment in breast cancer: a meta-analysis. J Natl Cancer Inst. 2005;97:188.
17. Xing Y, Foy M, Cox DD, Kuerer HM, Hunt KK, Cormier JN. Meta-analysis of sentinel lymph node biopsy after preoperative chemotherapy in patients with breast cancer. Br J Surg. 2006;93:539–46.
18. Lyman GH, Giuliano AE, Somerfield MR, et al. American Society of Clinical Oncology guideline recommendations for sentinel lymph node biopsy in early-stage breast cancer. J Clin Oncol. 2005;23:7703.

19. Mieog JS, van der Hage JA, van de Velde CJ. Preoperative chemotherapy for women with operable breast cancer. Cochrane Database Syst Rev. 2007;2007(2):CD005002.
20. Shannon C, Smith I. Is there still a role for neoadjuvant therapy in breast cancer? Crit Rev Oncol Hematol. 2003;45:77.
21. Mamtani A, Barrio AV, King TA, et al. How often does neoadjuvant chemotherapy avoid axillary dissection in patients with histologically confirmed nodal metastases? Results of a prospective study. Ann Surg Oncol. 2016;23:3467.
22. Early Breast Cancer Trialists' Collaborative Group (EBCTCG). Long-term outcomes for neoadjuvant versus adjuvant chemotherapy in early breast cancer: meta-analysis of individual patient data from ten randomised trials. Lancet Oncol. 2018;19:27.
23. Board of Directors, The American Society of Breast Surgeons. Performance and practice guidelines for the use of neoadjuvant systemic therapy in the management of breast cancer. American Society of Breast Surgeons; 2017.
24. Cavalcante FP, Millen EC, Zerwes FP, Novita GG. Role of axillary surgery after neoadjuvant chemotherapy. JCO Glob Oncol. 2020;6:238–41. Published at ascopubs.org/journal/go on February 19, 2020. https://doi.org/10.1200/JGO.19.00351.
25. van Ramshorst MS, van der Voort A, van Werkhoven ED, et al. Neoadjuvant chemotherapy with or without anthracyclines in the presence of dual HER2 blockade for HER2-positive breast cancer (TRAIN-2): a multicentre, open-label, randomised, phase 3 trial. Lancet Oncol. 2018;19:1630.
26. van der Voort A, van Ramshorst MS, van Werkhoven ED, et al. Three-year follow-up of neoadjuvant chemotherapy with or without anthracyclines in the presence of dual HER2-blockade for HER2-positive breast cancer (TRAIN-2): a randomized phase III trial. J Clin Oncol. 2020;38S:501.
27. National Comprehensive Cancer Network Clinical Practice Guidelines in Oncology. Breast Cancer Version 6.2020, September 8, 2020. www.nccn.org.
28. de Azambuja E, Holmes AP, Piccart-Gebhart M, Holmes E, Di Cosimo S, Swaby RF, et al. Lapatinib plus trastuzumab for patients with early breast cancer (NeoALTTO): survival outcomes of a randomised, open-label, multicentre, phase 3 trial and their association with pathological complete response. Lancet Oncol. 2014;15:1137–46.
29. Gianni L, Eiermann W, Semiglazov V, et al. Neoadjuvant chemotherapy with trastuzumab followed by adjuvant trastuzumab versus neoadjuvant chemotherapy alone, in patients with HER2-positive locally advanced breast cancer (the NOAH trial): a randomised controlled superiority trial with a parallel HER2-negative cohort. Lancet. 2010;375:377.
30. Gianni L, Eiermann W, Semiglazov V, et al. Neoadjuvant and adjuvant trastuzumab in patients with HER2-positive locally advanced breast cancer (NOAH): follow-up of a randomised controlled superiority trial with a parallel HER2-negative cohort. Lancet Oncol. 2014;15:640.
31. von Minckwitz G, Procter M, de Azambuja E, Zardavas D, Benyunes M, Viale G, et al. Adjuvant pertuzumab and trastuzumab in early HER2-positive breast cancer. N Engl J Med. 2017;377:122–31.
32. Schneeweiss A, Chia S, Hickish T, Harvey V, Eniu A, Waldron-Lynch M, Eng-Wong J, Kirk S, Cortés J. Long-term efficacy analysis of the randomised, phase II TRYPHAENA cardiac safety study: evaluating pertuzumab and trastuzumab plus standard neoadjuvant anthracycline-containing and anthracycline-free chemotherapy regimens in patients with HER2-positive early breast cancer. Eur J Cancer. 2018;89:27–35.
33. Chopra A, Wojtowicz M, Manikowski J, Maddineni B, Kirchner L, Panikkar R, Vogel V. Pathological complete response rate (pCR) in 33 women with triple negative breast cancer (TNBC) treated with a neoadjuvant carboplatin-based regimen. 2019 ASCO Annual Meeting Proceedings. Abstract No. e12099.
34. von Minckwitz G, et al. Neoadjuvant carboplatin in patients with triple-negative and HER2-positive early breast cancer (GeparSixto; GBG 66): a randomised phase 2 trial. Lancet Oncol. 2014;15:747–56.

35. Sikov WM, Berry DA, Perou CM, Singh B, Cirrincione CT, Tolaney SM, et al. Impact of the addition of carboplatin and/or bevacizumab to neoadjuvant once-per-week paclitaxel followed by dose-dense doxorubicin and cyclophosphamide on pathologic complete response rates in stage II to III triple-negative breast cancer: CALGB 40603 (Alliance). J Clin Oncol. 2015;33:13–21.
36. Gluz O, Kolberg-Liedtke C, Prat A, Christgen M, Gebauer D, Kates R, et al. Efficacy of deescalated chemotherapy according to PAM50 subtypes, immune and proliferation genes in triple-negative early breast cancer: primary translational analysis of the WSG-ADAPT-TN trial. Int J Cancer. 2020;146:262–71.
37. Schmid P, Cortes J, Pusztai L, McArthur H, Kümmel S, Bergh J, et al. Pembrolizumab for early triple-negative breast cancer. N Engl J Med. 2020;382:810–21.
38. Mittendorf EA, Zhang H, Barrios CH, Saji S, Jung KH, Hegg R. Neoadjuvant atezolizumab in combination with sequential nab-paclitaxel and anthracycline-based chemotherapy versus placebo and chemotherapy in patients with early-stage triple-negative breast cancer (IMpassion031): a randomised, double-blind, phase 3 trial. Lancet. 2020;396(10257):1090.
39. von Minckwitz G, Untch M, Blohmer J-U, et al. Definition and impact of pathologic complete response on prognosis after neoadjuvant chemotherapy in various intrinsic breast cancer subtypes. J Clin Oncol. 2012;30:1796–804.
40. Liedtke C, Mazouni C, Hess KR, André F, Tordai A, Mejia JA, Symmans WF, Gonzalez-Angulo AM, Hennessy B, Green M, Cristofanilli M, Hortobagyi GN, Pusztai L. Response to neoadjuvant therapy and long-term survival in patients with triple-negative breast cancer. J Clin Oncol. 2008;26:1275–81.
41. Cortazar P, Zhang L, Untch M, Mehta K, Costantino JP, Wolmark N, et al. Pathological complete response and long-term clinical benefit in breast cancer: the CTNeoBC pooled analysis. Lancet. 2014;384(9938):164–72. Erratum in: Lancet. 2019;393(10175):986.
42. von Minckwitz G, Huang CS, Mano MS, Loibl S, Mamounas EP, Untch M, et al. Trastuzumab emtansine for residual invasive HER2-positive breast cancer. N Engl J Med. 2019;380:617–28.
43. Aebi S, Gelber S, Anderson SJ, Láng I, Robidoux A, Martín M, et al. Chemotherapy for isolated locoregional recurrence of breast cancer (CALOR): a randomised trial. Lancet Oncol. 2014;15:156–63.
44. Masuda N, Lee S-J, Ohtani S, Im Y-H, Lee E-S, Yokota I, et al. Adjuvant capecitabine for breast cancer after preoperative chemotherapy. N Engl J Med. 2017;376:2147–59.
45. Schott AF, Roubidoux MA, Helvie MA, Hayes DF, Kleer CG, Newman LA, et al. Clinical and radiologic assessments to predict breast cancer pathologic complete response to neoadjuvant chemotherapy. Breast Cancer Res Treat. 2005;92:231–8.
46. Schott AF, Hayes DF. Defining the benefits of neoadjuvant chemotherapy for breast cancer. J Clin Oncol. 2012;30:1747–9.

Chapter 2
The Macroscopic and Microscopic Evaluation of Breast and Axillary Lymph Node Specimens Following Neoadjuvant Systemic Therapy for Breast Cancer

Gabrielle M. Baker

Macroscopic Examination of Breast Specimens Following NAST

Before embarking on the macroscopic examination of a specimen from a breast cancer patient treated with NAST, it is imperative to be aware of all relevant history. Relevant clinical history includes the initial clinical presentation, the type of systemic therapy that was employed, pre- and post-NAST imaging findings, and the presence and location(s) of biopsy clip(s). Relevant histologic information includes the histologic type and grade of the carcinoma present in pre-NAST tissue sampling, the receptor profile of the pre-treatment tumor(s) (i.e., the status of estrogen receptor [ER], progesterone receptor [PR], and human epidermal growth factor receptor 2 [HER2]), as well as the method and results of any pre-treatment lymph node evaluation. An incomplete understanding of the relevant history risks inadequate specimen evaluation that may result in a final pathology report that does not optimally reflect the true response to NAST.

The macroscopic appearance of tumor bed is variable, and the observations made on gross examination may not be concordant with the clinical and/or radiologic impression of response to NAST. The tumor bed may be notable for a softer texture than the surrounding fibrous parenchyma, whereas in other specimens it may appear fibrotic, resembling scarring suggestive of a prior surgical site. In some instances, changes consistent with tumor bed may be inapparent on gross examination [1–3]. Macroscopically evident foci of residual viable tumor may be tan-pink in appearance with a variably fleshy appearance [2, 4].

G. M. Baker (✉)
Department of Pathology, Beth Israel Deaconess Medical Center, Boston, MA, USA

Department of Pathology, Harvard Medical School, Boston, MA, USA
e-mail: gbaker1@bidmc.harvard.edu

A. Soran, F. Nakhlis (eds.), *Management of the Breast and Axilla in the Neoadjuvant Setting*, https://doi.org/10.1007/978-3-030-88020-0_2

For all cases with grossly identifiable residual tumor and/or changes consistent with tumor bed, relevant information to provide in the macroscopic description includes the size of candidate tumor bed and its distance to all margins as well as the dimensions of candidate residual tumor and its distance to all margins. If multiple foci of tumor bed and/or residual disease are identified, the distance between these foci should be clearly stated. As noted above, meticulous correlation with pre- and post-NAST clinical and imaging findings and the identification of any biopsy clips are important in all specimens.

Various patterns in the distribution of residual disease may be observed as a given tumor responds to treatment [3–7]. Rarely, a tumor may demonstrate continued growth during NAST. Specimens from patients exhibiting varying degrees of clinical and/or radiologic response to NAST may demonstrate scattered residual foci of tumor either approximating the pre-treatment area of disease or restricted to a smaller area within the pre-treatment tumor area; alternatively, a tumor may shrink concentrically with or without a change in cellularity. In patients exhibiting an excellent clinical response to NAST, tumor bed without evidence of residual viable tumor may be observed, and, in some cases, definitive tumor bed may not be identified on gross examination.

Given the inherent complexity of many post-NAST specimens and the awareness that the microscopic findings may not approximate the findings on clinical, radiologic, and/or gross examination, the creation of a specimen map may prove critical in determining the most appropriate American Joint Committee on Cancer (AJCC) Cancer Staging Manual's ypT stage and the Residual Cancer Burden (RCB) classification (see subsequent text for further discussion of these classification systems). A specimen map or diagram may take the form of a sketch or may be overlaid on a specimen photograph or radiograph (Fig. 2.1) [3, 4, 6].

In the absence of trial-based evidence, the Breast International Group-North American Breast Cancer Group and the authors of the RCB system have made the following suggestions for an approach to tissue sampling post-NAST [2–4, 6, 8]. If a specimen is subjectively "small" (<5 cm in greatest dimension or <30 g as defined by some authors), it may be submitted in its entirety for microscopic evaluation [4, 6]. Conversely, for larger specimens the largest cross-section of residual tumor bed and representation of tumor bed to all margins should be submitted; further sampling is appropriate to evaluate additional foci of potential residual disease. Additionally, if the residual tumor is "very large," five representative blocks of the region of interest per 1–2 cm of pre-NAST carcinoma size up to approximately 25 blocks of residual tumor tissue may be sufficient to determine appropriate AJCC ypTNM staging, RCB classification, and margin assessment [3, 6]. The United States Food and Drug Administration (FDA) has provided the guideline that at least one block of residual tumor per centimeter of pre-NAST tumor size *or* a minimum of ten blocks of residual tumor be submitted for microscopic evaluation, whichever guideline prompts submission of the greater number of tissue blocks [7]. Conversely, in the setting of stable disease or disease progression during NAST, the specimen may be grossed as a non-NAST specimen would be evaluated [1]. As it is imperative to identify microscopic changes consistent with tumor bed, if no definitive tumor

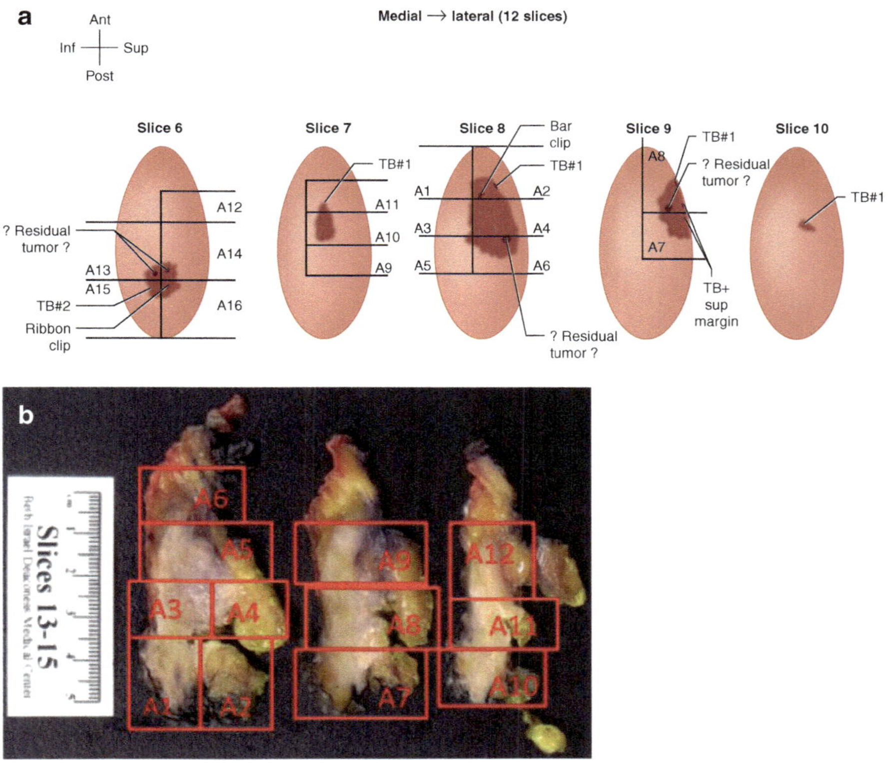

Fig. 2.1 As the gross and microscopic evaluation of post-NAST specimens may be challenging, the creation of a specimen map or diagram may be of great value in ensuring the appropriate AJCC ypT stage and RCB classification. (**a**) A specimen diagram may be in the form of a sketch or (**b**) may be superimposed on a specimen photograph or radiograph

bed and/or if no residual disease is identified on the initially submitted tissue sections, it is prudent to evaluate additional tissue. Regardless of the specimen size, a pragmatic and informed approach to tissue submission is advised rather than routine total tissue embedding or random tissue sampling [9, 10].

Microscopic Evaluation of Breast Specimens Following NAST

In keeping with the variable appearance of tumor bed on macroscopic examination, the microscopic manifestations of treatment effect on invasive carcinoma, in situ carcinoma, and the background breast parenchyma are also diverse.

Regarding alterations in the tumor bed stroma, varying degrees of edema, elastosis, hyalinization, and fibrosis as well as mucinous or myxoid change may be observed (Fig. 2.2) [1, 2, 4, 7]. A variably prominent chronic inflammatory cell infiltrate may be present including aggregates or sheets of foamy macrophages [1, 2, 7]. Stromal hemosiderin deposition and hemosiderin-laden macrophages may be seen, and an increase in the density of small-caliber vascular elements is often present [1, 2, 7]. Additionally, a paucity of pre-existing ducts and lobules is often

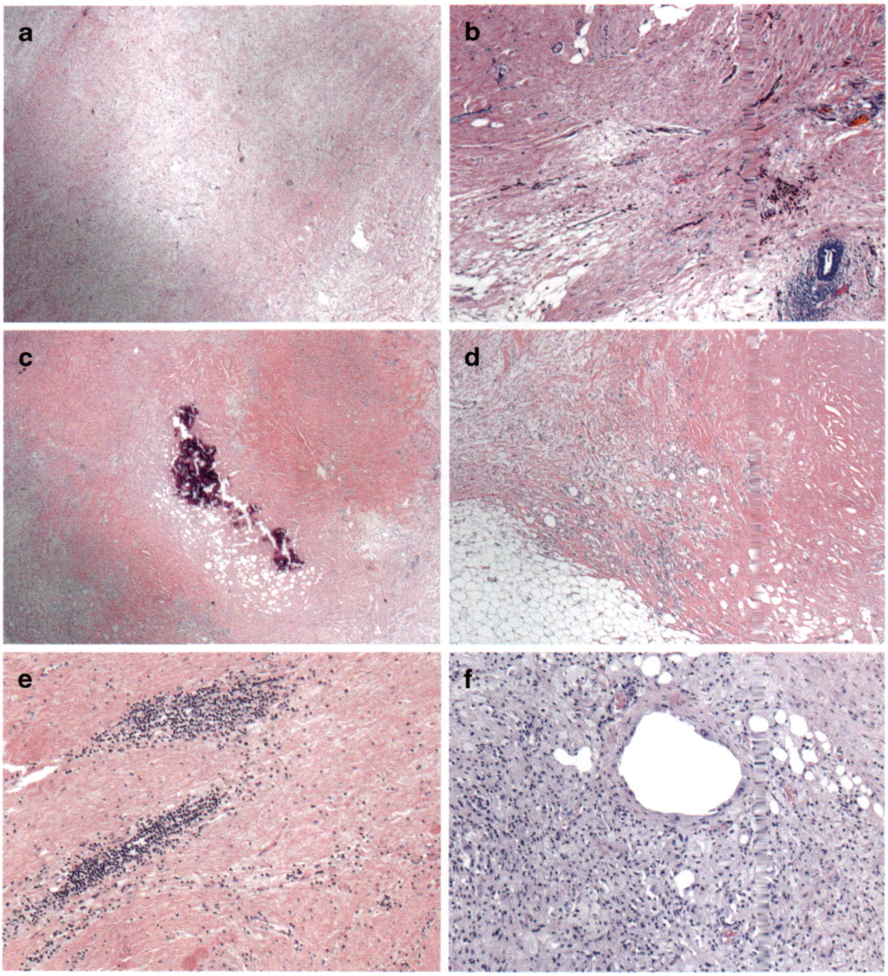

Fig. 2.2 The microscopic features of tumor bed post-NAST are diverse. (**a**) A paucity of normal pre-existing ducts and lobules is evident in this example and the stroma is notable for a loose quality. (**b**) Conspicuous hemosiderin deposition and an increase in the density of small-caliber vessels are noted. (**c**) This tumor bed demonstrates variable cellularity and areas of necrosis and calcifications are present. (**d**) Variable cellularity is noted with areas of increased cellularity and a myxoid appearance (upper left) adjacent to paucicellular, hyalinized areas. (**e**) Small aggregates of lymphocytes are present in this tumor bed as well as scattered macrophages, a subset of which is hemosiderin-laden. (**f**) In this example, aggregates of foamy macrophages are present adjacent to focal fat necrosis

noted within the tumor bed [1, 2, 7]. Whereas in some cases the delineation of tumor bed from the surrounding tissue may be readily apparent, in other instances the demarcation is more subtle and may merge inconspicuously with the adjacent normal tissue.

The primary manifestations of treatment effect on carcinoma are a reduction in tumor cellularity and/or tumor size [4, 6]. A diverse array of morphologic changes attributable to treatment effect may be observed in residual tumor cells (Fig. 2.3); less commonly the residual malignant cells may appear unaltered when compared to the pre-treatment biopsy specimen(s) [1, 2, 4, 5]. These alterations may manifest as either an increase or decrease in cell size and/or nuclear: cytoplasmic ratio. Additionally, variably marked cellular and nuclear pleomorphism may be observed as well as multinucleation and the presence of bizarre giant cell forms. The cytoplasm of residual tumor cells may appear hypereosinophilic or squamoid and variably conspicuous vacuolation may be present. In some cases, tumors with a "ductal"

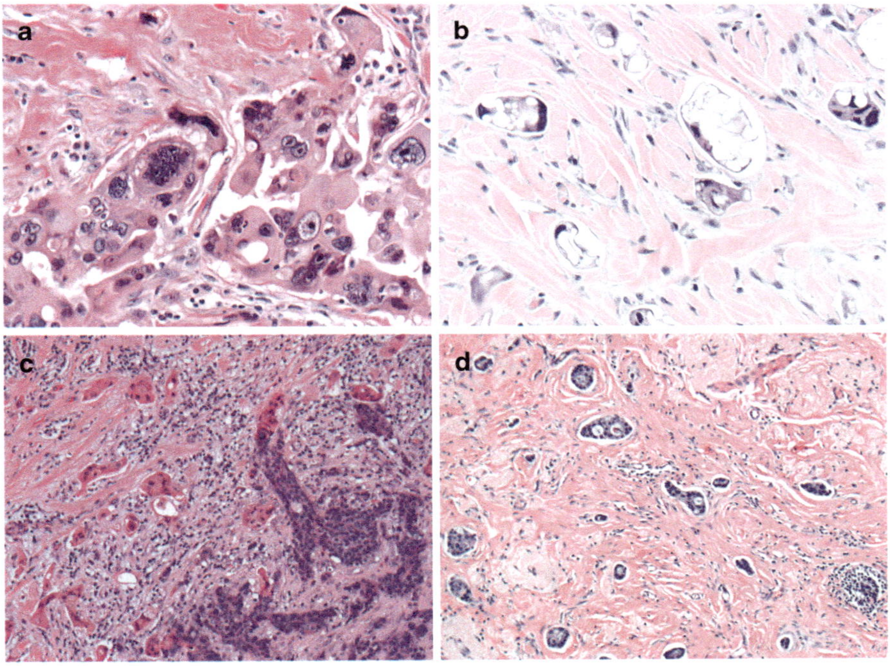

Fig. 2.3 A variety of histologic alterations attributable to treatment effect may be observed in residual invasive carcinoma post-NAST. (**a**) This example of residual invasive ductal carcinoma is notable for marked pleomorphism, multinucleation, and dense eosinophilic cytoplasm. (**b**) These singly dispersed residual invasive carcinoma cells demonstrate conspicuous cytoplasmic vacuolization. (**c**) A subset of these residual invasive carcinoma cells is notable for squamoid morphology; a non-brisk lymphocyte-predominant chronic inflammatory cell infiltrate is present in the associated stroma. (**d**) Conspicuous retraction artifact is present in association with this example of residual invasive carcinoma and may mimic lymphovascular invasion

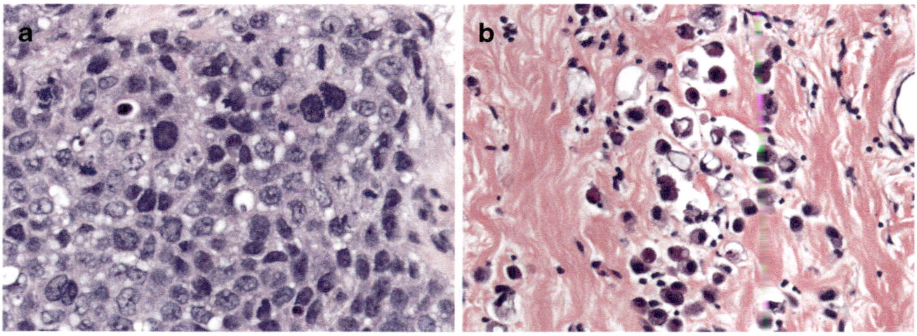

Fig. 2.4 The morphology of residual tumor post-NAST may differ from that noted in the pre-NAST biopsy specimen. In this example, the pre-NAST biopsy demonstrated a grade 3 invasive ductal carcinoma (**a**). The residual invasive carcinoma post-NAST was notable for a dyshesive, single cell pattern of invasion that in the non-NAST setting might suggest a diagnosis of invasive lobular carcinoma (**b**). Additionally, the conspicuous mitotic activity noted in the pre-NAST core needle biopsy (**a**) was not noted in the residual tumor post-NAST (**b**)

phenotype pre-NAST may appear strikingly dyshesive post-NAST (Fig. 2.4) [1, 6]; as this morphologic alteration is attributable to treatment effect, in most instances this should not prompt reclassifying a tumor as "lobular" post-NAST. Residual carcinoma cells may be notable for histiocytoid morphology such that evaluation of immunostains for cytokeratins (e.g., AE1/AE3) and histiocyte markers (e.g., CD68) may be prudent in order to accurately define the nature of the cells. In some cases, striking stromal retraction mimicking lymphovascular invasion may be present in association with the carcinoma necessitating the evaluation of endothelial markers such as D2–40 to accurately assess the location of the carcinoma cells [1, 2]. Residual carcinoma present within vascular spaces and residual carcinoma in situ may demonstrate the same spectrum of cytologic alterations as described above for residual invasive carcinoma.

Although many tumors maintain their pre-treatment histologic grade following NAST, a subset may be of higher grade (typically due to increased nuclear pleomorphism) or lower grade (most frequently due to reduced mitotic activity) post-treatment [1, 11]. Some authors and guidelines (including those provided by the College of American Pathologists) do recommend regrading a tumor post-NAST [11–13]; however, the significance of a change in histologic grade remains uncertain [6, 11]. If the histologic grade of a tumor post-NAST is different from that of a pre-NAST biopsy specimen, the inclusion of a comment regarding the pre-treatment grade in the final pathology report is worthy of consideration.

Uninvolved breast tissue frequently appears histologically unaltered post-NAST. The most common alterations that may be attributed to treatment effect are subtle and include lobular atrophy as well as increased prominence of myoepithelial cells and their associated basement membrane. Regarding the epithelial cells, cytoplasmic vacuolization and nuclear atypia akin to that seen post-radiation may be observed [1, 2]. Additionally, a variably conspicuous chronic inflammatory cell infiltrate may be present in the stroma.

Histologic Features of Primary Tumors Associated with Increased Rates of Pathologic Complete Response

Only a subset of all tumors treated with NAST undergo a pathologic complete response (pCR; see subsequent discussion regarding post-NAST classification systems and definitions of pCR). The rates of pCR depend not only on the treatment regimen employed but are also influenced by features of the primary tumor (Table 2.1). Features that have been identified to result in higher rates of pCR include triple-negative tumors (i.e., ER-negative, PR-negative, and HER2-negative) [14–18], HER2-positive tumors treated with anti-HER2 targeted therapy [18–20], the presence of a dense lymphocytic or lymphoplasmacytic infiltrate in association with the invasive carcinoma (see subsequent discussion of tumor-infiltrating lymphocytes) [21, 22], abundant tumor necrosis [23], high histologic grade, and high mitotic rate [2, 24]. In contrast, features of a primary tumor shown to have lower rates of pCR include ER positivity [15, 25–28], a lobular phenotype [27–32], and a low mitotic rate (Fig. 2.5) [33].

The Significance of Lymphovascular Invasion Following NAST

Most patients with lymphovascular invasion (LVI) post-NAST have residual invasive carcinoma in the breast and/or residual metastatic carcinoma in one or more lymph nodes [34–38]. Studies have demonstrated that residual LVI post-NAST is associated with worse prognosis [9, 34, 35, 39–41]. The clinical significance of residual LVI *only* post-NAST ("pure intralymphatic carcinoma"; i.e., neither residual invasive or in situ carcinoma present in the breast nor metastatic carcinoma in lymph nodes) is not well defined given its rarity. However, several studies have suggested that pure intralymphatic carcinoma post-NAST is associated with an adverse outcome [34–36]. In such a situation, it is incumbent upon the pathologist to ensure thorough evaluation of the tumor bed; additional sampling of the breast and/or axillary tissue may be prudent. As noted above, striking retraction artifact may be seen in association with residual carcinoma post-NAST such that use of immunohistochemistry (e.g., D2–40) may be appropriate to confirm an intralymphatic location.

Table 2.1 Features of primary tumors associated with increased rates of pCR

High histologic grade [2, 24]
High mitotic rate [2, 24]
Abundant tumor necrosis [23]
Presence of a dense lymphocytic or lymphoplasmacytic infiltrate [21, 22]
Triple negative tumors (i.e., ER-, PR-, HER2-) [14–18]
HER2+ tumors treated with anti-HER2 targeted therapy [18–20]

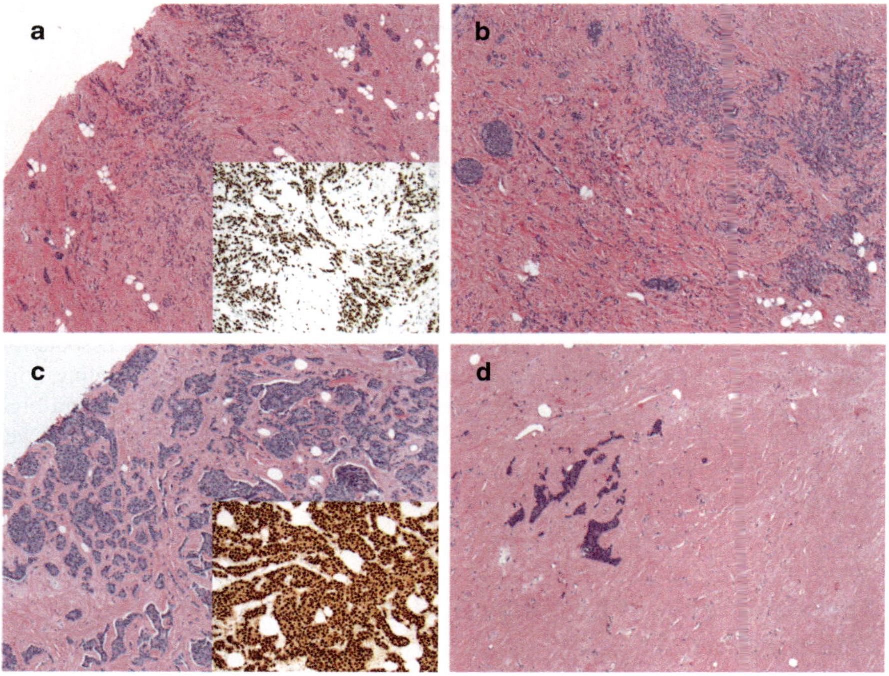

Fig. 2.5 Endocrine-only NAST infrequently results in a pCR. (**a**) A patient with a grade 1 invasive lobular carcinoma pre-NAST that was ER-positive (inset) was treated with an aromatase inhibitor; (**b**) no significant reduction in cellularity was noted post-NAST and no significant changes attributable to NAST were identified. (**c**) A patient with a grade 2 invasive ductal carcinoma pre-NAST that was ER-positive (inset) was treated with an aromatase inhibitor; (**d**) although residual invasive carcinoma was present post-NAST, a significant reduction in cellularity was noted and the stroma was notable for changes attributable to treatment effect (e.g., hyalinization)

The Significance of Residual Ductal Carcinoma In Situ Following NAST

In the absence of residual invasive carcinoma in the breast, the clinical significance of residual ductal carcinoma in situ (DCIS) remains a point of controversy. A pooled analysis led by the FDA of NAST trials with available long-term follow-up demonstrated that, in the absence of residual invasive carcinoma in the breast, similar event-free survival and overall survival was noted for patients with and without residual DCIS [26]. Similarly, in the absence of residual invasive carcinoma in the breast, a study from the MD Anderson Cancer Center did not find evidence that residual DCIS was associated with an increased risk of future distant relapse [42]. Although a study from the German and Austrian Breast Groups demonstrated that disease-free survival was significantly better for patients lacking residual invasive *and* in situ carcinoma compared to patients with residual carcinoma in situ, a statistically significant difference in overall survival was not identified [43]. The pathology report should state whether residual DCIS is present or absent, particularly if no residual invasive component is identified. As noted above, although the prognostic significance of residual DCIS remains uncertain, the FDA as well as most clinical trials and the majority of the existing classification systems do permit the presence of residual carcinoma in situ in classifying a patient as having achieved a pCR (see subsequent discussion regarding post-NAST classification systems and definitions of pCR).

Tumor-Infiltrating Lymphocytes and Their Significance in Tumors Treated with NAST

Recommendations for the evaluation of tumor-infiltrating lymphocytes (TIL) in breast cancer have been published by an international TIL working group [44]. TIL may be divided into intratumoral TIL and stromal TIL. Intratumoral TIL are present within tumor cell nests or are otherwise contiguous with the carcinoma cells, whereas stromal TIL are present in the stromal area between tumor cell nests and individual carcinoma cells [22]. Although both stromal and intratumor TIL may be evaluated, it is the stromal component that is regarded as the parameter of primary clinical importance [22]. All mononuclear cells (i.e., plasma cells as well as lymphocytes) are included in the assessment of TIL; neutrophils are excluded [22]. The assessment of stromal TIL requires an estimation of the percent stromal area within the area involved by invasive carcinoma that is occupied by TIL; of note, it is not an estimation of the percent of nuclei that belong to tumor cells versus TIL [21, 22]. Additionally, areas of necrosis and biopsy-related changes as well as DCIS and crush artifact should be excluded from the evaluation [22]. In the non-NAST as well as the post-NAST setting, TIL are to be averaged over the entirety of the examined tumor area and are evaluated as a continuous variable [22, 44, 45]. Recognizing that significant heterogeneity is often observed in the distribution of TIL, one is advised to not preferentially evaluate so-called hot spots [22, 44, 45]. Although no formal recommendations regarding the evaluation of TIL in the post-NAST setting were provided in the original publication from the international TIL working group, the following suggestions have been made and presume that TIL present in close proximity to the residual carcinoma have greater immunologic import than areas of mononuclear infiltrate distant to the residual carcinoma [46]. The area of tumor bed used to calculate the RCB may also be used to determine percent TIL [46], to include what has been termed an "invasive margin" which represents a 1 mm span encompassing the interface of residual invasive carcinoma and the adjacent uninvolved stroma [45, 47]. In keeping with the recommendations for evaluation of TIL in the non-NAST setting, these authors also recommend that in the absence of residual viable carcinoma cells, areas of fibrosis or hyalinization suggestive of treatment effect should not be evaluated for TIL; additionally, areas of necrosis should not be evaluated [46]. With regard to the evaluation of TIL in cases of pCR, one group has suggested evaluating the region of tissue demonstrating changes consistent with tumor bed [46]. Despite these suggestions, evidence-based recommendations regarding the percentage of TIL that has clinical or prognostic significance have yet to be established [45].

Evidence continues to accumulate that the presence of significant TIL is associated with increased rates of pCR and that TIL may be prognostic in at least some breast cancer subtypes [10, 21, 22, 46, 48–55]. Although some degree of TIL is present in the majority of breast cancers, a dense infiltrate is present in association with only a minority of tumors [56]. Tumors with a conspicuous mononuclear inflammatory cell infiltrate may be referred to as TIL-rich or lymphocyte-predominant breast cancer (LPBC) if the infiltrate occupies at least 50–60% of the stromal area; such tumors are most commonly either triple-negative or HER2-positive [10, 21, 45, 48, 51, 56–58].

Chemotherapy owes its efficacy, at least in part, to its ability to promote an anti-tumor immune response [59]. Whereas some studies have suggested that all LPBC are associated with an improved prognosis [21, 48, 57, 58], other studies have identified improved prognosis for LPBC that is triple-negative but not for LPBC that is hormone receptor-negative and HER2-positive [21, 48, 60–62]. For HER2-positive tumors, it has been suggested that the prognostic benefit of high TIL may be attributed primarily to the hormone receptor-negative status of the tumor rather than its HER2-positive status [60]. In support of this hypothesis, in a pooled analysis of six randomized trials, the German Breast Cancer Group observed that increased TIL was predictive of response to NAST in all molecular subtypes of breast cancer. However, although these authors noted a survival benefit for those patients with HER2-positive and triple-negative breast cancers, increased TIL was found to be an adverse prognostic factor for patients with breast cancers of the luminal molecular subtypes (i.e., hormone receptor-positive tumors) [49].

Several studies have sought to investigate the significance of TIL in association with residual disease post-NAST, including an evaluation of the change in TILs from the pre-NAST biopsy to the post-NAST excision [53, 59, 62–65]. A subset of these authors has noted that the specimens from patients who achieve a pCR frequently demonstrate a reduction in TIL [62, 63] and that greater reductions in the percentage of stromal TIL post-NAST were associated with increasing rates of pCR [62, 66]. These authors observed that the presence of a high percentage of TIL post-NAST was associated with a lack of pCR and a higher RCB class [62, 66]. Furthermore, one of these studies noted that high TIL post-NAST was associated with higher RCB class, whereas high TIL pre-NAST was not [62]. In contrast, with regard to TNBC, other studies have reported that high TIL in association with residual disease post-NAST was associated with a better prognosis including recurrence-free survival, metastasis-free survival, and overall survival as well as lower RCB score [46, 48, 53, 59, 67–71]. In summary, the significance of TIL in post-NAST specimens is complex and requires additional evaluation.

The Significance of Lymph Node Status Following NAST

Studies have demonstrated that residual metastatic carcinoma in lymph nodes post-NAST confers a worse prognosis, even for patients with no residual carcinoma in the breast. Compared to patients with no nodal involvement, it has been demonstrated that greater residual nodal disease burden post-NAST is associated with significantly worse disease-free survival and overall survival; these findings have been noted to be independent of the in-breast response [25, 43, 72–74].

A study from the MD Anderson Cancer Center evaluating patients with cytologically proven axillary nodal involvement pre-NAST demonstrated that the absence of residual axillary disease post-NAST was associated with improved recurrence-free survival and overall survival when compared to patients with residual axillary disease post-NAST [72]. Of note, within the subset of the patients who achieved complete regression of axillary disease in this study, no significant difference in recurrence-free survival or overall survival was noted when comparing those patients with residual in-breast disease to those patients who also achieved an in-breast complete response [72]. Additional studies have also demonstrated that patients with axillary disease pre-NAST who lack residual axillary disease post-NAST have an excellent prognosis even if residual disease is present within the breast [43, 72, 73, 75–78].

The existing data suggests that in the absence of residual metastatic carcinoma in axillary lymph nodes, patients with microscopic evidence of tumor regression within the axillary lymph nodes (see following discussion) have an intermediate outcome compared to those patients with residual viable metastatic carcinoma in lymph nodes and those with negative lymph nodes that lack microscopic evidence of tumor regression [79].

Macroscopic and Microscopic Evaluation of Lymph Node Specimens Following NAST

Regardless of whether a patient has been treated with NAST or not, axillary lymph nodes should be sectioned at ≤2 mm intervals; lymph nodes lacking grossly evident tumor should be submitted in their entirety for microscopic evaluation. Common microscopic changes attributable to treatment effect include lymphocyte depletion and areas of stromal fibrosis or hyalinization; areas of myxoid or mucinous change may also be noted (Fig. 2.6) [7, 79]. However, the absence of these findings does not definitively rule out the possibility that metastatic carcinoma was present in a given lymph node pre-NAST. Residual foci of metastatic carcinoma may exhibit the same spectrum of cytopathic changes as seen in residual tumor within the breast, including a reduction in tumor cellularity (see preceding discussion including Fig. 2.3). As may be observed in the breast, a heterogeneous response to treatment may be noted in the evaluated lymph nodes.

The presence of isolated tumor cells (ITCs; i.e., ≤0.2 mm and ≤200 cells) post-NAST precludes classification as a pCR [80]. Whereas per the AJCC, ITCs are staged as ypN0(i+) as in the non-NAST setting, the World Health Organization (WHO) recommends classifying lymph nodes with ITCs as node-positive; however, the WHO does not specify whether these lymph nodes should be classified as containing micrometastatic (i.e., >0.2–2 mm and/or >200 cells) or macrometastatic (i.e., >2 mm) carcinoma [81]. It is likely that at least a subset of the lymph nodes involved by residual metastatic carcinoma classified as ITCs or micrometastases post-NAST represent downstaging of lymph nodes with micro- and/or macrometastatic carcinoma pre-NAST [42, 80]. Additional investigation is needed to

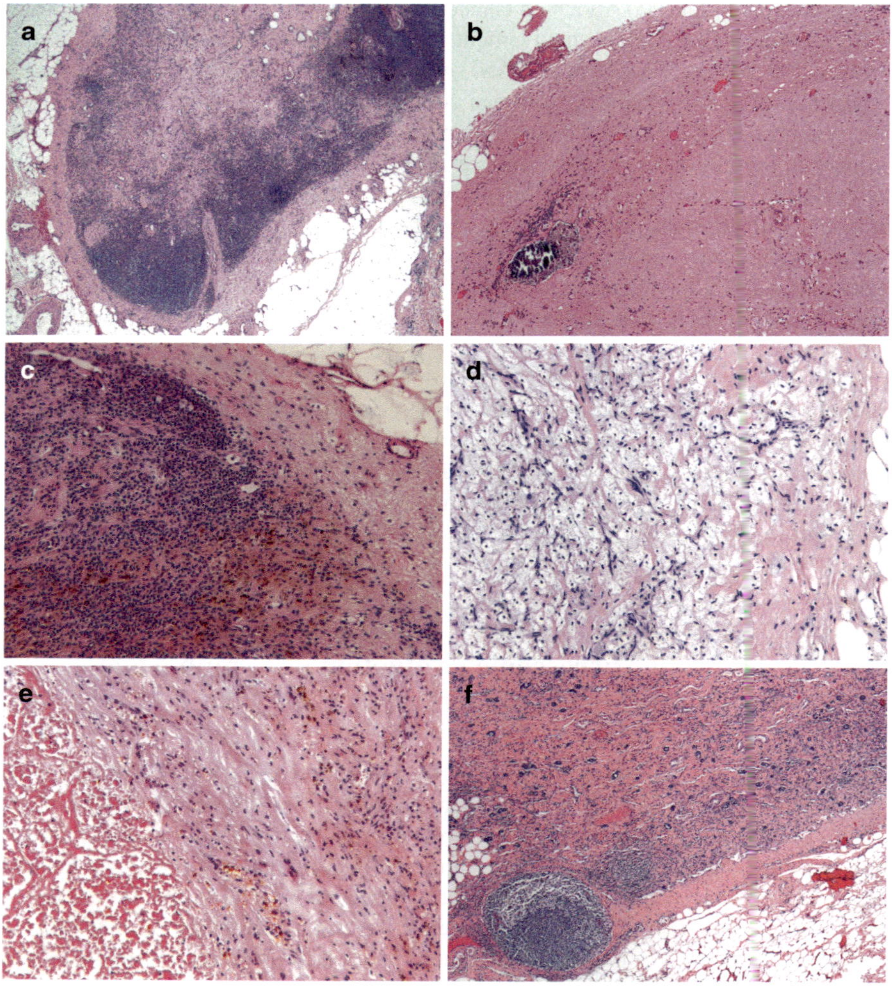

Fig. 2.6 The spectrum of changes seen in lymph nodes following NAST is similar to that seen in the breast. (**a**) At low power, this lymph node is notable for areas of lymphocyte depletion and stromal hyalinization, findings that may be attributed to NAST. (**b**) This lymph node is notable for diffuse lymphocyte depletion accompanied by stromal hyalinization; focal calcification in association with necroinflammatory debris is present (left lower). (**c**) Areas of hemosiderin deposition and hemosiderin-laden macrophages may also be a manifestation of treatment effect. (**d**) In this example, sheets of foamy macrophages were present throughout the lymph node which was also notable for lymphocyte depletion. (**e**) This lymph node was notable for hemosiderin deposition and necrotic tumor; no residual viable metastatic carcinoma was identified. (**f**) In addition to lymphocyte depletion and fibrosis, residual clusters of viable metastatic carcinoma are present throughout this lymph node

determine whether or not residual metastatic carcinoma classified as ITCs and/or micrometastases post-NAST has the same clinical significance as ITCs and/or micrometastatic carcinoma in the non-NAST setting or if their clinical significance more closely approximates that of macrometastatic carcinoma.

Information regarding lymph nodes that may be provided in the pathology report includes the total number of lymph nodes evaluated, the number of lymph nodes involved by residual viable metastatic carcinoma, the size of the largest residual metastatic focus, an enumeration of lymph nodes with macrometastases versus micrometastases versus ITCs, and the number of lymph nodes with and without metastatic carcinoma that demonstrate changes attributable to treatment effect. Additionally, the presence and extent of extranodal extension and the presence of carcinoma cells in the perinodal fibroadipose tissue should be documented as in the non-NAST setting.

With regard to pre-treatment sampling of lymph nodes, if a lymph node has been evaluated by fine needle aspiration or core needle biopsy, it is important to document whether or not changes attributable to a prior needling procedure are identified in the excision specimen; if a biopsy clip was placed in a lymph node pre-treatment, it should be clearly stated whether or not a clip and/or biopsy-related changes are noted. Although clips are frequently placed in a biopsied lymph node, standardized recommendations regarding this practice do not currently exist. It is important to note that if a lymph node containing metastatic carcinoma has been *excised* pre-NAST, the AJCC nodal stage (i.e., ypN) cannot be fully assessed and the RCB score is not evaluable [8].

Classification Systems Evaluating Specimens Following NAST

Multiple classification systems exist to evaluate response to NAST (Table 2.2). Although the majority of these systems require the absence of residual tumor in both the breast and axillary lymph nodes to be classified as pCR, the definition of what constitutes a pCR varies among systems, with some evaluating response in the breast only [1, 5, 8, 80, 82–86]. Most classification systems do permit the presence of residual carcinoma in situ in the designation of pCR [1, 5, 82, 85–88]. A subset of the systems does require access to the pre-treatment biopsy specimen in order to compare the cellularity of the tumor pre- and post-NAST [1, 5, 84, 85]. Only the Miller-Payne, Residual Cancer Burden, and American Joint Committee on Cancer systems will be discussed in further detail in this chapter.

The Miller-Payne system is based on the estimated reduction in tumor cellularity in the post-treatment surgical specimen compared to the pre-treatment core needle biopsy and is categorized into five grades [5]. The Miller-Payne system defines pCR as no residual invasive carcinoma although residual carcinoma in situ is permitted. Grade 1 corresponds to no observed reduction in overall cellularity; however,

Table 2.2 Representative classification systems to evaluate response to NAST

System	Does classification as pCR include response in breast *only* or both breast *and* lymph nodes?	Is residual carcinoma in situ permitted in classification as pCR?	Is the pre-NAST biopsy specimen required to evaluate response to NAST?
Regression of Sinn [83]	Both	No	Yes
National Surgical Adjuvant Breast and Bowel Project B-18 [81]	Breast only	Yes	No
Sataloff [84]	Both	Yes (Note: A minor component of residual *invasive* carcinoma is also permitted)	Yes
Chevallier [82]	Both	No	No
Pinder [1]	Both	Yes	Yes
Residual Disease in Breast and Nodes [85]	Both	Yes	No
Miller-Payne [5]	Breast only	Yes	Yes
Residual Cancer Burden [88]	Both	Yes	No
American Joint Committee on Cancer [80]	Both	Yes	No

cytologic alterations to individual cells may be noted. Grades 2, 3, and 4 correspond to increasing reductions in residual cellularity, and Grade 5 constitutes a pCR. Several significant limitations for this system exist including the requirement for access to the pre-treatment biopsy and the absence of formal guidelines regarding how to evaluate cellularity. Of greatest significance, the Miller-Payne system does not incorporate lymph node status in classification as pCR.

The RCB is a continuous variable generated via a calculator that is freely available online and defines four categories of response to treatment [8]. The RCB score and class generated by this calculator have been demonstrated to correlate with patient outcome (i.e., distant relapse-free survival) in all breast cancer subtypes [43, 89, 90]. The RCB defines pCR as the absence of residual invasive carcinoma in the breast and no carcinoma in lymph nodes; residual carcinoma in situ is permitted. RCB-0 corresponds to a pCR; RCB classes I, II, and III are gradations of partial responses ranging from minimal to extensive residual disease. Of note, the assessment of RCB score and class must be determined via the online calculator; it is not a subjective assessment rendered by the pathologist.

To determine the RCB score and class, the following parameters are evaluated: the size of the tumor bed in two dimensions, the total percent tumor cellularity within the tumor bed (carcinoma in situ and invasive carcinoma including tumor in vascular spaces), the percent of overall tumor cellularity that is carcinoma in situ,

Table 2.3 Parameters required to calculate the Residual Cancer Burden

Parameters to calculate the Residual Cancer Burden (see text for details)
Primary tumor bed area
Total residual cancer cellularity (as percentage of primary tumor bed area)
Percentage of total residual cancer cellularity that is carcinoma in situ
Number of lymph nodes with residual metastatic carcinoma
Diameter of largest lymph node metastasis

and the tumor burden in lymph nodes (including the total number of lymph nodes with residual viable carcinoma and the size of the largest metastasis) (Table 2.3). Of note with regard to calculating the RCB, the term "tumor bed" refers to the area of breast parenchyma that contains residual invasive carcinoma and may not correspond to the entire area of tissue exhibiting changes attributable to treatment effect. The assessment of residual tumor cellularity is averaged over the entirety of the area containing residual *invasive* carcinoma (i.e., the tumor bed); so-called hot spots with greater residual cellularity are not preferentially evaluated [4, 6, 89]. This represents an important clarification as significant heterogeneity in residual cellularity is often observed. The RCB website provides a helpful guide for estimating cancer cellularity that aids in preventing significant under- or overestimate of percent cellularity post-NAST. Of note, modest differences in the estimated percent cellularity do not significantly affect the calculated RCB score and class. As discussed earlier, given that the extent of residual nodal disease represents the most significant histologic parameter regarding prognosis, this factor is weighted accordingly in the RCB calculator. The implications of this weighting are such that an accurate assessment of lymph node status is more significant than a modest degree of interobserver variability in the assessment of residual tumor cellularity in the breast [8, 89]. It is important to note that the RCB score cannot be calculated if a positive axillary lymph node was *excised* pre-treatment; however, evaluation by fine needle aspiration or core needle biopsy only does not preclude RCB calculation. Of note, the RCB classification system does not require access to the pre-treatment biopsy to assess response to NAST.

The AJCC Cancer Staging Manual's method of staging post-NAST (i.e., ypTNM) is similar to staging in the non-NAST setting (i.e., pTNM) wherein the anatomic staging is based on the extent of disease present in the breast, in lymph nodes, and at distant sites [80]. As in the non-NAST setting, the use of the (m) modifier denotes the presence of multiple foci of residual invasive carcinoma in the breast. Per the AJCC, a pCR is defined as no residual invasive carcinoma in the breast (residual carcinoma in situ is permitted) and no residual metastatic carcinoma in lymph nodes; the presence of residual carcinoma in vessels only does preclude classification as a pCR. The ypT stage is based on the maximum linear extent of the largest focus of residual invasive carcinoma, and the ypN stage is based on the largest contiguous deposit of residual viable metastatic carcinoma. The 8th Edition of the AJCC Cancer Staging Manual clarifies that treatment-related fibrosis adjacent to and/or between foci of residual invasive carcinoma in the breast or residual metastatic carcinoma in lymph nodes is *not* included in the measurements that determine the ypT and ypN stages. Given this update in how residual nodal deposits are measured and are therefore classified as macrometastases versus micrometastases versus ITCs, although the ypN stage is based on the largest contiguous residual metastatic deposit, if multiple foci of residual metastatic carcinoma are present in a given lymph node, an explanatory comment may be informative in conveying the extent of residual viable metastatic carcinoma. Of note, the AJCC system does not incorporate assessment of cellularity in the evaluation of response to NAST and does not require access to the pre-NAST core needle biopsy specimen.

Similar to the RCB classification as noted above, *excision* of a positive lymph node pre-NAST does preclude definitive assignment of the ypN stage [80]. If no additional lymph nodes are removed post-NAST *or* additional lymph nodes are removed post-NAST and no residual metastatic disease is identified, the nodal stage may be rendered as ypNX with an explanatory comment. If additional positive lymph nodes are removed post-NAST, one may provide the ypN stage based on the lymph nodes evaluated post-NAST and provide an explanatory comment about the excision of positive lymph node(s) pre-NAST. Regardless of whether or not lymph nodes with or without metastatic disease were excised pre-NAST, it is recommended that the pathology report clearly states the breakdown of macrometastases versus micrometastases versus isolated tumor cells for the positive lymph nodes excised post-NAST.

In addition to the anatomic staging (i.e., [y]pTNM) assessed in prior editions, the 8th Edition of the AJCC introduced Clinical and Pathological Prognostic Stages that incorporate biologic factors (e.g., tumor grade and ER, PR, and HER2 status) in addition to the anatomic (y)pTNM staging in order to more accurately assess a patient's prognosis. However, the authors of the AJCC 8th Edition stated that the newly defined Pathological Prognostic Stage was not to be applied to the post-NAST setting [80]. A recent publication sought to evaluate whether the Pathological Prognostic Stage could be applied to the post-NAST setting in order to stratify survival outcomes for the increasing subset of patients who are treated with NAST [91]. Leveraging a previously developed system that incorporates clinical, histologic, and biologic factors to stratify prognosis (i.e., Neo-Bioscore), these authors confirmed that biologic factors and anatomic stage are important for assessing prognosis in patients treated with NAST, and, although further study is warranted, their results suggest that the AJCC 8th Edition's Pathological Prognostic Stage is applicable to the post-NAST setting [91, 92].

Clarifications Regarding Reporting and Staging, Including AJCC 8th Edition Updates

For specimens containing gross residual disease post-NAST, although the microscopic findings may closely correlate with the gross examination, additional microscopic foci of residual invasive carcinoma may be noted within and/or beyond the grossly identified area(s) of treatment effect. Similarly, for specimens without grossly evident residual disease, including from patients with clinical and/or radiologic evidence of a complete response, microscopic residual disease within and/or beyond areas of treatment effect may be noted. For specimens in which no residual carcinoma is identified microscopically, it is critical to identify histologic changes consistent with tumor bed before classifying a patient as having achieved a pCR, which is defined as either ypT0N0 or ypTisN0 [26, 43, 80]. As in the non-NAST setting, consideration for additional tissue sampling may be appropriate depending upon the microscopic findings in the initially submitted tissue, and, as in all cases, correlation with radiologic and clinical findings is imperative. Explanatory comments may be of great value in conveying how the ypT and/or ypN stages were determined for a given case as these specimens may be complicated and challenging to evaluate. Additional information that may be provided in the pathology report to convey extent and distribution of residual disease includes the number of discrete residual foci, the total approximate span of residual carcinoma, and the number of tissue blocks with residual disease [11].

Multiple foci of invasive carcinoma need not have been demonstrated histologically, radiographically, or clinically pre-treatment to merit the use of the (m) modifier signifying the presence of multiple foci of residual invasive carcinoma post-NAST [80, 93]. For patients with a single focus of invasive carcinoma pre-treatment, multiple smaller foci of residual invasive carcinoma may persist post-NAST; a subset of such cases may merit the (m) modifier. It may serve as a pragmatic general guideline to regard multiple areas of residual invasive carcinoma as discrete foci if the distance separating them is greater than the largest single dimension of the candidate foci [94]. As the potential for significant subjectivity exists with regard to interpreting these specimens, explanatory notes may be provided in the pathology report in order to clarify how the assessment was made. An explanatory comment may also prove informative if the discrete foci demonstrate markedly different cellularity estimates.

As noted above, the largest contiguous focus of residual invasive carcinoma determines the ypT stage; if multiple foci of residual invasive carcinoma are present, their dimensions should not be added together to determine the ypT stage or to calculate the RCB score [80]. In the AJCC 8th Edition, it is the largest contiguous focus of residual viable invasive carcinoma in the breast and the largest contiguous focus of residual viable metastatic carcinoma in a lymph node that determines the ypT and ypN stage, respectively; intervening areas of tumor bed and treatment effect are excluded from these measurements [80]. To calculate the RCB score, the largest residual discrete area of residual invasive carcinoma in two dimensions *including* the tumor bed stroma is measured [8]. As noted previously, if a lymph node *containing* metastatic carcinoma was excised pre-NAST, the ypN stage cannot be assessed and the RCB score cannot be calculated [8]. Data elements required for the RCB classification and AJCC ypTNM staging are provided in Table 2.4.

The presence of lymphovascular invasion *only* post-NAST (i.e., no residual invasive or in situ carcinoma identified in the breast following adequate tissue sampling and no metastatic carcinoma identified in any of the evaluated lymph nodes) is

Table 2.4 Data elements to calculate the Residual Cancer Burden and to determine the AJCC ypTNM stage

Data Element	Residual Cancer Burden [88]	AJCC 8th Edition [80]
Definition of pCR	RCB-0	ypT0N0 *or* ypTisN0 Note: ypN0(i+) is *not* considered a pCR
Residual Tumor Size	Largest area containing residual invasive carcinoma (if multicentric residual invasive carcinoma present, the largest area is used to calculate RCB)	Largest contiguous focus of residual viable invasive carcinoma, *excluding* treatment-related fibrosis
Cellularity	Percentage of the tumor bed area containing carcinoma (invasive, in situ, and intravascular disease) *and* percentage of the total residual carcinoma that is in situ	Not evaluated
Multifocality of residual invasive carcinoma	Not evaluated	Use of the "m" modifier denotes the presence of multiple residual invasive foci (as in the non-NAST setting)
Number of lymph nodes with metastatic tumor	Yes, required to calculate RCB	Yes, required for ypN stage
Size of lymph node metastasis	Diameter of largest metastasis, *including* treatment-related fibrosis present in association with and/or between metastatic deposits	Diameter of largest contiguous focus of residual viable metastatic carcinoma *excluding* treatment-related fibrosis present in association with and/or between metastatic deposits
Does *excision* of a positive lymph node pre-NAST preclude determination of RCB or ypTNM stage?	Yes	Yes (see text for additional recommendations)
Distant metastasis	Not evaluated	If distant metastasis (c/pM1) is present pre-NAST, the patient is staged as c/pM1 post-NAST *regardless* of response to NAST

uncommon and should not be classified as a pCR; an attempt to calculate RCB is not appropriate in this scenario. Such residual disease may be staged as ypTX with an explanatory comment [4, 6, 35]. Alternatively, the AJCC suggests assigning such residual disease as ypT0 with an explicit comment that the patient should not be regarded as having achieved a pCR [80]. Outside of the setting of a clinical trial, it is not currently recommended either to approximate the span of LVI as an estimate of residual disease or to report the distance of intravascular tumor to specimen margins.

If a patient was diagnosed with inflammatory breast cancer pre-NAST, that clinical diagnosis is retained post-NAST regardless of the response to therapy [80]. The ypT may be reported based on the extent of residual disease; however, a note should be made of the pre-treatment c/pT4d classification. In the same way, if a patient has been diagnosed with distant metastasis pre-NAST, the patient remains classified as M1 regardless of response to NAST [80].

Consensus guidelines now exist for acceptable margin widths for invasive carcinoma in the non-NAST setting and for ductal carcinoma in situ [95, 96]; however, the optimal margin width for residual invasive carcinoma and ductal carcinoma in situ post-NAST is not yet resolved [37, 97–99]. A recent retrospective evaluation of a cohort of breast cancer patients treated with NAST (patients receiving endocrine-only therapy were excluded) and breast-conserving therapy evaluated the relationship between reported margin width and local recurrence and survival: the authors found no association between margin width and local recurrence free-survival, disease-free survival, and overall survival suggesting that, as in the non-NAST setting, a "no-ink-on-tumor" margin may be acceptable in at least a subset of patients [97]. Some authors have suggested that the presence of tumor bed and changes consistent with treatment effect at inked specimen margins should be reported; however, the clinical significance of this finding has not yet been determined [4, 6].

Reassessment of ER, PR, and HER2 Post-NAST

Most breast carcinomas maintain their pre-treatment ER, PR, and HER2 status post-NAST. However, a subset does demonstrate altered ER, PR, and/or HER2 status post-NAST. Two meta-analyses identified the following frequency of discordant results: 13% and 18% for ER, 32% and 26% for PR, and 9% and 6% for HER2 [100, 101]. These altered profiles may be due to a variety of factors including the inherent heterogeneity of a given tumor and therapy-related effects. For example, loss of PR expression may be observed following treatment with aromatase inhibitors, and loss of HER2 overexpression may be observed following HER2-targeted therapy. Repeat evaluation of ER, PR, and HER2 is routinely performed on residual invasive carcinoma at the author's institution; however, such policies are variable among institutions. Although uniform guidelines and recommendations regarding the evaluation of ER, PR, and HER2 post-NAST are not yet formalized, the College of American Pathologists does recommend repeat evaluation of any markers (i.e., ER, PR, and/or HER2) that were negative pre-NAST [11]. Assessing a change in proliferation index as evaluated by Ki67 has been proposed as an ancillary method of evaluating response to treatment in addition to the assessment of mitotic rate necessary to provide a histologic grade. However, this is not currently recommended in routine practice in either the NAST or non-NAST settings due, at least in part, to the lack of standardization in the evaluation of Ki67 [80, 102–108].

Conclusion

The macroscopic and microscopic evaluation of breast and axillary lymph node specimens from patients treated with NAST presents unique challenges in addition to those routinely encountered in the non-NAST setting. This chapter seeks to provide pragmatic guidance for the evaluation of these specimens with particular attention to the standardization of reporting the pathologic findings. A thorough understanding of the pre- and post-NAST clinical, radiologic, and histologic findings is crucial in accurately assessing response to treatment which has immediate prognostic implications for individual patients and will, in turn, facilitate more meaningful comparisons among ongoing and future clinical trials, thereby benefiting current and future breast cancer patients as a whole.

References

1. Pinder SE, et al. Laboratory handling and histology reporting of breast specimens from patients who have received neoadjuvant chemotherapy. Histopathology. 2007;50(4):409–17. ISSN 0309-0167. Disponível em: https://www.ncbi.nlm.nih.gov/pubmed/17448015.
2. Sahoo S, Lester SC. Pathology of breast carcinomas after neoadjuvant chemotherapy: an overview with recommendations on specimen processing and reporting. Arch Pathol Lab Med. 2009;133(4):633–42. ISSN 1543-2165. Disponível em: https://www.ncbi.nlm.nih.gov/pubmed/19391665.
3. Bossuyt V, Symmans WF. Standardizing of pathology in patients receiving neoadjuvant chemotherapy. Ann Surg Oncol. 2016;23(10):3153–61. ISSN 1534-4681. Disponível em: https://www.ncbi.nlm.nih.gov/pubmed/27380637.
4. Bossuyt V, et al. Recommendations for standardized pathological characterization of residual disease for neoadjuvant clinical trials of breast cancer by the BIG-NABCG collaboration. Ann Oncol. 2015;26(7):1280–91. ISSN 1569-8041. Disponível em: https://www.ncbi.nlm.nih.gov/pubmed/26019189.
5. Ogston KN, et al. A new histological grading system to assess response of breast cancers to primary chemotherapy: prognostic significance and survival. Breast. 2003;12(5):320–7. ISSN 0960-9776. Disponível em: https://www.ncbi.nlm.nih.gov/pubmed/14659147.
6. Provenzano E, et al. Standardization of pathologic evaluation and reporting of postneoadjuvant specimens in clinical trials of breast cancer: recommendations from an international working group. Mod Pathol. 2015;28(9):1185–201. ISSN 1530-0285. Disponível em: https://www.ncbi.nlm.nih.gov/pubmed/26205180.
7. U.S. Department of Health and Human Services, Food and Drug Administration, Center for Drug Evaluation and Research (CDER). Guidance for industry: pathological complete response in neoadjuvant treatment of high-risk early-stage breast cancer use as an endpoint to support accelerated approval. October 2014. fda.gov.
8. Residual Cancer Burden calculator and associated documents (Guide for Measuring Cancer Cellularity, Examples of Gross and Microscopic Evaluation, Pathology Protocol for Macroscopic and Microscopic Assessment of RCB). Disponível em: http://www3.mdanderson.org/app/medcalc/index.cfm?pagename=jsconvert3. Acesso em: January [illegible].
9. Tamura N, et al. Tumor histology in lymph vessels and lymph nodes for the accurate prediction of outcome among breast cancer patients treated with neoadjuvant chemotherapy. Cancer Sci. 2009;100(10):1823–33. ISSN 1349-7006. Disponível em: https://www.ncbi.nlm.nih.gov/pubmed/19604245.
10. Würfel F, et al. TILGen: a program to investigate immune targets in breast cancer patients – first results on the influence of tumor-infiltrating lymphocytes. Breast Care (Basel). 2018;13(1):8–14. ISSN 1661-3791. Disponível em: https://www.ncbi.nlm.nih.gov/pubmed/29950961.
11. Fitzgibbons PL, et al. Protocol for the examination of specimens from patients with invasive carcinoma of the breast. College of American Pathologists; 2017.
12. Brain E, et al. Long-term prognostic and predictive factors in 107 stage II/III breast cancer patients treated with anthracycline-based neoadjuvant chemotherapy. Br J Cancer.

1997;75(9):1360–7. ISSN 0007-0920. Disponível em: https://www.ncbi.nlm.nih.gov/pubmed/9155059.
13. Corben AD, et al. Pathologic response and long-term follow-up in breast cancer patients treated with neoadjuvant chemotherapy: a comparison between classifications and their practical application. Arch Pathol Lab Med. 2013;137(8):1074–82. ISSN 1543-2165. Disponível em: https://www.ncbi.nlm.nih.gov/pubmed/23899063.
14. Kuerer HM, et al. Clinical course of breast cancer patients with complete pathologic primary tumor and axillary lymph node response to doxorubicin-based neoadjuvant chemotherapy. J Clin Oncol. 1999;17(2):460–9. ISSN 0732-183X. Disponível em: https://www.ncbi.nlm.nih.gov/pubmed/10080586.
15. Rouzier R, et al. Nomograms to predict pathologic complete response and metastasis-free survival after preoperative chemotherapy for breast cancer. J Clin Oncol. 2005;23(33):8331–9. ISSN 0732-183X. Disponível em: https://www.ncbi.nlm.nih.gov/pubmed/16293864.
16. Liedtke C, et al. Response to neoadjuvant therapy and long-term survival in patients with triple-negative breast cancer. J Clin Oncol. 2008;26(8):1275–81. ISSN 1527-7755. Disponível em: https://www.ncbi.nlm.nih.gov/pubmed/18250347.
17. Silver DP, et al. Efficacy of neoadjuvant Cisplatin in triple-negative breast cancer. J Clin Oncol. 2010;28(7):1145–53. ISSN 1527-7755. Disponível em: https://www.ncbi.nlm.nih.gov/pubmed/20100965.
18. King TA, Morrow M. Surgical issues in patients with breast cancer receiving neoadjuvant chemotherapy. Nat Rev Clin Oncol. 2015;12(6):335–43. ISSN 1759-4782. Disponível em: https://www.ncbi.nlm.nih.gov/pubmed/25850554.
19. Gianni L, et al. Neoadjuvant chemotherapy with trastuzumab followed by adjuvant trastuzumab versus neoadjuvant chemotherapy alone, in patients with HER2-positive locally advanced breast cancer (the NOAH trial): a randomised controlled superiority trial with a parallel HER2-negative cohort. Lancet. 2010;375(9712):377–84. ISSN 1474-547X. Disponível em: https://www.ncbi.nlm.nih.gov/pubmed/20113825.
20. Buzdar AU, et al. Significantly higher pathologic complete remission rate after neoadjuvant therapy with trastuzumab, paclitaxel, and epirubicin chemotherapy: results of a randomized trial in human epidermal growth factor receptor 2-positive operable breast cancer. J Clin Oncol. 2005;23(16):3676–85. ISSN 0732-183X. Disponível em: https://www.ncbi.nlm.nih.gov/pubmed/15738535.
21. Denkert C, et al. Tumor-associated lymphocytes as an independent predictor of response to neoadjuvant chemotherapy in breast cancer. J Clin Oncol. 2010;28(1):105–13. ISSN 1527-7755. Disponível em: https://www.ncbi.nlm.nih.gov/pubmed/19917869.
22. Salgado R, et al. Tumor-infiltrating lymphocytes and associations with pathological complete response and event-free survival in HER2-positive early-stage breast cancer treated with lapatinib and trastuzumab: a secondary analysis of the NeoALTTO trial. JAMA Oncol. 2015;1(4):448–54. ISSN 2374-2445. Disponível em: https://www.ncbi.nlm.nih.gov/pubmed/26181252.
23. Pu RT, et al. Pathologic features of breast cancer associated with complete response to neoadjuvant chemotherapy: importance of tumor necrosis. Am J Surg Pathol. 2005;29(3):354–8. ISSN 0147-5185. Disponível em: https://www.ncbi.nlm.nih.gov/pubmed/15725804.
24. Fisher B, et al. Effect of preoperative chemotherapy on the outcome of women with operable breast cancer. J Clin Oncol. 1998;16(8):2672–85. ISSN 0732-183X. Disponível em: https://www.ncbi.nlm.nih.gov/pubmed/9704717.
25. Bear HD, et al. Sequential preoperative or postoperative docetaxel added to preoperative doxorubicin plus cyclophosphamide for operable breast cancer: National Surgical Adjuvant Breast and Bowel Project Protocol B-27. J Clin Oncol. 2006;24(13):2019–27. ISSN 1527-7755. Disponível em: https://www.ncbi.nlm.nih.gov/pubmed/16606972.
26. Cortazar P, et al. Pathological complete response and long-term clinical benefit in breast cancer: the CTNeoBC pooled analysis. Lancet. 2014;384(9938):164–72. ISSN 1474-547X. Disponível em: https://www.ncbi.nlm.nih.gov/pubmed/24529560.

27. Delpech Y, et al. Clinical benefit from neoadjuvant chemotherapy in oestrogen receptor-positive invasive ductal and lobular carcinomas. Br J Cancer. 2013;108(2):285–91. ISSN 1532-1827. Disponível em: https://www.ncbi.nlm.nih.gov/pubmed/23299541.
28. Petruolo OA, et al. Standard pathologic features can be used to identify a subset of estrogen receptor-positive, HER2 negative patients likely to benefit from neoadjuvant chemotherapy. Ann Surg Oncol. 2017;24(9):2556–62. ISSN 1534-4681. Disponível em: https://www.ncbi.nlm.nih.gov/pubmed/28560596.
29. Cristofanilli M, et al. Invasive lobular carcinoma classic type: response to primary chemotherapy and survival outcomes. J Clin Oncol. 2005;23(1):41–8. ISSN 0732-183X. Disponível em: https://www.ncbi.nlm.nih.gov/pubmed/15625359.
30. Riba LA, et al. Characterizing response to neoadjuvant chemotherapy in invasive lobular breast carcinoma. J Surg Res. 2019;233:436–43. ISSN 1095-8673. Disponível em: https://www.ncbi.nlm.nih.gov/pubmed/30502283.
31. Truin W, et al. Differences in response and surgical management with neoadjuvant chemotherapy in invasive lobular versus ductal breast cancer. Ann Surg Oncol. 2016;23(1):51–7. ISSN 1534-4681. Disponível em: https://www.ncbi.nlm.nih.gov/pubmed/25980321.
32. Marmor S, et al. Relative effectiveness of adjuvant chemotherapy for invasive lobular compared with invasive ductal carcinoma of the breast. Cancer. 2017;123(16):3015–21. ISSN 1097-0142. Disponível em: https://www.ncbi.nlm.nih.gov/pubmed/28382636.
33. Matsubara N, et al. Different prognostic significance of Ki-67 change between pre- and post-neoadjuvant chemotherapy in various subtypes of breast cancer. Breast Cancer Res Treat. 2013;137(1):203–12. ISSN 1573-7217. Disponível em: https://www.ncbi.nlm.nih.gov/pubmed/23184081.
34. Rabban JT, et al. Pure and predominantly pure intralymphatic breast carcinoma after neoadjuvant chemotherapy: an unusual and adverse pattern of residual disease. Am J Surg Pathol. 2009;33(2):256–63. ISSN 1532-0979. Disponível em: https://www.ncbi.nlm.nih.gov/pubmed/18936689.
35. Cheng E, et al. Residual pure intralymphatic breast carcinoma following neoadjuvant chemotherapy is indicative of poor clinical outcome, even in node-negative patients. Am J Surg Pathol. 2017;41(9):1275–82. ISSN 1532-0979. Disponível em: https://www.ncbi.nlm.nih.gov/pubmed/28654428.
36. Mc G, Sc L. Lymph-vascular invasion in the absence of stroll invasion after neoadjuvant therapy: a rare pattern of residual carcinoma that lacks an AJCC/UICC T category. San Antonio Breast Cancer Symposium; 2016.
37. Chen AM, et al. Breast conservation after neoadjuvant chemotherapy: the MD Anderson cancer center experience. J Clin Oncol. 2004;22(12):2303–12. ISSN 0732-183X. Disponível em: https://www.ncbi.nlm.nih.gov/pubmed/15197191.
38. Sharkey FE, et al. Effects of preoperative chemotherapy on the morphology of resectable breast carcinoma. Mod Pathol. 1996;9(9):893–900. ISSN 0893-3952. Disponível em: https://www.ncbi.nlm.nih.gov/pubmed/8878021.
39. Liu YL, et al. Lymphovascular invasion is an independent predictor of survival in breast cancer after neoadjuvant chemotherapy. Breast Cancer Res Treat. 2016;157(3):555–64. ISSN 1573-7217. Disponível em: https://www.ncbi.nlm.nih.gov/pubmed/27225388.
40. Uematsu T, et al. Is lymphovascular invasion degree one of the important factors to predict neoadjuvant chemotherapy efficacy in breast cancer? Breast Cancer. 2011;18(4):309–13. ISSN 1880-4233. Disponível em: https://www.ncbi.nlm.nih.gov/pubmed/20574730.
41. Caudle AS, et al. Local-regional control according to surrogate markers of breast cancer subtypes and response to neoadjuvant chemotherapy in breast cancer patients undergoing breast conserving therapy. Breast Cancer Res. 2012;14(3):R83. ISSN 1465-542X. Disponível em: https://www.ncbi.nlm.nih.gov/pubmed/22621334.
42. Mazouni C, et al. Residual ductal carcinoma in situ in patients with complete eradication of invasive breast cancer after neoadjuvant chemotherapy does not adversely affect patient outcome. J Clin Oncol. 2007;25(19):2650–5. ISSN 1527-7755. Disponível em: https://www.ncbi.nlm.nih.gov/pubmed/17602071.

43. Von Minckwitz G, et al. Definition and impact of pathologic complete response on prognosis after neoadjuvant chemotherapy in various intrinsic breast cancer subtypes. J Clin Oncol. 2012;30(15):1796–804. ISSN 1527-7755. Disponível em: https://www.ncbi.nlm.nih.gov/pubmed/22508812.
44. Salgado R, et al. The evaluation of tumor-infiltrating lymphocytes (TILs) in breast cancer: recommendations by an International TILs Working Group 2014. Ann Oncol. 2015;26(2):259–71. ISSN 1569-8041. Disponível em: https://www.ncbi.nlm.nih.gov/pubmed/25214542.
45. Hendry S, et al. Assessing tumor-infiltrating lymphocytes in solid tumors: a practical review for pathologists and proposal for a standardized method from the International Immunooncology Biomarkers Working Group: Part 1: assessing the host immune response, TILs in invasive breast carcinoma and ductal carcinoma in situ, metastatic tumor deposits and areas for further research. Adv Anat Pathol. 2017;24(5):235–51. ISSN 1533-4031. Disponível em: https://www.ncbi.nlm.nih.gov/pubmed/28777142.
46. Dieci MV, et al. Update on tumor-infiltrating lymphocytes (TILs) in breast cancer, including recommendations to assess TILs in residual disease after neoadjuvant therapy and in carcinoma in situ: a report of the International Immuno-Oncology Biomarker Working Group on Breast Cancer. Semin Cancer Biol. 2018;52(Pt 2):16–25. ISSN 1096-3650. Disponível em: https://www.ncbi.nlm.nih.gov/pubmed/29024776.
47. Mlecnik B, et al. The tumor microenvironment and Immunoscore are critical determinants of dissemination to distant metastasis. Sci Transl Med. 2016;8(327):327ra26. ISSN 1946-6242. Disponível em: https://www.ncbi.nlm.nih.gov/pubmed/26912905.
48. Loi S, et al. Prognostic and predictive value of tumor-infiltrating lymphocytes in a phase III randomized adjuvant breast cancer trial in node-positive breast cancer comparing the addition of docetaxel to doxorubicin with doxorubicin-based chemotherapy: BIG 02-98. J Clin Oncol. 2013;31(7):860–7. ISSN 1527-7755. Disponível em: https://www.ncbi.nlm.nih.gov/pubmed/23341518.
49. Denkert C, et al. Tumour-infiltrating lymphocytes and prognosis in different subtypes of breast cancer: a pooled analysis of 3771 patients treated with neoadjuvant therapy. Lancet Oncol. 2018;19(1):40–50. ISSN 1474-5488. Disponível em: https://www.ncbi.nlm.nih.gov/pubmed/29233559.
50. Yang X, et al. Evaluation of the predictive and prognostic values of stromal tumor-infiltrating lymphocytes in HER2-positive breast cancers treated with neoadjuvant chemotherapy. Target Oncol. 2018;13(6):757–67. ISSN 1776-260X. Disponível em: https://www.ncbi.nlm.nih.gov/pubmed/30406444.
51. Hwang HW, et al. A nomogram to predict pathologic complete response (pCR) and the value of tumor-infiltrating lymphocytes (TILs) for prediction of response to neoadjuvant chemotherapy (NAC) in breast cancer patients. Breast Cancer Res Treat. 2019;173(2):255–66. ISSN 1573-7217. Disponível em: https://www.ncbi.nlm.nih.gov/pubmed/30324273.
52. Ruan M, et al. Predictive value of tumor-infiltrating lymphocytes to pathological complete response in neoadjuvant treated triple-negative breast cancers. Diagn Pathol. 2018;13(1):66. ISSN 1746-1596. Disponível em: https://www.ncbi.nlm.nih.gov/pubmed/30170605.
53. Luen SJ, et al. Prognostic implications of residual disease tumor-infiltrating lymphocytes and residual cancer burden in triple negative breast cancer patients after neo-adjuvant chemotherapy. Ann Oncol. 2019;30(2):236–42. ISSN 1569-8041. Disponível em: https://www.ncbi.nlm.nih.gov/pubmed/30590484.
54. Zhang L, Wang XI, Zhang S. Tumor-infiltrating lymphocyte volume is a better predictor of neoadjuvant therapy response and overall survival in triple-negative invasive breast cancer. Hum Pathol. 2018;80:47–54. ISSN 1532-8392. Disponível em: https://www.ncbi.nlm.nih.gov/pubmed/29883779.
55. Labrosse J, et al. Chemosensitivity, tumor infiltrating lymphocytes (TILs), and survival of postpartum PABC patients treated by neoadjuvant chemotherapy. Breast. 2018;42:61–7. ISSN 1532-3080. Disponível em: https://www.ncbi.nlm.nih.gov/pubmed/30179779.
56. Stanton SE, Adams S, Disis ML. Variation in the incidence and magnitude of tumor-infiltrating lymphocytes in breast cancer subtypes: a systematic review. JAMA Oncol.

2016;2(10):1354–60. ISSN 2374-2445. Disponível em: https://www.ncbi.nlm.nih.gov/pubmed/27355489.
57. Dieci MV, et al. Prognostic and predictive value of tumor-infiltrating lymphocytes in two phase III randomized adjuvant breast cancer trials. Ann Oncol. 2015;26(8):1698–704. ISSN 1569-8041. Disponível em: https://www.ncbi.nlm.nih.gov/pubmed/259953[illegible].
58. Issa-Nummer Y, et al. Prospective validation of immunological infiltrate for prediction of response to neoadjuvant chemotherapy in HER2-negative breast cancer--a substudy of the neoadjuvant GeparQuinto trial. PLoS One. 2013;8(12):e79775. ISSN 1932-6203. Disponível em: https://www.ncbi.nlm.nih.gov/pubmed/24312450.
59. Dieci MV, et al. Prognostic value of tumor-infiltrating lymphocytes on residual disease after primary chemotherapy for triple-negative breast cancer: a retrospective multicenter study. Ann Oncol. 2014;25(3):611–8. ISSN 1569-8041. Disponível em: https://www.ncbi.nlm.nih.gov/pubmed/24401929.
60. Liu S, et al. CD8+ lymphocyte infiltration is an independent favorable prognostic indicator in basal-like breast cancer. Breast Cancer Res. 2012;14(2):R48. ISSN 1465-542X. Disponível em: https://www.ncbi.nlm.nih.gov/pubmed/22420471.
61. Loi S, et al. Tumor infiltrating lymphocytes are prognostic in triple negative breast cancer and predictive for trastuzumab benefit in early breast cancer: results from the FinHER trial. Ann Oncol. 2014;25(8):1544–50. ISSN 1569-8041. Disponível em: https://www.ncbi.nlm.nih.gov/pubmed/24608200.
62. Hamy AS, et al. Stromal lymphocyte infiltration after neoadjuvant chemotherapy is associated with aggressive residual disease and lower disease-free survival in HER2-positive breast cancer. Ann Oncol. 2017;28(9):2233–40. ISSN 1569-8041. Disponível em: https://www.ncbi.nlm.nih.gov/pubmed/28911063.
63. Ali HR, et al. Computational pathology of pre-treatment biopsies identifies lymphocyte density as a predictor of response to neoadjuvant chemotherapy in breast cancer. Breast Cancer Res. 2016;18(1):21. ISSN 1465-542X. Disponível em: https://www.ncbi.nlm.nih.gov/pubmed/26882907.
64. Ladoire S, et al. Pathologic complete response to neoadjuvant chemotherapy of breast carcinoma is associated with the disappearance of tumor-infiltrating foxp3+ regulatory T cells. Clin Cancer Res. 2008;14(8):2413–20. ISSN 1078-0432. Disponível em: https://www.ncbi.nlm.nih.gov/pubmed/18413832.
65. Pelekanou V, et al. Tumor-infiltrating lymphocytes and PD-L1 expression in pre- and post-treatment breast cancers in the SWOG S0800 phase II neoadjuvant chemotherapy trial. Mol Cancer Ther. 2018;17(6):1324–31. ISSN 1538-8514. Disponível em: https://www.ncbi.nlm.nih.gov/pubmed/29588392.
66. García-Martínez E, et al. Tumor-infiltrating immune cell profiles and their change after neoadjuvant chemotherapy predict response and prognosis of breast cancer. Breast Cancer Res. 2014;16(6):488. ISSN 1465-542X. Disponível em: https://www.ncbi.nlm.nih.gov/pubmed/25432519.
67. Loi S, et al. RAS/MAPK activation is associated with reduced tumor-infiltrating lymphocytes in triple-negative breast cancer: therapeutic cooperation between MEK and PD-1/PD-L1 immune checkpoint inhibitors. Clin Cancer Res. 2016;22(6):1499–509. ISSN 1078-0432. Disponível em: https://www.ncbi.nlm.nih.gov/pubmed/26515496.
68. Miyashita M, et al. Prognostic significance of tumor-infiltrating CD8+ and FOXP3+ lymphocytes in residual tumors and alterations in these parameters after neoadjuvant chemotherapy in triple-negative breast cancer: a retrospective multicenter study. Breast Cancer Res. 2015;17:124. ISSN 1465-542X. Disponível em: https://www.ncbi.nlm.nih.gov/pubmed/26341640.
69. Gennari R, et al. Pilot study of the mechanism of action of preoperative trastuzumab in patients with primary operable breast tumors overexpressing HER2. Clin Cancer Res. 2004;10(17):5650–5. ISSN 1078-0432. Disponível em: https://www.ncbi.nlm.nih.gov/pubmed/15355889.

70. Demaria S, et al. Development of tumor-infiltrating lymphocytes in breast cancer after neoadjuvant paclitaxel chemotherapy. Clin Cancer Res. 2001;7(10):3025–30. ISSN 1078-0432. Disponível em: https://www.ncbi.nlm.nih.gov/pubmed/11595690.
71. Bianchini G, Gianni L. The immune system and response to HER2-targeted treatment in breast cancer. Lancet Oncol. 2014;15(2):e58–68. ISSN 1474-5488. Disponível em: https://www.ncbi.nlm.nih.gov/pubmed/24480556.
72. Hennessy BT, et al. Outcome after pathologic complete eradication of cytologically proven breast cancer axillary node metastases following primary chemotherapy. J Clin Oncol. 2005;23(36):9304–11. ISSN 0732-183X. Disponível em: https://www.ncbi.nlm.nih.gov/pubmed/16361629.
73. Mccready DR, et al. The prognostic significance of lymph node metastases after preoperative chemotherapy for locally advanced breast cancer. Arch Surg. 1989;124(1):21–5. ISSN 0004-0010. Disponível em: https://www.ncbi.nlm.nih.gov/pubmed/2910244.
74. Kuerer HM, et al. Residual metastatic axillary lymph nodes following neoadjuvant chemotherapy predict disease-free survival in patients with locally advanced breast cancer. Am J Surg. 1998;176(6):502–9. ISSN 0002-9610. Disponível em: https://www.ncbi.nlm.nih.gov/pubmed/9926779.
75. Rastogi P, et al. Preoperative chemotherapy: updates of National Surgical Adjuvant Breast and Bowel Project Protocols B-18 and B-27. J Clin Oncol. 2008;26(5):778–85. ISSN 1527-7755. Disponível em: https://www.ncbi.nlm.nih.gov/pubmed/18258986.
76. Rouzier R, et al. Incidence and prognostic significance of complete axillary downstaging after primary chemotherapy in breast cancer patients with T1 to T3 tumors and cytologically proven axillary metastatic lymph nodes. J Clin Oncol. 2002;20(5):1304–10. ISSN 0732-183X. Disponível em: https://www.ncbi.nlm.nih.gov/pubmed/11870173.
77. Buchholz TA, et al. Predictors of local-regional recurrence after neoadjuvant chemotherapy and mastectomy without radiation. J Clin Oncol. 2002;20(1):17–23. ISSN 0732-183X. Disponível em: https://www.ncbi.nlm.nih.gov/pubmed/11773149.
78. Klauber-Demore N, et al. Size of residual lymph node metastasis after neoadjuvant chemotherapy in locally advanced breast cancer patients is prognostic. Ann Surg Oncol. 2006;13(5):685–91. ISSN 1068-9265. Disponível em: https://www.ncbi.nlm.nih.gov/pubmed/16523367.
79. Newman LA, et al. Histopathologic evidence of tumor regression in the axillary lymph nodes of patients treated with preoperative chemotherapy correlates with breast cancer outcome. Ann Surg Oncol. 2003;10(7):734–9. ISSN 1068-9265. Disponível em: https://www.ncbi.nlm.nih.gov/pubmed/12900363.
80. American Joint Committee on Cancer (AJCC). AJCC cancer staging manual. 8th ed. New York: Springer; 2017.
81. Lakhani EI Sr, Schnitt SJS, et al. WHO classification of tumors of the breast. 4th ed. Lyon: International Agency for Research on Cancer; 2012. ISBN 978-92-832-2433-4.
82. Wolmark N, et al. Preoperative chemotherapy in patients with operable breast cancer: nine-year results from National Surgical Adjuvant Breast and Bowel Project B-18. J Natl Cancer Inst Monogr. 2001;(30):96–102. ISSN 1052-6773. Disponível em: https://www.ncbi.nlm.nih.gov/pubmed/11773300.
83. Chevallier B, et al. Lenograstim prevents morbidity from intensive induction chemotherapy in the treatment of inflammatory breast cancer. J Clin Oncol. 1995;13(7):1564–71. ISSN 0732-183X. Disponível em: https://www.ncbi.nlm.nih.gov/pubmed/7541448.
84. Sinn HP, et al. [Histologic regression of breast cancer after primary (neoadjuvant) chemotherapy]. Geburtshilfe Frauenheilkd. 1994;54(10):552–8. ISSN 0016-5751. Disponível em: https://www.ncbi.nlm.nih.gov/pubmed/8001751.
85. Sataloff DM, et al. Pathologic response to induction chemotherapy in locally advanced carcinoma of the breast: a determinant of outcome. J Am Coll Surg. 1995;180(3):297–306. ISSN 1072-7515. Disponível em: https://www.ncbi.nlm.nih.gov/pubmed/7874340.

86. Chollet P, et al. A new prognostic classification after primary chemotherapy for breast cancer: residual disease in breast and nodes (RDBN). Cancer J. 2008;14(2):128–32. ISSN 1528-9117. Disponível em: https://www.ncbi.nlm.nih.gov/pubmed/18391619.
87. Tordai A, et al. Evaluation of biological pathways involved in chemotherapy response in breast cancer. Breast Cancer Res. 2008;10(2):R37. ISSN 1465-542X. Disponível em: https://www.ncbi.nlm.nih.gov/pubmed/18445275.
88. Pilewskie M, Morrow M. Axillary nodal management following neoadjuvant chemotherapy: a review. JAMA Oncol. 2017;3(4):549–55. ISSN 2374-2445. Disponível em: https://www.ncbi.nlm.nih.gov/pubmed/27918753.
89. Symmans WF, et al. Measurement of residual breast cancer burden to predict survival after neoadjuvant chemotherapy. J Clin Oncol. 2007;25(28):4414–22. ISSN 1527-7755. Disponível em: https://www.ncbi.nlm.nih.gov/pubmed/17785706.
90. Symmans WF, et al. Long-term prognostic risk after neoadjuvant chemotherapy associated with residual cancer burden and breast cancer subtype. J Clin Oncol. 2017;35(10):1049–60. ISSN 1527-7755. Disponível em: https://www.ncbi.nlm.nih.gov/pubmed/28135148.
91. Yi M, et al. Staging for breast cancer patients receiving neoadjuvant chemotherapy: utility of incorporating biologic factors. Ann Surg Oncol. 2020;27(2):359–66. ISSN 1534-4681. Disponível em: https://www.ncbi.nlm.nih.gov/pubmed/31667721.
92. Mittendorf EA, et al. The neo-bioscore update for staging breast cancer treated with neoadjuvant chemotherapy: incorporation of prognostic biologic factors into staging after treatment. JAMA Oncol. 2016;2(7):929–36. ISSN 2374-2445. Disponível em: https://www.ncbi.nlm.nih.gov/pubmed/26986538.
93. Giuliano AE, et al. Breast Cancer-Major changes in the American Joint Committee on Cancer eighth edition cancer staging manual. CA Cancer J Clin. 2017;67(4):290–303. ISSN 1542-4863. Disponível em: https://www.ncbi.nlm.nih.gov/pubmed/28294295.
94. Baker GM, King TA, Schnitt SJ. Evaluation of breast and axillary lymph node specimens in breast cancer patients treated with neoadjuvant systemic therapy. Adv Anat Pathol. 2019;26(4):221–34. ISSN 1533-4031. Disponível em: https://www.ncbi.nlm.nih.gov/pubmed/31149907.
95. Moran MS, et al. Society of Surgical Oncology-American Society for Radiation Oncology consensus guideline on margins for breast-conserving surgery with whole-breast irradiation in stages I and II invasive breast cancer. J Clin Oncol. 2014;32(14):1507–15. ISSN 1527-7755. Disponível em: https://www.ncbi.nlm.nih.gov/pubmed/24516019.
96. Morrow M, et al. Society of Surgical Oncology-American Society for Radiation Oncology-American Society of Clinical Oncology consensus guideline on margins for breast-conserving surgery with whole-breast irradiation in ductal carcinoma in situ. J Clin Oncol. 2016;34(33):4040–6. ISSN 1527-7755. Disponível em: https://www.ncbi.nlm.nih.gov/pubmed/27528719.
97. Choi J, et al. Margins in breast-conserving surgery after neoadjuvant therapy. Ann Surg Oncol. 2018;25(12):3541–7. ISSN 1534-4681. Disponível em: https://www.ncbi.nlm.nih.gov/pubmed/30128902.
98. Rouzier R, et al. Primary chemotherapy for operable breast cancer: incidence and prognostic significance of ipsilateral breast tumor recurrence after breast-conserving surgery. J Clin Oncol. 2001;19(18):3828–35. ISSN 0732-183X. Disponível em: https://www.ncbi.nlm.nih.gov/pubmed/11559720.
99. Jwa E, et al. Locoregional recurrence by tumor biology in breast cancer patients after preoperative chemotherapy and breast conservation treatment. Cancer Res Treat. 2016;48(4):1363–72. ISSN 2005-9256. Disponível em: https://www.ncbi.nlm.nih.gov/pubmed/26910473.
100. Jabbour MN, Massad CY, Boulos FI. Variability in hormone and growth factor receptor expression in primary versus recurrent, metastatic, and post-neoadjuvant breast carcinoma. Breast Cancer Res Treat. 2012;135(1):29–37. ISSN 1573-7217. Disponível em: https://www.ncbi.nlm.nih.gov/pubmed/22484731.

101. Zhang N, et al. The hormonal receptor status in breast cancer can be altered by neoadjuvant chemotherapy: a meta-analysis. Cancer Invest. 2011;29(9):594–8. ISSN 1532-4192. Disponível em: https://www.ncbi.nlm.nih.gov/pubmed/22011281.
102. Polley MY, et al. An international Ki67 reproducibility study. J Natl Cancer Inst. 2013;105(24):1897–906. ISSN 1460-2105. Disponível em: https://www.ncbi.nlm.nih.gov/pubmed/24203987.
103. Denkert C, et al. Ki67 levels as predictive and prognostic parameters in pretherapeutic breast cancer core biopsies: a translational investigation in the neoadjuvant GeparTrio trial. Ann Oncol. 2013;24(11):2786–93. ISSN 1569-8041. Disponível em: https://www.ncbi.nlm.nih.gov/pubmed/23970015.
104. Denkert C, et al. Strategies for developing Ki67 as a useful biomarker in breast cancer. Breast. 2015;24(Suppl 2):S67–72. ISSN 1532-3080. Disponível em: https://www.ncbi.nlm.nih.gov/pubmed/26283598.
105. Polley MY, et al. An international study to increase concordance in Ki67 scoring. Mod Pathol. 2015;28(6):778–86. ISSN 1530-0285. Disponível em: https://www.ncbi.nlm.nih.gov/pubmed/25698062.
106. Coates AS, et al. Tailoring therapies--improving the management of early breast cancer: St Gallen International Expert Consensus on the primary therapy of early breast cancer 2015. Ann Oncol. 2015;26(8):1533–46. ISSN 1569-8041. Disponível em: https://www.ncbi.nlm.nih.gov/pubmed/25939896.
107. Chen R, et al. Assessment of the predictive role of pretreatment Ki-67 and Ki-67 changes in breast cancer patients receiving neoadjuvant chemotherapy according to the molecular classification: a retrospective study of 1010 patients. Breast Cancer Res Treat. 2018;170(1):35–43. ISSN 1573-7217. Disponível em: https://www.ncbi.nlm.nih.gov/pubmed/29480449.
108. Cabrera-Galeana P, et al. Ki67 changes identify worse outcomes in residual breast cancer tumors after neoadjuvant chemotherapy. Oncologist. 2018;23(6):670–8. ISSN 1549-490X. Disponível em: https://www.ncbi.nlm.nih.gov/pubmed/29490940.

Part II
Pre- and Post-neoadjuvant Systemic Therapy Imaging Considerations

Chapter 3
Radiology Case Presentations in Neoadjuvant Setting

Uzma Waheed and Margarita Zuley

Case 1 This woman presented with an area of palpable concern in her right breast. She underwent ultrasound-guided core biopsy which revealed right invasive ductal carcinoma, nuclear grade 3 (ER/PR-positive, HER-2 negative, Ki-67 30%). Clinical stage IA (T1, N0, M0). She received four cycles of T/C systemic therapy with incomplete response (Figs. 3.1, 3.2, 3.3, 3.4, 3.5, and 3.6).

Case 2 This woman presented for mammographic screening which detected left breast invasive ductal carcinoma (nuclear grade 2, ER/PR-negative, Her2-positive, Ki-67 30%). Following NST with six cycles of TCH-P therapy, she achieved a complete imaging response with pathologic complete response (pCR) verified at surgery, ypT0N0 (Figs. 3.7, 3.8, 3.9, 3.10, and 3.11).

Case 3 This woman had a right breast mass detected on screening mammography, core biopsy-proven TN IDC. She received NST with A/C/T and post-therapy imaging revealed a partial response. This study shows how partial disease can have persistent kinetics (blue on kinetic color overlay) identified on MRI similar to fibrosis; tumor enhancement kinetics after treatment may also be below the kinetic threshold on MRI. Indeed, in this case, residual disease was found at surgery measuring 1.1 cm similar to that reported on posttreatment US and MRI.

U. Waheed (✉)
Breast Imaging Division, Department of Radiology, Stanford University, Palo Alto, CA, USA
e-mail: uzmaw@stanford.edu

M. Zuley
Breast Imaging Division, Department of Radiology, University of Pittsburgh Medical Center, Pittsburgh, PA, USA
e-mail: zuleyml@upmc.edu

A. Soran, F. Nakhlis (eds.), *Management of the Breast and Axilla in the Neoadjuvant Setting*, https://doi.org/10.1007/978-3-030-88020-0_3

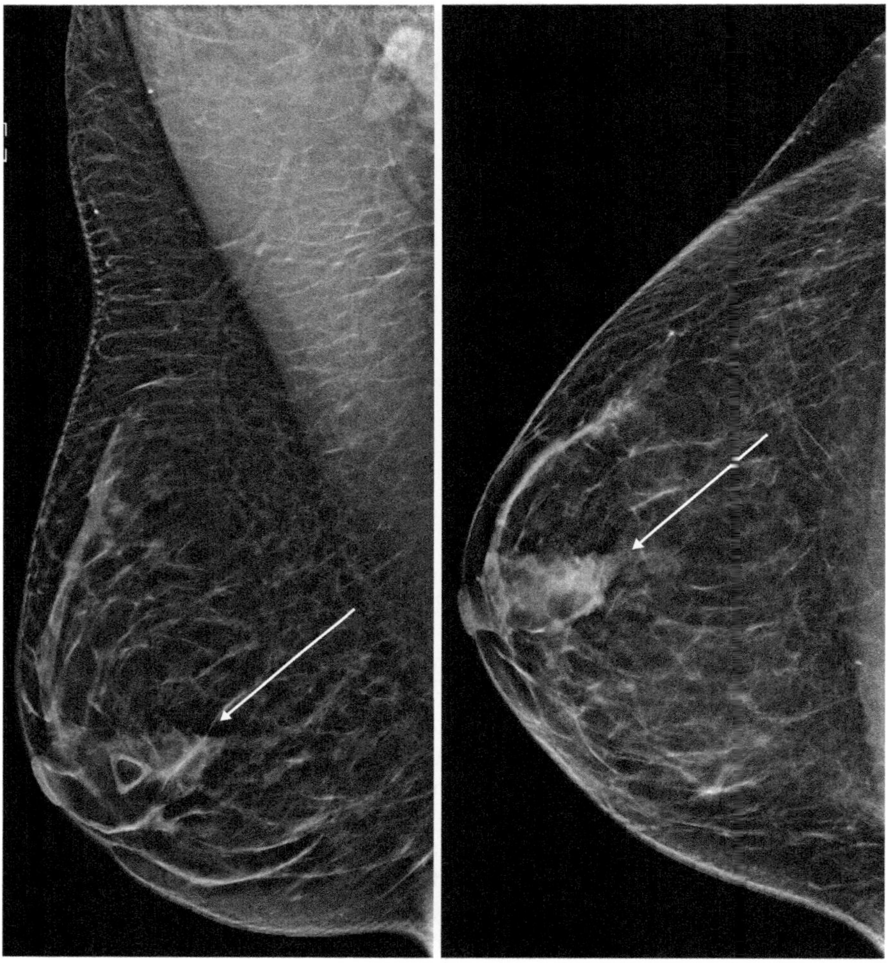

Fig. 3.1 Digital mammogram with tomosynthesis including mediolateral oblique (MLO, left) and craniocaudal (CC, right) shows an irregular dense mass (arrow) with an overlying triangular marker on the MLO view denoting the corresponding area of palpable concern

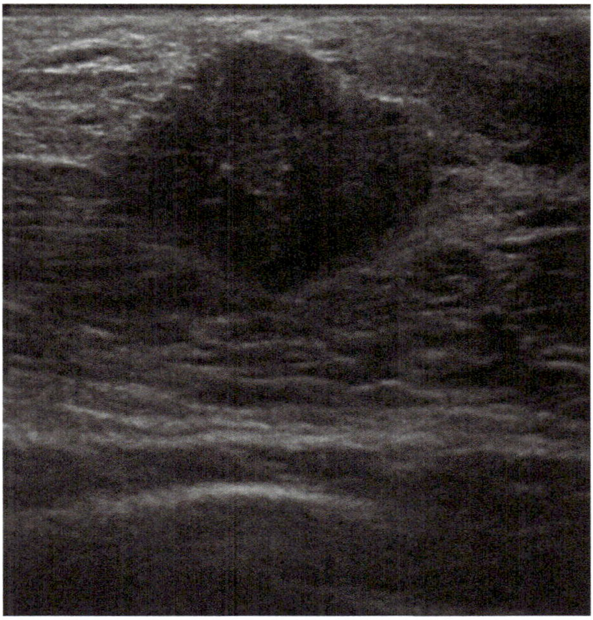

Fig. 3.2 Grayscale ultrasound (US) shows an oval mass with irregular and indistinct margins (arrow) and no posterior features

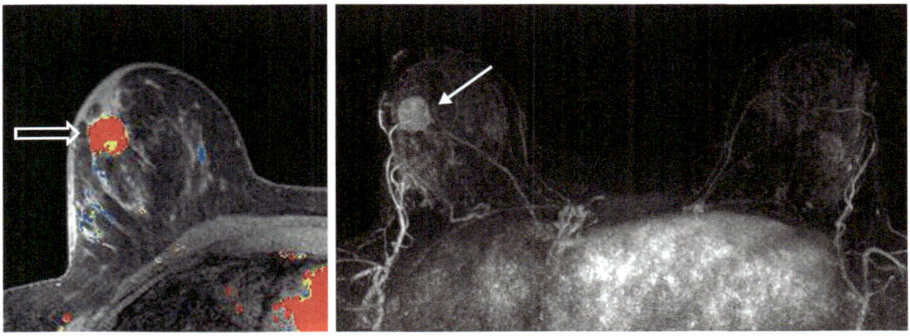

Fig. 3.3 Axial T1 post-contrast fat saturation (left) and MIP (maximum intensity projection) post-processed image (right) show an irregular homogenously enhancing mass (arrow) with washout kinetics (open arrow)

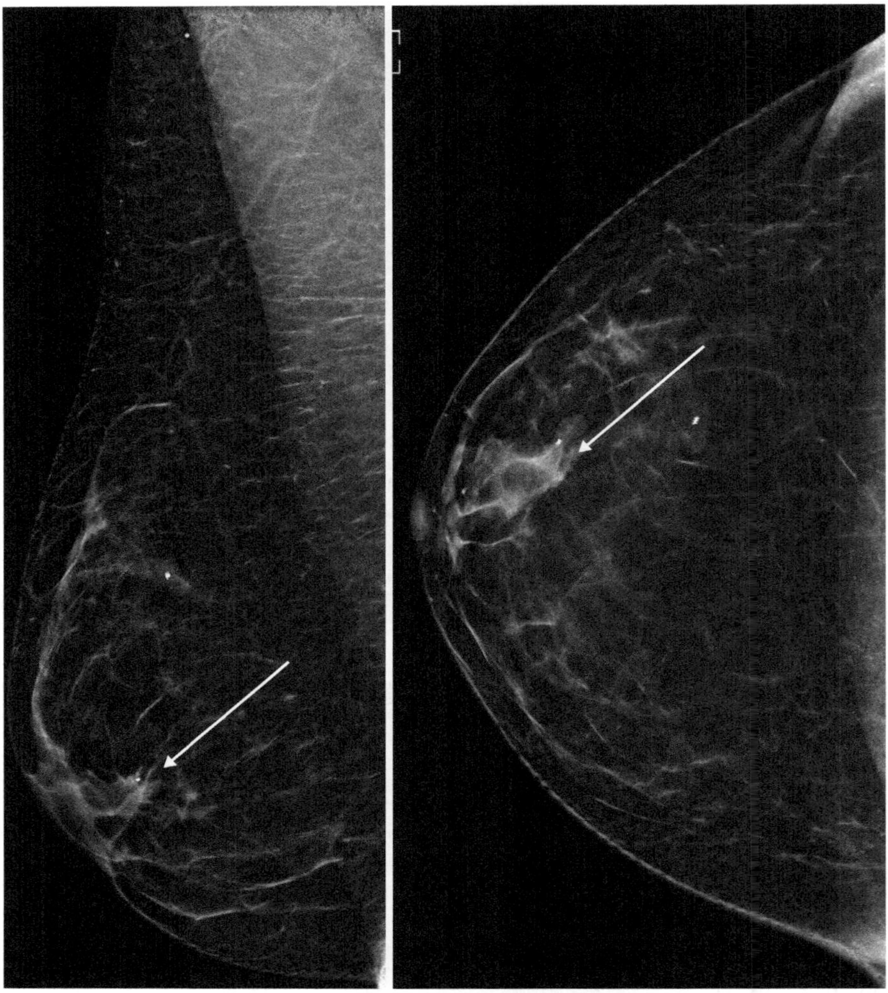

Fig. 3.4 Following NST digital mammogram (MG) with tomosynthesis including MLO (right) and CC (left) views showed the mass has decreased in size; there is associated architectural distortion (best seen on the MLO view) which can be seen with treatment-related fibrosis but is difficult to delineate from residual disease on MG and US

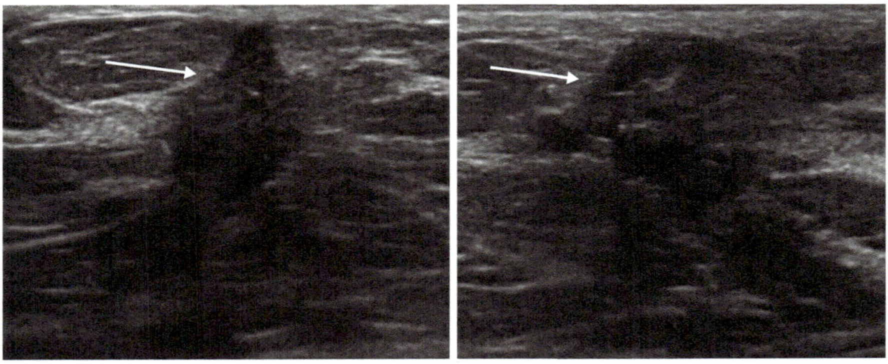

Fig. 3.5 Grayscale ultrasound shows incomplete response to NST with a small residual hypoechoic mass with angular and irregular margins (arrow)

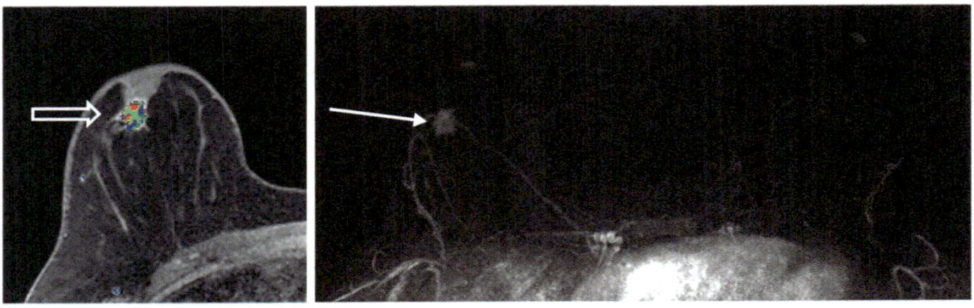

Fig. 3.6 Axial T1 post-contrast fat saturation (left) and MIP (maximum intensity projection) post-processed image (right) show a small residual right breast mass at the site of core biopsy proven IDC (arrow). The kinetic color overlay shows heterogeneous mixed kinetics (open arrow), compared to the homogenous washout kinetics on pretreatment MRI

T2N0 screen detected TN breast cancer 7/28/20 (Figs. 3.12, 3.13, 3.14, 3.15, 3.16, 3.17, and 3.18).

Case 4 This 57-year-old woman was diagnosed with screen detected left IDC at the 12:00 position (nuclear grade 3, ER/PR-negative, HER-2-negative by FISH, Ki-67 greater than 90% with lymphovascular invasion) (Fig. 3.19). Left axillary node biopsy CNB showed metastatic carcinoma (Fig. 3.20). She completed 4 cycles of Adriamycin and Cytoxan and then completed 12 cycles of Taxol and carboplatin. Following NST, complete response was proven in the breast and lymph node (Figs. 3.21, 3.22, and 3.23).

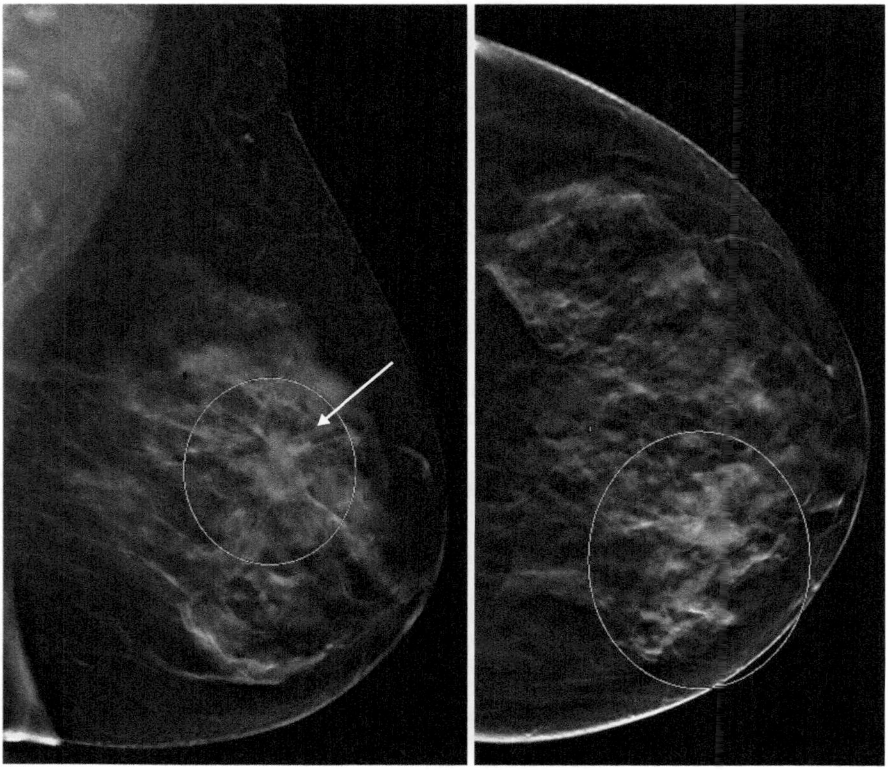

Fig. 3.7 Digital MG with tomosynthesis including MLO and CC views shows an irregular mass (circle) with architectural distortion (arrow) in the medial left breast

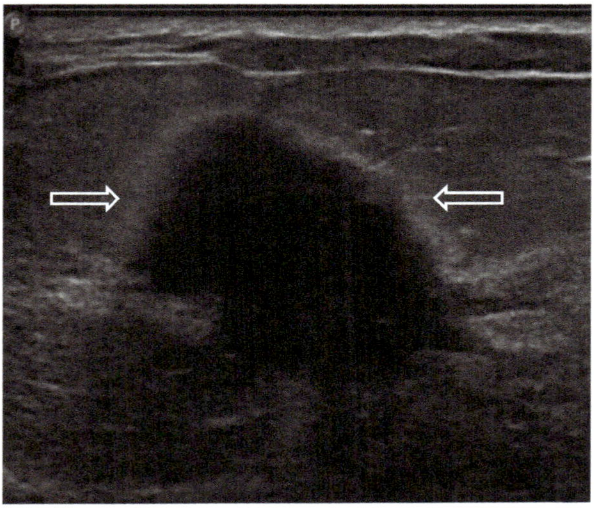

Fig. 3.8 Grayscale ultrasound shows an irregular hypoechoic mass with a peripheral echogenic rim (open arrows) corresponding to tumor infiltration

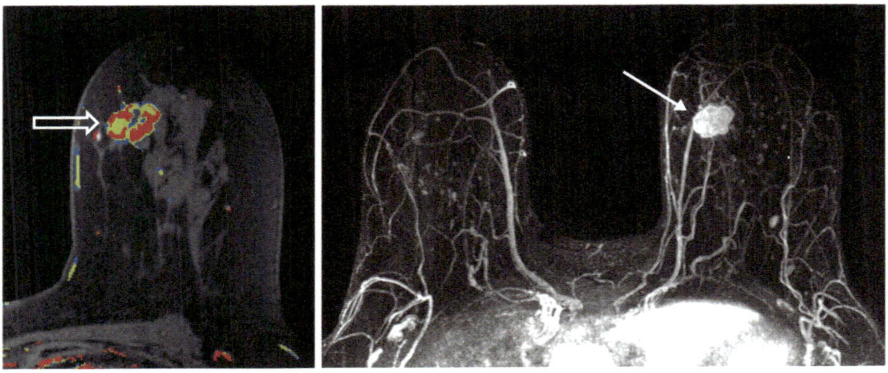

Fig. 3.9 Pretreatment axial T1 post-contrast fat saturation (left) and MIP (maximum intensity projection) post-processed image (right) show an irregular homogenously enhancing mass in the medial left breast (arrow). The mass demonstrated predominant washout kinetics (open arrow)

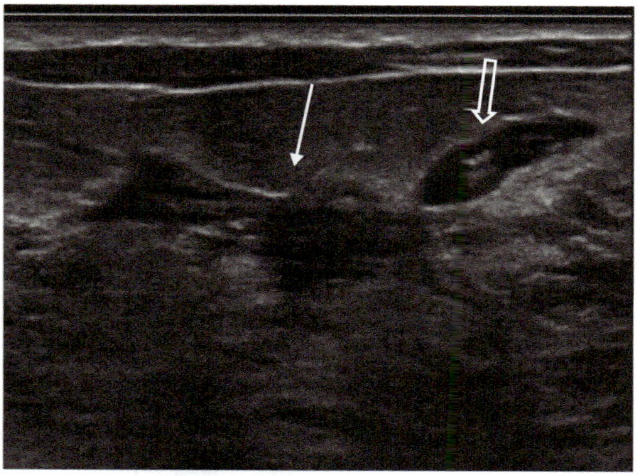

Fig. 3.10 Post-NST grayscale US shows a residual parallel hypoechoic mass-like area (arrow); it is difficult to assess residual disease versus treatment-related fibrosis within this area. The hydrophilic clip from previous CNB is identified nearby (open arrow)

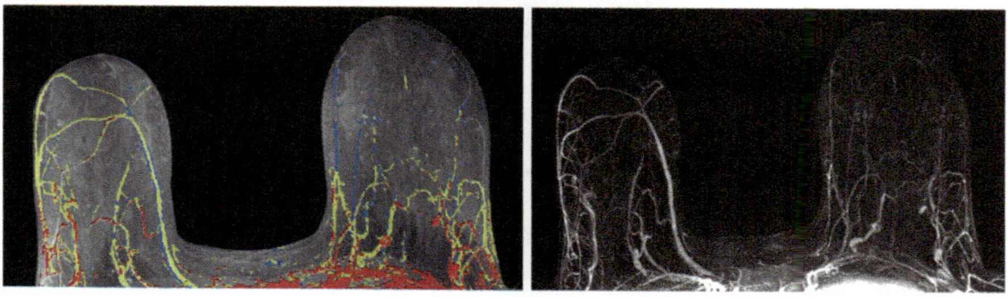

Fig. 3.11 Post-NST MIP MRI with (left) and without (right) kinetic overlay shows no residual enhancing mass or NME consistent with a complete imaging response and strongly favoring treatment-related fibrosis rather than residual disease at the aforementioned hypoechoic mass-like area (Fig. 3.10) identified on US

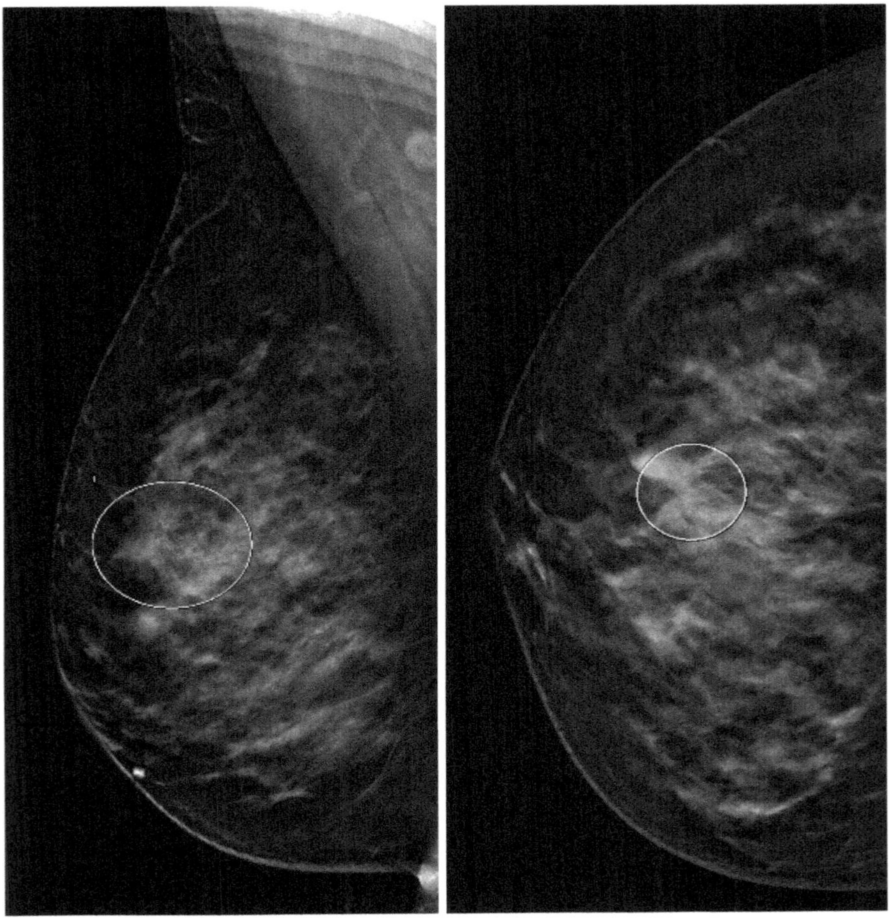

Fig. 3.12 MLO (left) and CC (right) digital MG views with tomosynthesis show heterogeneously dense breast tissue; a focal asymmetry with subtle architectural distortion was identified, best seen on the tomosynthesis image slices (circle)

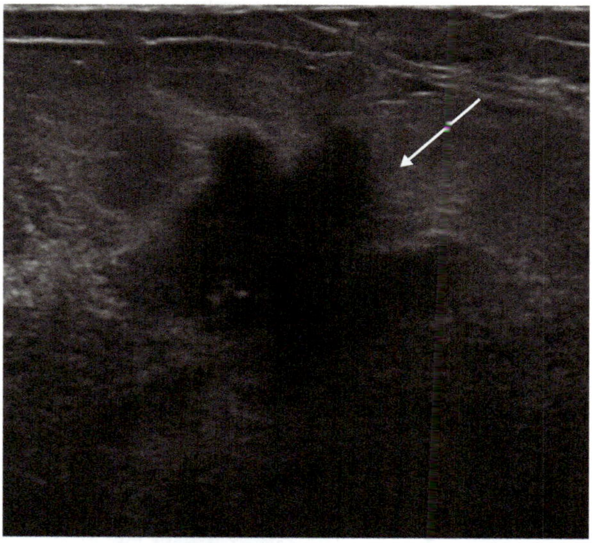

Fig. 3.13 Grayscale ultrasound shows a corresponding irregular hypoechoic mass (arrow)

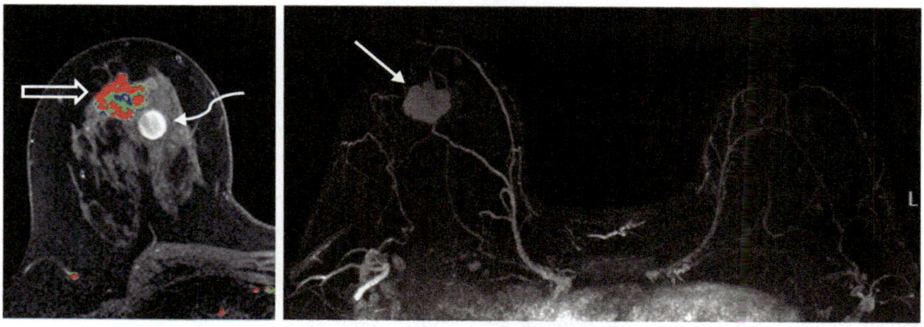

Fig. 3.14 Pretreatment axial T1 post-contrast fat saturation image with kinetic color overlay (left) and MIP (right) images show a corresponding irregular homogenously enhancing mass in the right breast (arrow) with washout predominant kinetics (noted in red, open arrow). A benign round proteinaceous cyst is incidentally noted (curved arrow)

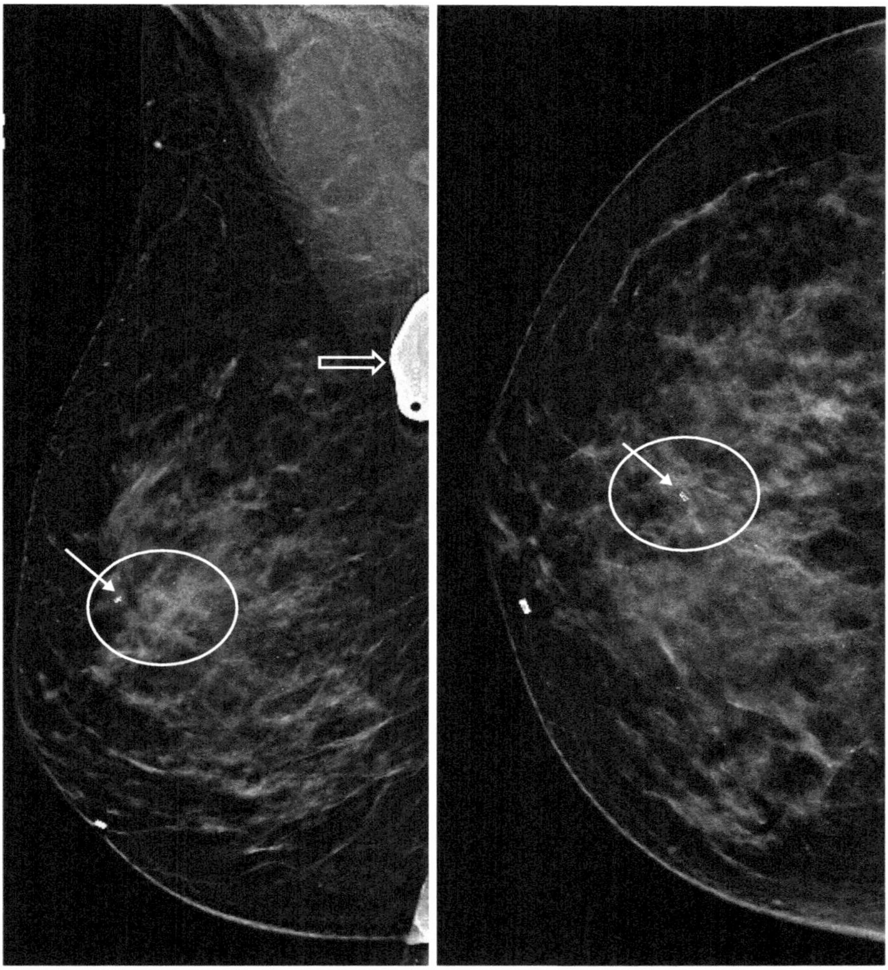

Fig. 3.15 MLO (right) and CC (left) MG images following NST show the clip from previous CNB (arrow) with subtle architectural distortion (circle) at the site of known malignancy. The patient has an infusion port overlying the pectoralis muscle on the MLO view (open arrow)

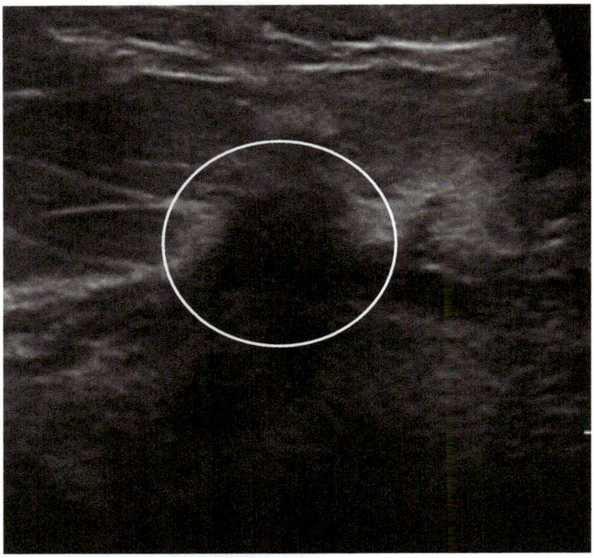

Fig. 3.16 Grayscale US shows a residual hypoechoic mass at the site of known malignancy (circle)

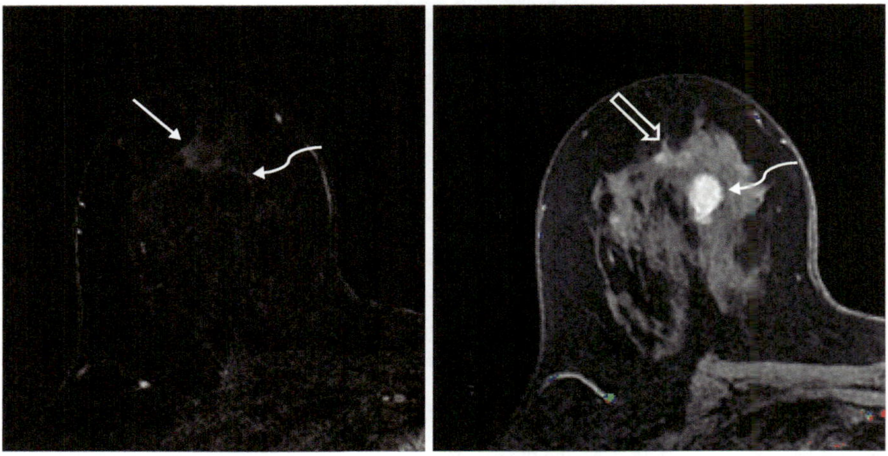

Fig. 3.17 Post-NST MRI including axial T1 post-contrast subtraction (left) and T1 post-contrast FS with color overlay (right) shows a subtle residual irregular heterogeneously enhancing mass at the site of incompletely treated malignancy (arrow); this does not meet the threshold for kinetic analysis (open arrow). The incidental non-enhancing benign proteinaceous cyst is again noted (curved arrow)

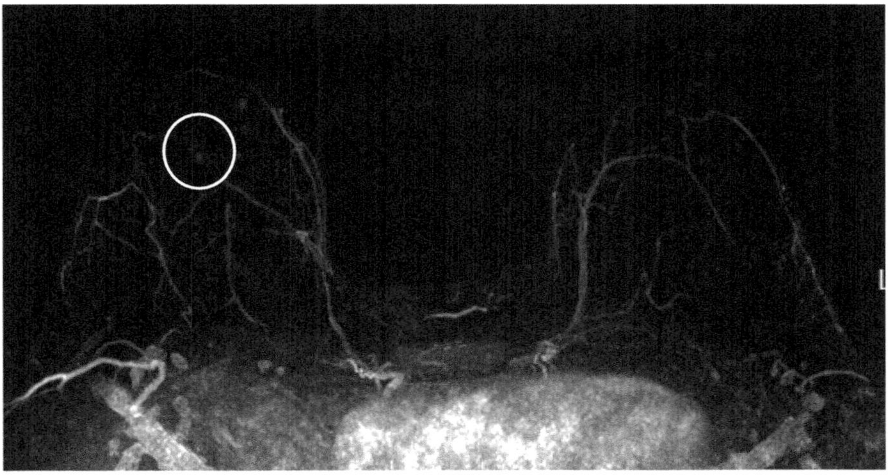

Fig. 3.18 Post-NST MIP shows only stippled enhancement at site of incompletely treated malignancy (circle)

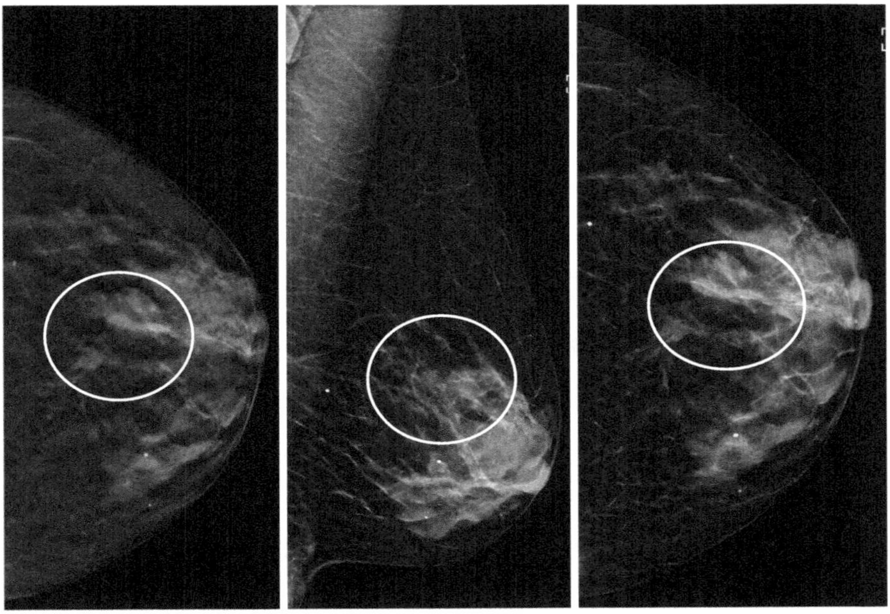

Fig. 3.19 CC tomosynthesis slice (left), MLO (center), and CC (right) images show two nearly contiguous irregular masses (best seen on CC images) in the left breast

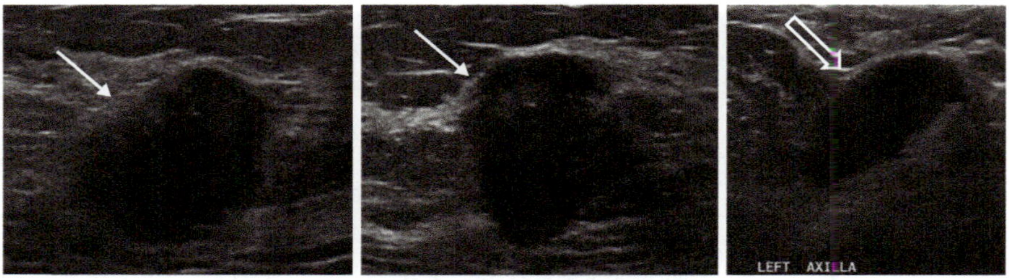

Fig. 3.20 Grayscale US images show an irregular nonparallel mass in the breast (arrow). An abnormally enlarged left axillary lymph node shows complete absence of the normal central hilum (open arrow) and CNB confirmed metastatic carcinoma

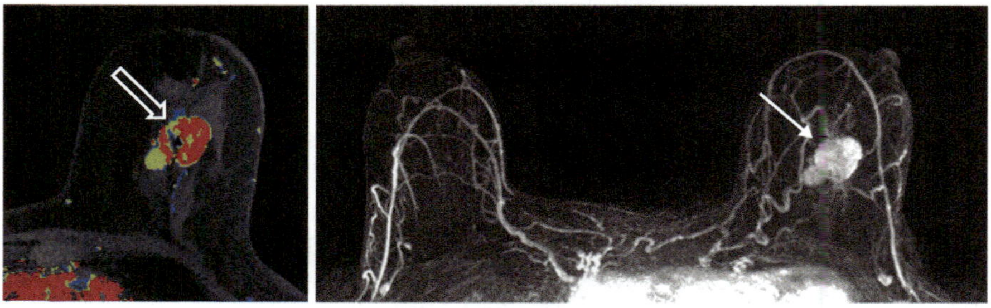

Fig. 3.21 Pretreatment axial T1 post-contrast fat saturation with color overlay (left) and MIP (right) images show a bilobed irregular mass (arrow) with predominant washout kinetics (open arrow)

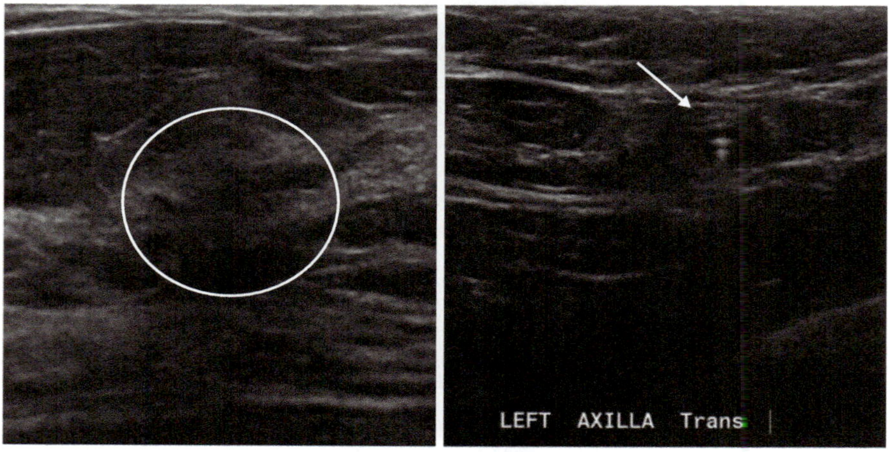

Fig. 3.22 Grayscale US of the breast (left) and axilla (right) shows subtle architectural distortion without a residual mass at the site known malignancy (circle). The proven metastatic lymph node has a normal size and morphology after NST (arrow denotes the clip from CNB)

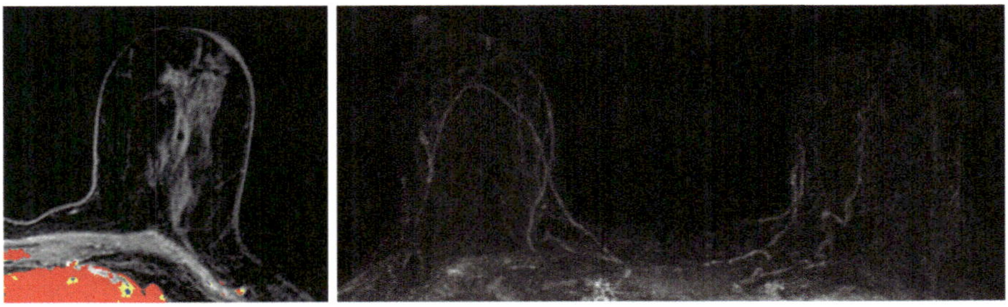

Fig. 3.23 Post-NST T1 post-contrast FS with color overlay (left) and axial MIP (right) images show a complete imaging response to NST with no residual enhancing mass or non-mass enhancement (NME)

Chapter 4
Imaging of the Axilla and Approaches to Node-Negative Versus Node-Positive Disease at Presentation

Leah H. Portnow, Allyson L. Chesebro, and Eva C. Gombos

When to Image the Axilla

Imaging of the axilla usually is performed when patients present with symptoms in the axilla or when they are recently diagnosed with breast cancer. Imaging is also utilized to guide axillary procedures for diagnosis and surgical management. The axillary area is included within the field of view on chest CT, PET/CT, or chest and shoulder MR exams and may incidentally reveal axillary findings that necessitate further targeted work-up.

Differential diagnosis of axillary findings is extensive. Findings typically fall into the following groups: benign and malignant primary axillary neoplasms, including breast cancer, sarcomas, granular cell tumor, schwannoma, etc.; skin lesions; congenital and developmental anomalies; infectious, inflammatory, and metastatic lymphadenopathy; lymphopoietic diseases; and postoperative changes. Accessory breast tissue in the axilla may contain all the pathologies that can occur in other areas of breast tissue. Extra-axillary masses can also grow or protrude into the axillary area.

In the USA, imaging evaluation of a palpable breast or axillary findings in women over the age of 30 years starts with a mammogram, with marking the skin over the area of concern and a subsequent targeted ultrasound (US) [1]. In younger patients, imaging begins with US [1].

Staging of the axilla is an important step in patients with invasive breast cancer as the status of a patient's axillary lymph nodes is a very important prognostic factor. Imaging assessment of the axilla has a key role in treatment planning [2, 3]. If

L. H. Portnow (✉) · A. L. Chesebro · E. C. Gombos
Breast Imaging Division, Department of Radiology, Brigham and Women's Hospital, Dana-Farber Cancer Institute, Boston, MA, USA
e-mail: lportnow@bwh.harvard.edu; achesebro@bwh.harvard.edu; egombos@bwh.harvard.edu

A. Soran, F. Nakhlis (eds.), *Management of the Breast and Axilla in the Neoadjuvant Setting*, https://doi.org/10.1007/978-3-030-88020-0_4

clinically indicated, imaging evaluation of the axilla usually starts with US, frequently followed by US-guided sampling of abnormal appearing lymph nodes and possible post-procedural clip marker placement. Routine axillary US in patients presenting with ductal carcinoma in situ (DCIS) is not recommended [4].

Until recently, patients with positive axillary lymph nodes, regardless of the receipt of neoadjuvant systemic therapy, were managed with complete axillary lymph node dissection (ALND). ALND causes frequent, significant disruption to the lymphatic system and a high risk for lymphedema, which is a substantial morbidity affecting the patients' quality of life. The incidence of lymphedema in patients undergoing ALND compared to sentinel lymph node biopsy (SLNB) is much higher (13–19.9% vs. 3–5.6%) [5, 6].

The published results from the American College of Surgeons Oncology Group (ACOSOG) Z0011 trial led to a major shift in the understanding and surgical management of the axilla. This multicenter, prospective randomized-controlled trial showed that patients with a clinical stage T1 or 2 breast cancer, clinical node-negative (cN0) disease, and one or two metastatic nodes on SLNB could be spared a complete ALND [7]. This, as well as better understanding of underlying tumor biology as in the prognostic implications of achieving a complete pathologic response in the axilla after neoadjuvant chemotherapy (NACT) in patients with cN1 disease at diagnosis, has led to further research on de-escalation of axillary surgery (see Section "Response to Neoadjuvant Chemotherapy").

However, patients with palpable lymph nodes, which are considered clinically positive, may still be treated with ALND, particularly if they have residual disease present after preoperative systemic therapy.

Axillary evaluation with imaging can identify patients with a high nodal tumor burden in whom SLNB would be inappropriate and who should undergo an ALND. According to National Comprehensive Cancer Network (NCCN) guidelines, patients with palpable lymphadenopathy should undergo an axillary US [8].

Axillary imaging also affects decisions on NACT. In patients with locally advanced disease or known node-positive disease, axillary lymph node evaluation is useful in monitoring overall response to NACT.

Mammography

A normal lymph node has a reniform shape with a radiolucent, fatty hilum (Fig. 4.1). Increased density, obliterated hilum, focally or diffusely thickened cortex, or increased size of a node on mammography is concerning for involvement by disease (Fig. 4.2). Abnormal appearing lymph nodes may be seen both in benign processes and in malignant neoplasms; thus, a tissue diagnosis remains the gold standard in confirming the axillary nodal status.

Assessment of nodal disease burden to guide multidisciplinary treatment decisions is the most critical role of axillary imaging and typically is completed with axillary US and US-guided biopsy, and when concerned for extensive nodal burden,

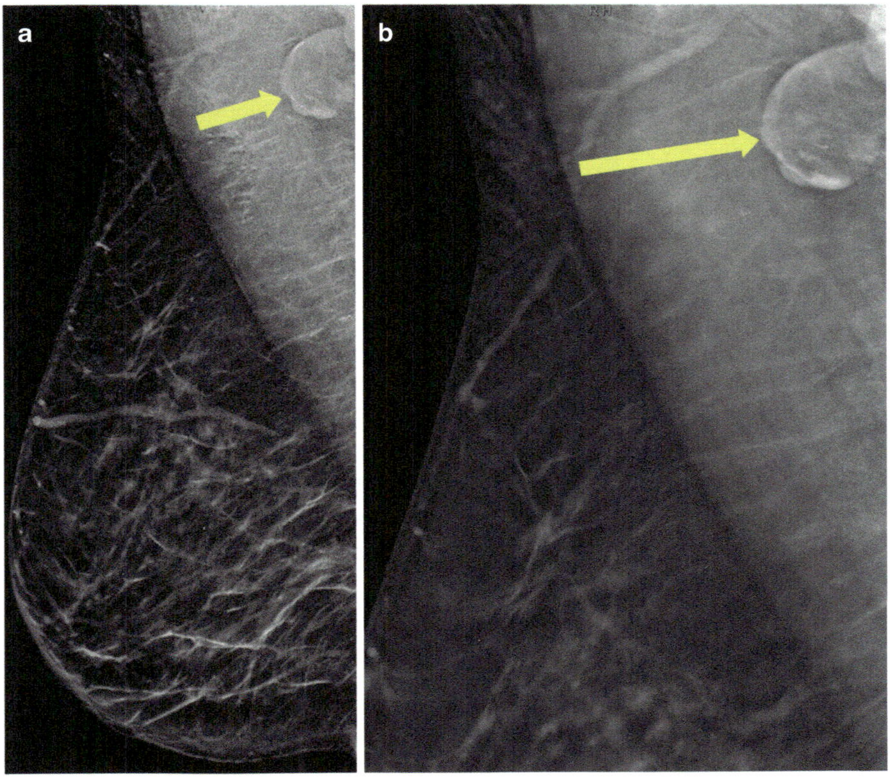

Fig. 4.1 Benign axillary lymph node on mammogram. A 46-year-old asymptomatic woman with a screening mammogram. (**a**) Right mediolateral oblique (MLO) view demonstrates a normal axillary lymph node (arrow) with a reniform shape, circumscribed margins, and thin homogeneous cortex. (**b**) The preserved fatty hilum can be better appreciated on a zoomed-in tomosynthesis view (arrow). Note that although the long axis of the lymph node is over 2 cm, fatty replacement and normal architecture confirm its benign nature. The lymph node is stable in comparison to mammograms from prior years and similar lymph nodes are present in the contralateral axilla (not shown)

possibly magnetic resonance imaging (MRI) [9]. Nevertheless, digital mammography or digital breast tomosynthesis (DBT) is the first step and the first recommended imaging modality in women with newly diagnosed breast cancer. Axillary lymph nodes are evident at routine mammography in about half of the patients. However, axillary visualization is usually limited to level I lymph nodes, and even with special views, deeper level I or level II nodes may not be included within the mammogram. Even without mammographically visibly enlarged lymph nodes, with bulky lymphadenopathy, trabecular or skin thickening is often seen by mammography.

Calcifications within axillary lymph nodes can be detected by mammography. Antiperspirants on the skin surface may mimic calcifications. The patient may be recalled from screening mammography for additional diagnostic imaging. A repeat

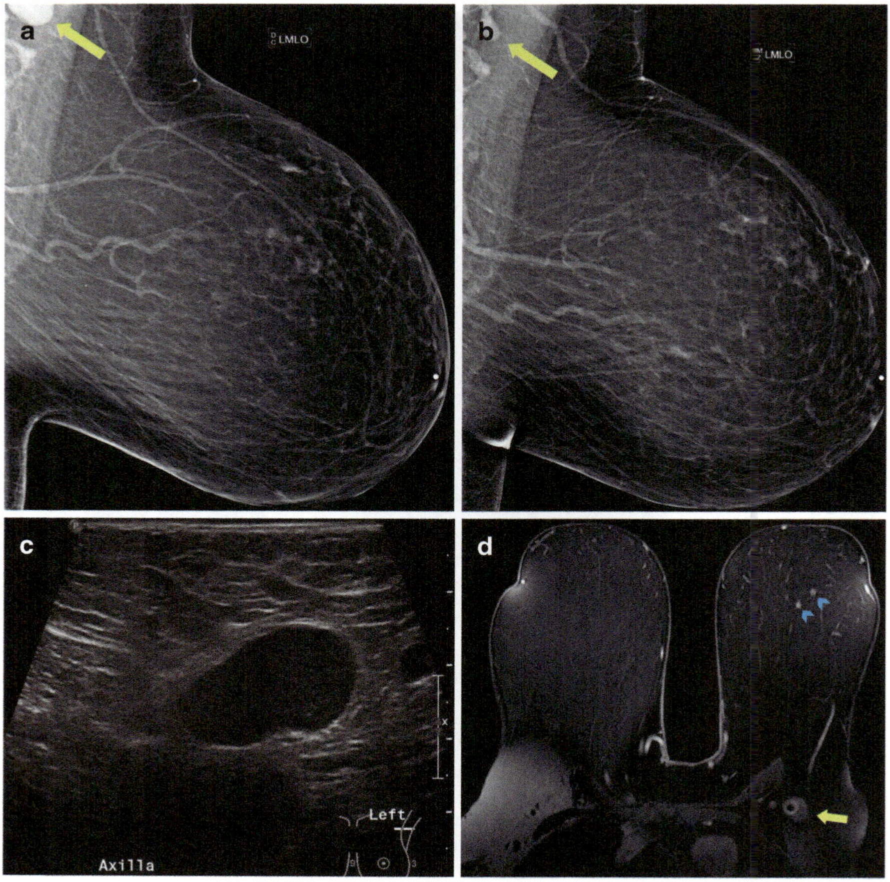

Fig. 4.2 Metastatic axillary lymph node on mammogram. A 64-year-old asymptomatic woman with a screening mammogram. (**a**) Left MLO view shows a high density, enlarged lymph node at the edge of the image (arrow). No suspicious mammographic finding is with the breast. (**b**) For comparison, the left MLO 1 year prior showed a normal appearance of the axillary lymph node (arrow). (**c**) Targeted axillary ultrasound shows the oval, enlarged, hypoechoic lymph node with obliteration of its fatty hilum. Subsequent ultrasound-guided biopsy revealed metastatic adenocarcinoma from a breast primary. (**d**) Breast MRI was requested for detection of the primary tumor and revealed two subcentimeter irregular masses with spiculated margins (arrowheads). The final histopathology revealed grade 2 invasive lobular carcinoma ER+/HER2-neu−. The biopsied level I axillary lymph node contains a susceptibility artifact due to a high-visibility biopsy marker (arrow)

mediolateral oblique (MLO) view after cleaning the skin of the axilla is performed to show that the densities are no longer present on the images or to confirm that they are indeed located within a lymph node or within the axillary tissue. The widespread use of DBT can make it easier to localize the high-density particles/calcifications on the skin surface versus within a lymph node on either screening or diagnostic imaging.

The differential diagnosis of calcified lymph nodes includes granulomatous infections, prior gold therapy for rheumatoid arthritis, collagen vascular disease, and metastasis from breast or other cancers (e.g., thyroid cancer). Calcifications within lymph nodes can be due to metastatic breast cancer, and frequently the morphology of the calcifications resembles that of the primary tumor [10].

Mammography may suggest extranodal/extracapsular extension (Fig. 4.3). Extranodal extension is defined as invasive cancer growing through the nodal capsule into the perinodal fatty tissue by invading the lymph node capsule [11]. Lymph nodes with indistinct or spiculated margins are suspicious for extranodal extension. There is an association between the presence of extranodal extension and worse outcomes as it was demonstrated by multiple studies [11–16].

For the node-positive patients treated with NACT, restaging of the axilla may include mammography, US, and MRI. Posttreatment size of axillary lymph nodes and, if placed, location of axillary clips may be documented by mammography and aid in treatment decisions for patients.

Following axillary surgery, multiple findings can be seen in the axilla. Postsurgical changes are related to hematoma, seroma, tissue disruption, and edema, which evolve with time. Mammographic images may show site of postoperative fluid collections seen as an ill-defined mass or area of increased density, distortion, skin and trabecular thickening, and fat necrosis. Mammography may also detect an axillary recurrence before symptoms occur.

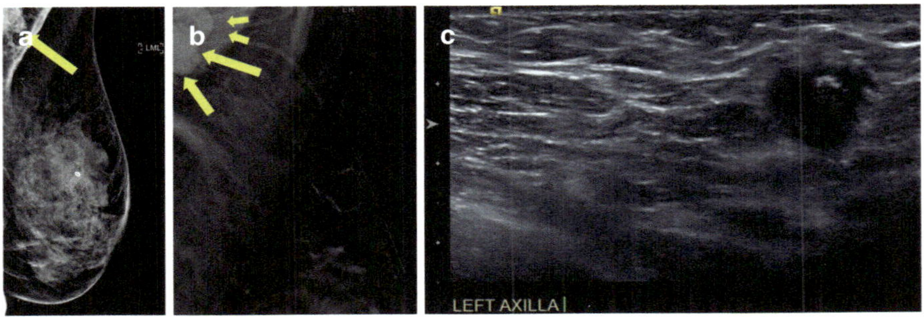

Fig. 4.3 Extranodal extension. A 69-year-old woman with grade 2 HER2 + invasive ductal carcinoma on her diagnostic mammogram. (**a**) Left medial-lateral (ML) view demonstrates an upper breast grade 2, HER2-neu+ invasive ductal carcinoma (indicated by a Tumark® Q) and multiple enlarged axillary lymph nodes with indistinct margins (arrow). (**b**) Zoomed-in tomosynthesis view shows indistinct lymph node margins (arrows) and stranding of the surrounding axillary fat, consistent with fat infiltration by the tumor. (**c**) Targeted axillary ultrasound shows an irregular mass with indistinct margins and no recognizable lymph node architecture. The patient underwent 6 months of preoperative chemotherapy and subsequent left axillary lymph node dissection and lumpectomy. Histopathology of the axillary tissue showed metastatic carcinoma in four of ten lymph nodes (4/10) with a 20% reduction in tumor cellularity, extranodal extension up to 0.6 cm, and perineural invasion. There was a 20% reduction in tumor cellularity

Ultrasound

Ultrasonography is the modality of choice for imaging axillary lymph nodes. Axillary sonography is performed with the same high-frequency transducer used for imaging of the breast. The patient lies supine or in a contralateral decubitus position with the ipsilateral arm raised over the head in an abducted, externally rotated position. Level I lymph nodes (lateral and inferior to the pectoralis minor muscle) are routinely imaged with US. Images of the lymph node with grayscale sonography are documented in orthogonal planes, which are two perpendicular planes defined as either transverse and longitudinal or radial and anti-radial. Color Doppler images should be taken with low velocity and low wall filter settings in order to detect non-hilar blood flow [17].

Cortical morphologic features, rather than size criteria, are important predictors of metastasis to axillary lymph nodes [18, 19]. A systematic review found that sonography of nonpalpable lymph nodes based on size (>5 mm) had a sensitivity of 48.8–87.1% and a specificity of 55.6–97.3% [19]. Sensitivity increased to 54.7–92.3% and specificity to 80.4–97.1% when morphologic characteristics (round, hypoechoic, eccentric cortical thickening, loss of central hilum, lobulation) are used in interpretation of sonography of nonpalpable lymph nodes [19].

A normal axillary lymph node is characterized by a reniform or oval shape; a uniform, hypoechoic cortical thickness less than 3 mm; a central hyperechoic hilum; and smooth, circumscribed margins (Fig. 4.4). Features of axillary lymph nodes that increase suspicion for malignancy include round shape, cortical thickening greater than or equal to 3 mm, loss of hyperechoic hilum, and focal or eccentric cortical bulging [18, 20] (Fig. 4.5). On color Doppler US, metastatic axillary lymph nodes are more likely to show increased peripheral or cortical blood flow than benign axillary lymph nodes [17, 19] (Fig. 4.5). Non-hilar blood flow on color Doppler has a positive predictive value of 78% in patients with known, ipsilateral primary breast cancer [20]. Sometimes, microcalcifications can be seen within the lymph node, which should correlate in appearance with microcalcifications associated with the primary breast cancer [21].

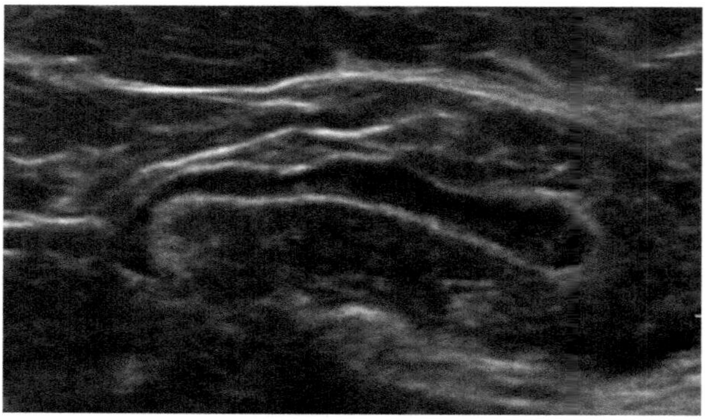

Fig. 4.4 Normal axillary lymph node on ultrasound. A 44-year-old woman with a palpable, normal-appearing right axillary lymph node demonstrating reniform shape, central hyperechoic fatty hilum, and thin, symmetric hypoechoic cortex

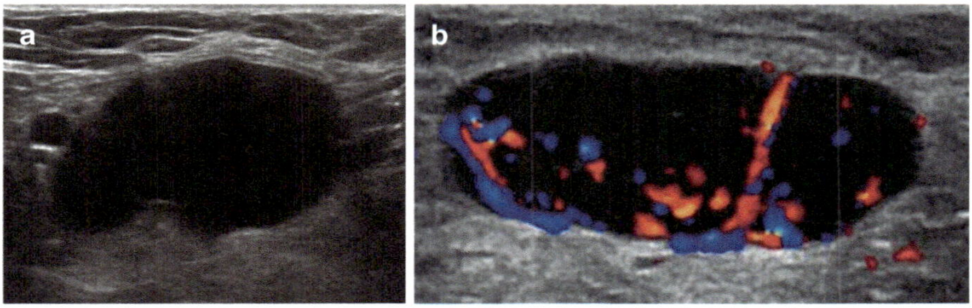

Fig. 4.5 Abnormal axillary lymph node on ultrasound. A 49-year-old woman with a history of right triple-negative breast cancer metastatic to the right axilla. The woman was treated with mastectomy and ALND 15 months prior to her ultrasound. (**a**) Right axillary ultrasound demonstrates a morphologically abnormal axillary lymph node with markedly increased hypoechoic cortical thickening and flattening of the central hyperechoic fatty hilum. (**b**) Right axillary color Doppler ultrasound demonstrates that the abnormal lymph node has marked cortical Doppler flow

Breast MRI

Contrast-enhanced breast MRI is not the primary tool to evaluate the axilla. Breast MRI is often used for high-risk screening, diagnostic problem-solving, extent of disease work-up in biopsy-proven cancer, and evaluation of response to neoadjuvant treatment. However, MRI provides a more global view of the bilateral axillae than either mammography or US. This cross-sectional imaging modality allows for evaluation of some level 1, level 2, and level 3 axillary lymph nodes [22]. Level 1 lymph nodes are lateral to the pectoralis minor, level II lymph nodes are central and either behind the pectoralis minor or between the pectoralis major and minor known as the Rotter's nodes, and level III axillary lymph nodes are medial to the pectoralis minor. Due to pulsation artifact from the heart in the left to right phase-encoding direction, parts of the axillae may be obscured [21].

As on axillary US, normal lymph nodes are reniform shaped and have circumscribed margins with a fatty hilum (Fig. 4.6). The fatty hilum can often be seen best on T1 pre-contrast non-fat-saturated sequences [22]. The lymph node cortex is T2 intermediate to high in signal. Lymph nodes are highly vascular and demonstrate T1 post-contrast homogeneous or rim enhancement with rapid uptake and washout kinetics. Since normal lymph nodes have a type III washout kinetic curve, kinetics alone are not useful for determining malignancy [21].

Differential diagnosis of morphologically abnormal axillary lymph nodes includes metastatic breast cancer, leukemia/lymphoma, lung, thyroid, GI, and ovarian cancer. Benign enlargement occurs in infection and inflammatory conditions such as rheumatoid arthritis, systemic lupus erythematosus, psoriatic arthritis, and sarcoid. Similar to mammography or US, the key finding of abnormality in axillary lymph nodes is the loss of its reniform shape and increased cortical thickness (Fig. 4.7). Malignant lymph nodes are rounded and enlarged or with a long-to-short axis ratio less than 2, develop cortical thickening that may be eccentric, and have

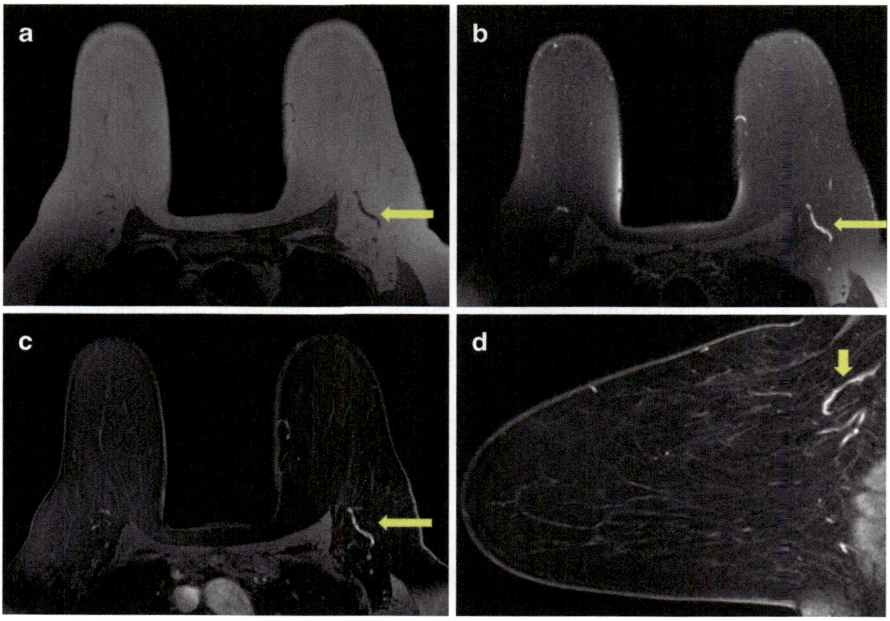

Fig. 4.6 Normal axillary lymph node on MRI. A 71-year-old woman with newly diagnosed invasive lobular carcinoma has a diagnostic breast MRI for extent of disease. A morphologically normal left axillary lymph node with a reniform, thin cortex is (**a**) hypointense on pre-contrast T1 non-fat-saturated axial image, (**b**) T2 hyperintense on T2/STIR axial image, and T1 hyperintense on (**c**) axial and (**d**) sagittal T1 post-contrast fat-saturated images

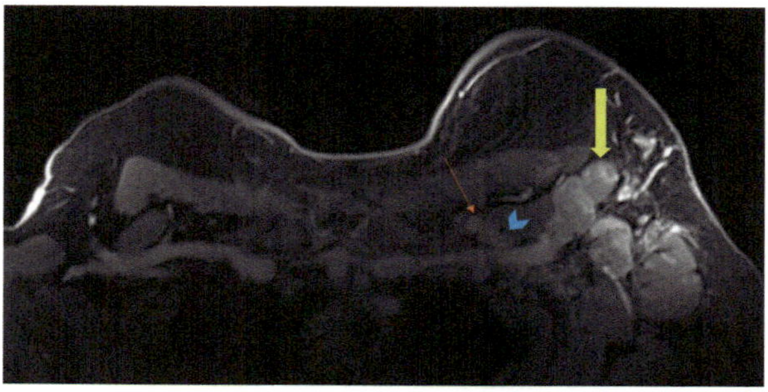

Fig. 4.7 Abnormal axillary lymph node on MRI. A 33-year-old woman with inflammatory breast cancer demonstrates morphologically abnormal axillary lymphadenopathy. The metastatic lymph nodes are rounded and enlarged and demonstrate heterogeneous enhancement on T1 post-contrast fat-saturated images at axillary level 1 (thick arrow), level 2 (arrowhead), and level 3 (thin arrow)

obliteration of its fatty hilum. The nodes develop heterogeneous enhancement, but if totally replaced by tumor, can diffusely enhance [22]. If extranodal extension occurs, the lymph node margins become irregular [22]. Baltzer et al. [23] reviewed 56 patients with primary breast cancer who underwent breast MRI to determine predictors of lymph node metastasis. The most significant predictors of metastasis

($p < 0.001$) were presence of an irregular margin, an inhomogeneously thickened cortex, perifocal edema (prolonged T2 relaxation times/T2 hyperintensity of soft tissues surrounding the lymph node), and asymmetry to the contralateral axilla [23]. Prolonged T2* relaxation times, a paramagnetic quantitative characteristic that takes into account magnetic field inhomogeneities in addition to T2 relaxation time and is not performed under standard MRI protocols, correlates with metastasis [24].

No consensus has been reached on morphologic characterization to distinguish between benign and malignant nodes. Even with high spatial resolution on a 7-tesla magnet, morphologic criteria may not determine malignancy without sampling. Cortical thickness greater than or equal to 3 mm has been demonstrated to have a sensitivity of 88% and specificity of 32% and, if less than 3 mm, a high negative predictive value of 91% [24].

Despite the lack of consensus on imaging characteristics of malignant lymph nodes, if a radiologist suspects the lymph node to be abnormal due to marked cortical thickness, lack of a fatty hilum, or asymmetry when compared to the contralateral breast on standard MRI, especially in the setting of known cancer, targeted US and US-guided fine needle aspiration (FNA) or large core needle biopsy (LCNB) is standard practice.

Ultrasound-Guided Diagnostic Interventions

Ultrasonography is the modality of choice for performing image-guided interventions on axillary lymph nodes.

Axillary lymph nodes can be sampled preoperatively either with percutaneous US-guided fine needle aspiration (FNA) or large core needle biopsy (LCNB) to determine if the lymph node is metastatic or benign. There is no clear advantage of either technique over the other.

If LCNB is utilized, a "no throw"/"open trough" technique (Fig. 4.8) should be employed, usually with a 14-gauge needle, to avoid damage to the surrounding axillary artery and vein while safely allowing appropriate needle excursion [20, 25]. If a "no throw"/"open trough" device is not available or the lymph node is sufficiently large to avoid damage to the surrounding tissue, then a "throw" device, also usually a 14-gauge needle, could be utilized (Fig. 4.9). The negative predictive value (NPV) and sensitivity of LCNB is 89% and 94%, respectively [20].

FNA is usually performed with a 25- to 20-gauge needle attached to a syringe with a small amount of suction (Fig. 4.10). This technique necessitates a competent cytopathologist to interpret the sample. The NPV, sensitivity, specificity, and positive predictive value (PPV) of FNA are reported as 80.5%, 80%, 85.7%, and 85.2% in one study [26]. In another study [27], the sensitivity of FNA was 80% for indeterminate and suspicious lymph nodes, but increased to 93% when only suspicious lymph nodes were evaluated.

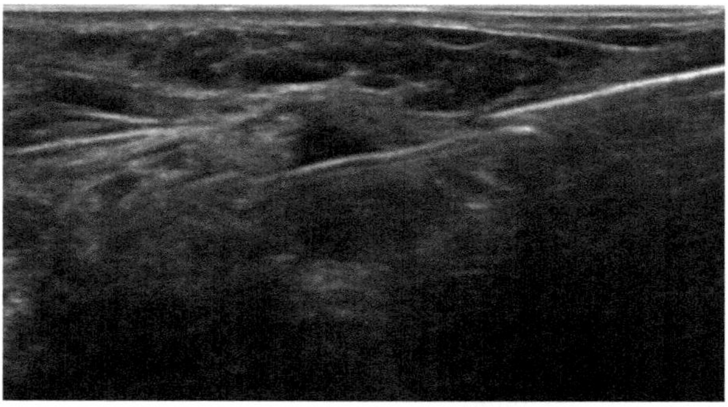

Fig. 4.8 Ultrasound-guided large core needle biopsy with a "no-throw" device. A 64-year-old woman with a history of right breast cancer treated with lumpectomy and radiation therapy and axillary node dissection 30 years prior to her ultrasound. Right axillary LCNB was performed with a no-throw device. The device was kept parallel to the chest wall with the axillary lymph node seen within the open bowl of the needle and the tip just distal to the lymph node

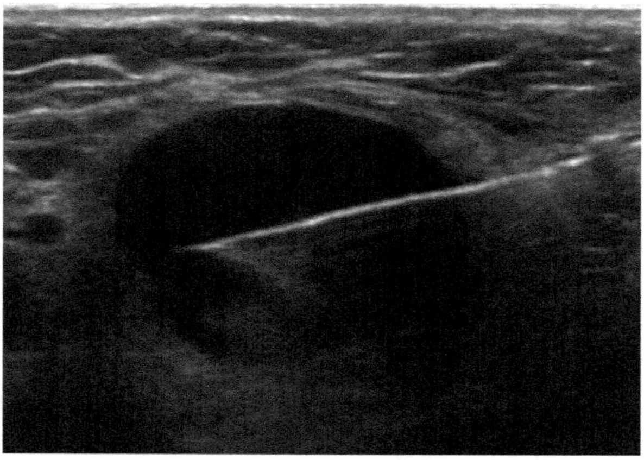

Fig. 4.9 Ultrasound-guided large core needle biopsy with a "throw" device. A 49-year-old woman with a history of right triple-negative breast cancer metastatic to the right axilla. The woman was treated with mastectomy and ALND 15 months prior to her ultrasound. Right axillary LCNB was performed with a throw device given the large size of the lymph node and the markedly increased cortical thickness. The biopsy device was kept parallel to the chest wall and the distal tip of the device remained entirely within the lymph node

In a direct comparison of the FNA and LCNB, there is no significant difference in the sensitivity of LCNB (82%) versus FNA (75%) with an equivalent specificity of 100% [28]. However, the cost of LCNB is significantly higher than FNA [28]. Neither LCNB nor FNA alleviates the need for axillary surgery, but can guide upfront management in whether to pursue neoadjuvant chemotherapy or perform more or less extensive surgical evaluation.

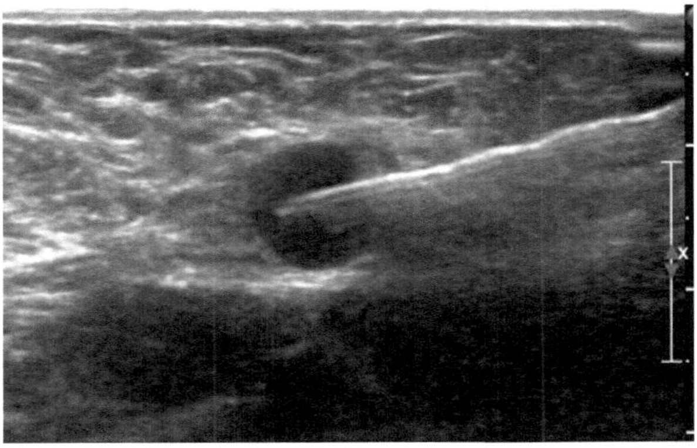

Fig. 4.10 Ultrasound-guided fine needle aspiration. A 57-year-old woman with history of metastatic non-small cell lung cancer with enlarged right axillary lymph nodes. Right axillary fine needle aspiration with a 20-gauge needle attached to a 5-cc syringe was performed. The needle was kept parallel to the chest wall

Assessment of Concordance

Once the lymph node has been sampled, pathology results are considered definitive. If insufficient cells are within the sample, a repeat FNA or LCNB can be performed. If a lymph node has been sampled and lymphocytes are noted by the cytologist or pathologist, either a negative or positive biopsy result should be considered concordant.

Response to Neoadjuvant Chemotherapy

NACT response in a lymph node is especially relevant given the results of the prospective trials ACOSOG Z1071, SENTINA, and SN FNAC. Initially, the ACOSOG Z0011 and the AMAROS trials revealed that limiting the extent of axillary surgery in patients with cT1-T2N0 disease undergoing upfront surgery and found to have low-volume nodal disease (up to two positive sentinel nodes) led to similar overall survival and disease-free survival as more extensive surgery [29–31]. Understandably, these critically important data are not applicable to the neoadjuvant setting. As such, the ACOSOG Z1071 and SENTINA trials evaluated axillary management in patients with larger primary tumors up to T4 and nodal disease up to cN2 who received NAC [32–34]. Although the initial false-negative rates (FNR) with SLNB were 12.6% in Z1071, the FNR safety threshold of 10% determining that SLNB is appropriate for axillary staging was met in subset analyses. Safety thresholds were met when three or more sentinel nodes were retrieved, both radiotracer and blue dye were used intraoperatively to detect the sentinel nodes, and when initially sampled, biopsy proven to be positive at diagnosis node was retrieved in addition to or as part of the three or more sentinel nodes [34]. Since one method to obtain the 10% safety threshold includes removal of the biopsy-proven metastatic lymph node, known as targeted axillary dissection (TAD) [32–37], axillary US evaluation after NACT is often performed [38].

Upon receiving NACT, the patient's axillary lymph nodes may result in progression, stability, partial response, or complete response. Axillary lymph nodes that have increased in size or cortical thickness and have loss of their fatty hilum are considered to have progressed, no change is considered stable, and decrease in size is considered partial response (Fig. 4.11). Complete response is normalization of the lymph node with a cortical thickness <3 mm, reniform shape, and normal fatty hilum or the absence of the lymph node entirely (Fig. 4.12).

The use of TAD has become mainstream at some institutions. Diagnostic evaluation of abnormal axillary lymph nodes requires documentation of location, depth, and number. At the time of lymph node sampling, a high US visibility biopsy marker is placed within the sampled lymph node. After NACT, axillary US is performed to determine response. In radiographic partial or complete response, the sampled lymph node may be difficult to detect, but the clip is often still visible. Localization of the sampled node and/or associated clip is performed prior to surgery. Selective removal of the sampled node along with at least three sentinel nodes has reduced the FNR to 7% [36]. In addition, the sampled node is often not the sentinel node in 23% of cases [36], so its direct removal is important. NCCN guidelines note that SLNB may be performed if only one or two sentinel lymph nodes or the clip-containing lymph node does not have metastasis [8].

Localization

The decision to perform TAD with the clipping of lymph nodes is institution-dependent. Many institutions prefer mapping with dual tracer and blue dye and retrieving three or more sentinel nodes at the time of surgery, which together achieves an FNR of 9.1% [34]. These institutions prefer not to clip the axillary lymph node. If the institution uses the TAD method, the radiologist localizes the biopsy-proven-positive, clipped axillary lymph node prior to surgery.

Similar to localization of the primary breast malignancy, axillary lymph nodes may be localized by a variety of methods. Given the far superior and lateral location of the axilla, US-guided localization is preferred. The localizing device should be placed within the nodal cortex, which acts as an anchor.

Traditionally, localization was performed with a wire [39]. A preloaded needle introducer and wire anchor was first implemented in the mid-1970s [40]. The wire ranges in length from 3 to 15 cm [40]. It is placed within the lymph node, with the 2-cm-thick reinforced segment through the cortex and the tip just beyond the target. Care to avoid axillary vasculature is paramount. Limitations of the wire include compromised cosmesis and extent of surgical dissection because the surgeon may need to dissect along the wire tract in order to retrieve the wire in its entirety and coordinating of the localization procedure to the day of surgery as is typically the practice in the USA [40]. Technical difficulties may occur related to its axillary location.

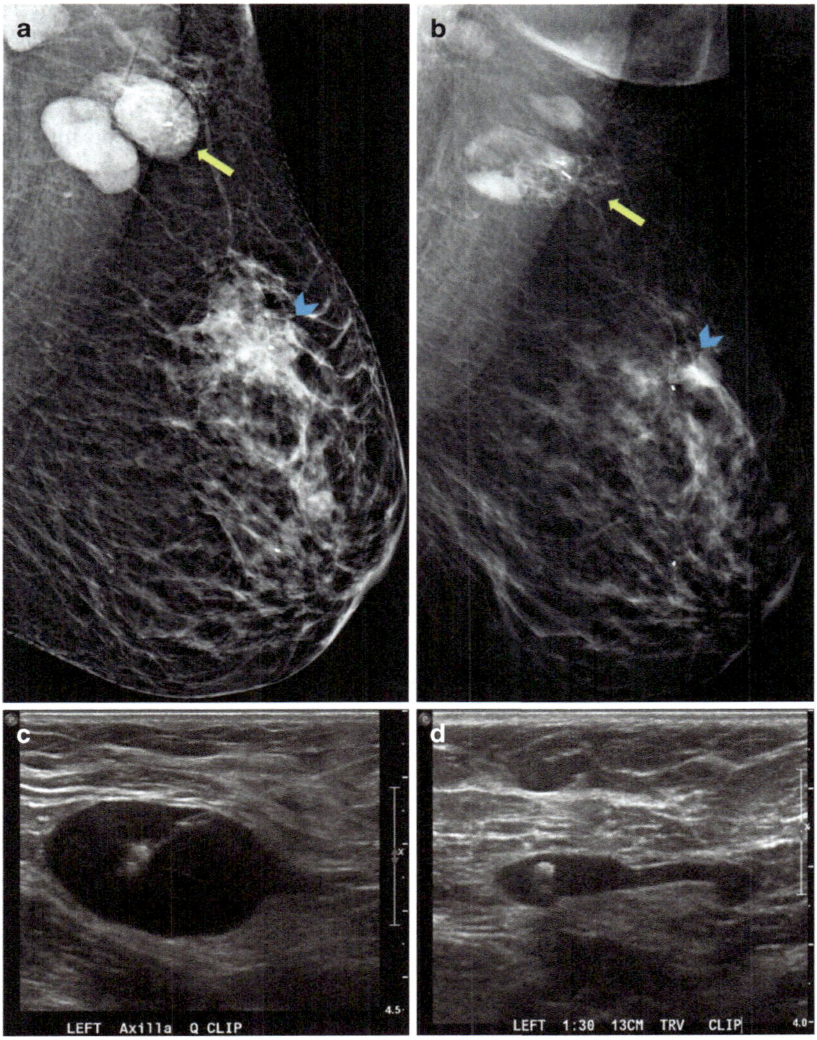

Fig. 4.11 Radiographic partial response after neoadjuvant chemotherapy. A 48-year-old woman with left invasive ductal carcinoma and axillary lymph node metastasis. (**a**) Left MLO view demonstrates multiple high-density, enlarged axillary lymph nodes with no fatty hilum, one of which was sampled, as indicated by a Tumark Q biopsy marker (arrow). A high-density asymmetry containing a cork marker is the primary tumor (arrowhead). (**b**) After 4 months of neoadjuvant chemotherapy, left MLO view shows that the lymph nodes remain prominent but have decreased in size. A radioseed is now within the sampled and clipped abnormal node in anticipation of surgery (arrow). The cancer has also decreased in size and density (arrowhead). (**c**) Left axillary ultrasound demonstrates an oval, hypoechoic abnormal lymph node with complete replacement of its fatty hilum. Cortical thickness measures 1.9 cm. An echogenic biopsy marker is present within the node. (**d**) After 4 months of neoadjuvant chemotherapy, the axillary lymph node remains abnormal, although its size has decreased and its reniform contour is better visualized. Cortical thickness now measures 0.6 cm. Upon sentinel lymph node biopsy, this clipped and radioseed-localized node was a sentinel lymph node and pathologically negative for metastasis

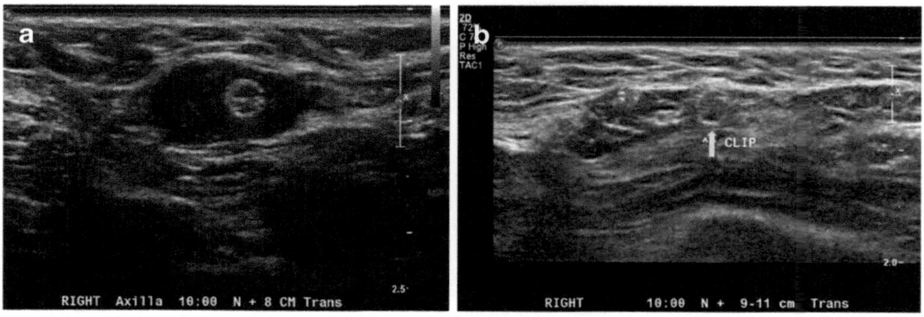

Fig. 4.12 Radiographic complete response after neoadjuvant chemotherapy. A 46-year-old woman with right invasive ductal carcinoma and axillary lymph node metastasis. (**a**) Right axillary ultrasound demonstrates an oval, hypoechoic abnormal lymph node with complete replacement of its fatty hilum. Cortical thickness measures 0.8 cm. An echogenic biopsy marker is present within the node. (**b**) After 6 months of neoadjuvant chemotherapy, the lymph node is no longer visualized and only the echogenic biopsy marker is present (arrow)

Newer, non-wire methods allow for uncoupling of the localization procedure and surgical date to improve workflow. However, repositioning cannot be performed, and none of these techniques are MRI-compatible.

Radioseeds were first reported as a localization technique in 1999 [40]. A radioseed is a 5-mm oblong titanium capsule containing a tungsten rod coated with I-125 [0.075–0.3 mCi], which has a long half-life of 59 days [40, 41]. The radioseed is manually placed or comes in a preloaded needle sheath that is occluded by bone wax [40]. The radiologist guides the radioseed to the desired location, directly in the axillary lymph node cortex or at the clip (Fig. 4.13). The radioseed is then deployed by advancing a stilette and extruding the seed. Radioseed use is overseen by the Nuclear Regulatory Commission, which requires radioseed placement within 5–7 days of surgery [40, 42]. Limitations include the requirement of authorized user status for the radiologist and careful tracking of the radioseed from acquisition, deployment, surgical excision, storage, and disposal [40, 42]. In the operating room, the radioseed is detected using a gamma probe set for I-125.

The SAVI SCOUT® is an alternative method first used in 2016 utilizing non-radioactive micro-impulse radar localization (Fig. 4.14). A preloaded 12-mm reflector composed of an infrared light receptor, resistor switch, and two antennae is deployed through a needle sheath directly through the target. Limitations include limited ability to reposition, inability to place deeper than a 6-cm limit of detection, nickel composition with concerns for nickel allergy, and issues with detection if older lights emit infrared radiation [40]. A handpiece and console system emits pulses of infrared light and radar wave signal, receiving signals from the reflect to provide localization to the surgeon [40, 43, 44].

Magnetic tracers such as Magseed® have also been approved for localization since 2016. A 5-mm stainless steel implantable seed containing a magnetic iron alloy can be placed up to 30 days before surgery [40, 45]. A needle sheath containing the Magseed® is used for deploying the tracer. The detector probe magnetizes the iron and detects its magnetization in the operating room.

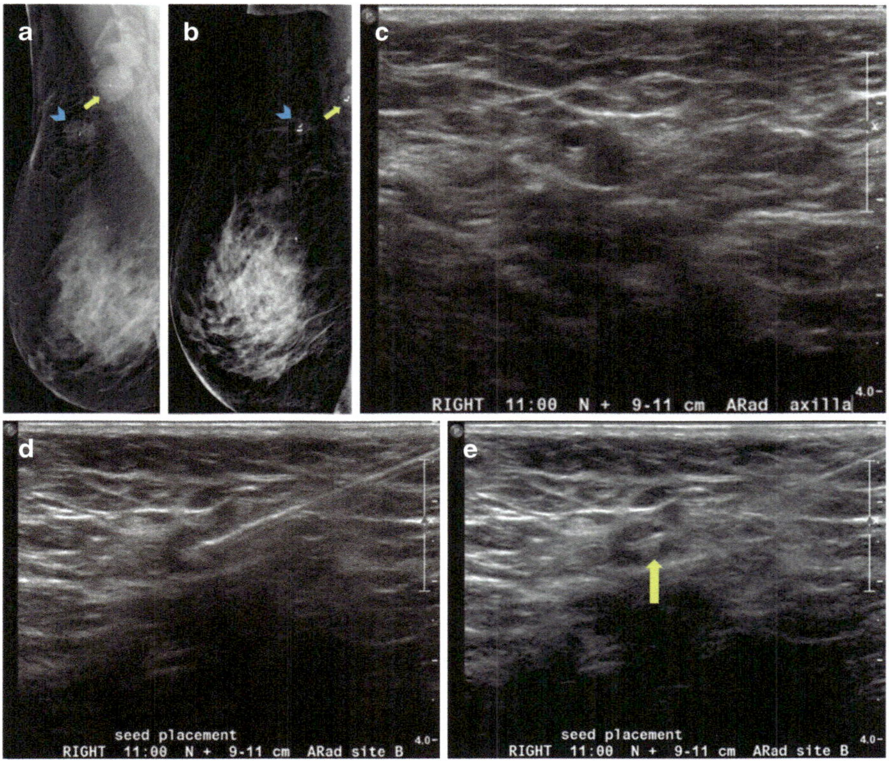

Fig. 4.13 Radioseed localization. A 49-year-old woman with right invasive ductal carcinoma and axillary lymph node metastasis. (**a**) Right MLO view demonstrates an upper breast posterior depth tumor (arrowhead) containing a ribbon marker and morphologically abnormal axillary lymph node (arrow) containing an open coil marker. (**b**) After 4 months of neoadjuvant chemotherapy, right ML view demonstrates that the tumor (arrowhead) and lymph node (arrow) have decreased in size. A radioseed is within the cortex next to the open coil marker. Right axillary ultrasound demonstrates radioseed placement: (**c**) An axillary lymph node containing an echogenic biopsy marker is noted. (**d**) A needle sheath containing the radioseed is placed within the cortex of the lymph node. (**e**) The radioseed (arrow) has now been deployed with the lymph node

Axillary lymph node tattooing is not yet widely used, but is currently being studied. At the time of sampling, either activated charcoal (Charcotrace™) or non-India ink (Spot™) tattooing can be placed on the surface of the sampled lymph node cortex [46–49]. A tuberculin syringe with ranges of 0.1–1.0 mL of ink placed has been reported [47, 49, 50]. Minimal risks, including ink migration to an adjacent lymph node and surrounding vessels, have been reported [46, 48].

Finally, radiofrequency identification tags measure up to 12 mm and allow for unique identification of multiple lesions in the same breast [40]. Its detector probe system is yet to be FDA-approved for operating room use. This cannot be used in patients with cardiac devices.

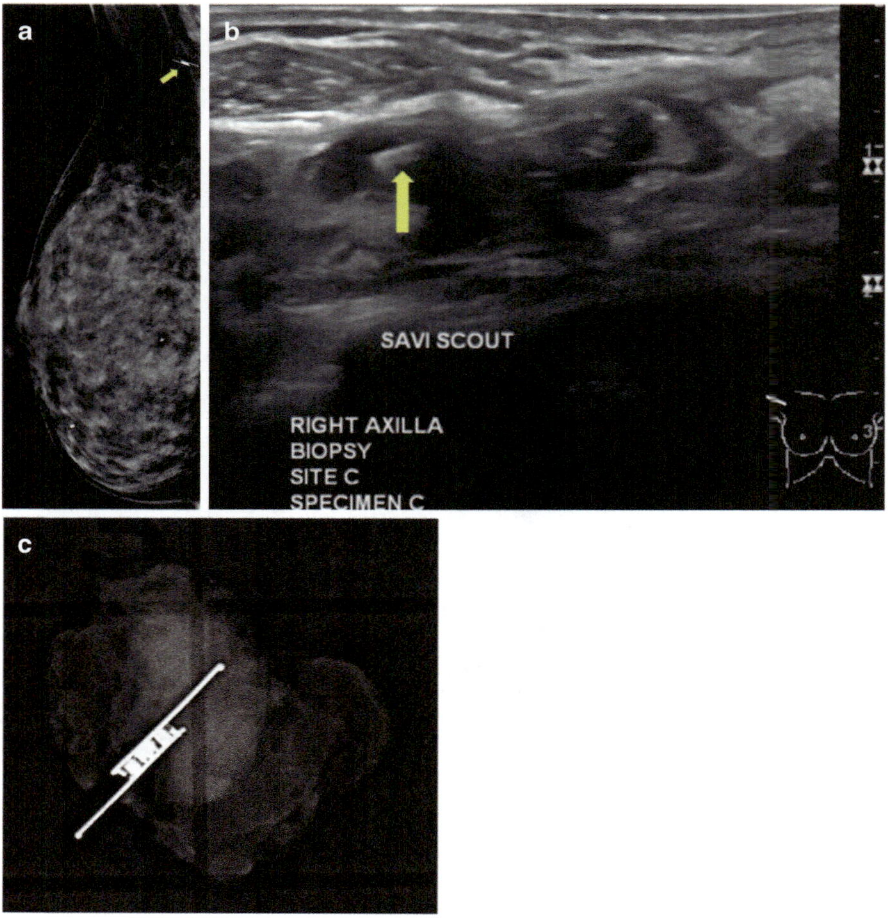

Fig. 4.14 SAVI SCOUT® localization. A 47-year-old woman with right multifocal breast cancer. (**a**) Right MLO view demonstrates an upper breast middle depth top-hat biopsy marker at the site of invasive ductal carcinoma and a lower breast posterior depth hourglass marker at the site of invasive lobular carcinoma. A retroareolar breast cork marker notes the site of a complex sclerosing lesion. A SAVI SCOUT® (arrow) is present within an axillary lymph node that was sampled positive for metastases. (**b**) Right axillary ultrasound demonstrates an abnormal lymph node with a thickened cortex. The echogenic linear structure corresponds to the SAVI SCOUT® (arrow). (**c**) A magnified specimen radiograph after surgery shows the high-density lymph node and SAVI SCOUT® with its two antennae in more detail

Conclusion

Imaging and imaging-guided procedures define axillary lymph node status prior to definitive surgical resection. The presence of axillary lymph node metastasis has implications for neoadjuvant treatment, overall management, and prognosis of the patient's breast cancer. Although lymph nodes present on mammography and MRI may have features that suggest malignancy, ultrasound is the most accurate imaging modality to evaluate the axilla. Ultrasound should be performed any time there is suspicion for axillary lymph node involvement. If suspicious cortical morphologic features (round shape, cortical thickening greater than or equal to 3 mm, focal or eccentric cortical bulging, loss of hyperechoic hilum, and non-hilar color Doppler blood flow) are present, ultrasound-guided fine needle aspiration or large core needle biopsy should be performed.

In the neoadjuvant setting, breast cancer patients with nodal disease up to cN2 who have partial or complete imaging response will undergo sentinel lymph node biopsy. Some institutions prefer the use of dual radiotracer and blue dye with retrieval of three or more sentinel nodes at the time of surgery to achieve an acceptable false-negative rate. Other institutions prefer targeted axillary dissection, which includes sentinel lymph node biopsy with specific retrieval of the sampled lymph node that is clipped at the time of biopsy and localized prior to surgery. Placement of a high-ultrasound visible clip within the nodal cortex is preferred. Multiple localization methods exist. The traditional wire and non-wire radioseed and SAVI SCOUT® methods have become mainstream for localization of the sampled node, each with its own pros and cons of use. Magseed®, axillary lymph node tattooing, and radiofrequency identification tags are still being researched for widespread use in the axilla as alternative means of localization.

References

1. Moy L, Heller SL, Bailey L. ACR appropriateness criteria® palpable breast masses. Available at https://acsearch.acr.org/docs/69495/Narrative/. American College of Radiology. Accessed 25 Nov 2020.
2. Krishnamurthy S, Bevers T, Kuerer HM, Smith B, Yang WT. Paradigm shifts in breast care delivery: impact of imaging in a multidisciplinary environment. AJR Am J Roentgenol. 2017;208(2):248–55. https://doi.org/10.2214/AJR.16.17130.
3. Verheuvel NC, Voogd AC, Tjan-Heijnen VCG, Siesling S, Roumen RMH. Different outcome in node-positive breast cancer patients found by axillary ultrasound or sentinel node procedure. Breast Cancer Res Treat. 2017;165(3):555–63. https://doi.org/10.1007/s10549-017-4342-1.
4. Ansari B, Boughey JC, Adamczyk DL, Degnim AC, Jakub JW, Morton MJ. Should axillary ultrasound be used in patients with a preoperative diagnosis of ductal carcinoma in situ? Am J Surg. 2012;204(3):290–3.
5. DiSipio T, Rye S, Newman B, Hayes S. Incidence of unilateral arm lymphedema after breast cancer: a systematic review and meta-analysis. Lancet Oncol. 2013;14:500–15.
6. Johnson AR, Kimball S, Epstein S, et al. Lymphedema incidence after axillary lymph node dissection: quantifying the impact of radiation and the lymphatic microsurgical preventive healing approach. Ann Plast Surg. 2019;82(4S Suppl 3):S234–41. https://doi.org/10.1097/sap.0000000000001864.
7. Giuliano AE, McCall L, Beitsch P, et al. Locoregional recurrence after sentinel lymph node dissection with and without axillary dissection in patients with sentinel lymph node metastases. The American College of Surgeons Oncology Group Z0011 Randomized Trial. Ann Surg. 2010;252(3):426–32.

8. NCCN clinical practice guidelines in oncology (NCCN guidelines®) breast cancer version 6.2020 — September 8, 2020 NCCN.org. Available at https://www.nccn.org/professionals/physician_gls/pdf/breast.pdf
9. Yoshimura G, Sakurai T, Oura S, Suzuma T, Tamaki T, Umemura T, Kokawa Y, Yang Q. Evaluation of axillary lymph node status in breast cancer with MRI. Breast Cancer. 1999;6(3):249–58. https://doi.org/10.1007/BF02967179.
10. Raza S. Axillary adenopathy. In: Berg WA, Birdwell RL, Kennedy A, Parlinson ET, Gombos E, Green G, Kettler M, Raza S, Wang S-C, editors. Diagnostic imaging: breast. AMIRSYS; 2006. IV.3.30.
11. Fisher ER, Gregorio RM, Redmond C, Kim WS, Fisher B. Pathologic findings from the national surgical adjuvant breast project. (Protocol no. 4). III. The significance of extranodal extension of axillary metastases. Am J Clin Pathol. 1976;65:439–44. https://doi.org/10.1093/ajcp/65.4.439.
12. Mambo NC, Gallagher HS. Carcinoma of the breast: the prognostic significance of extranodal extension of axillary disease. Cancer. 1977;39:2280–5.
13. Donegan WL, Stine SB, Samter TG. Implications of extracapsular nodal metastases for treatment and prognosis of breast cancer. Cancer. 1993;72:778–82.
14. Fisher BJ, Perera FE, Cooke AL, Opeitum A, Dar AR, Venkatesan VM, Stitt L, Radwan JS. Extracapsular axillary node extension in patients receiving adjuvant systemic therapy: an indication for radiotherapy? Int J Radiat Oncol Biol Phys. 1997;38:551–9. https://doi.org/10.1016/S0360-3016(97)89483-7.
15. Hetelekidis S, Schnitt SJ, Silver B, Manola J, Bornstein BA, Nixon AJ, Recht A, Gelman R, Harris JR, Connolly JL. The significance of extracapsular extension of axillary lymph node metastases in early-stage breast cancer. Int J Radiat Oncol Biol Phys. 2000;46:31–4. https://doi.org/10.1016/S0360-3016(99)00424-1.
16. Neri A, Marrelli D, Roviello F, De Stefano A, Guarnieri A, Pallucca E, Pinto E. Prognostic value of extracapsular extension of axillary lymph node metastases in T1 to T3 breast cancer. Ann Surg Oncol. 2005;12:246–53. https://doi.org/10.1245/ASO.2005.02.029.
17. Yang WT, Chang J, Metreweli C. Patients with breast cancer: differences in color Doppler flow and gray-scale US features of benign and malignant axillary lymph nodes. Radiology. 2000;215(2):568–73. https://doi.org/10.1148/radiology.215.2.r00ap20568.
18. Bedi DG, Krishnamurthy R, Krishnamurthy S, et al. Cortical morphologic features of axillary lymph nodes as a predictor of metastasis in breast cancer: in vitro sonographic study. AJR Am J Roentgenol. 2008;191:646–52. https://doi.org/10.2214/AJR.07.2460.
19. Alvarez S, Añorbe E, Alcorta P, López F, Alonos I, Cortés J. Role of sonography in the diagnosis of axillary lymph node metastases in breast cancer: a systematic review. AJR Am J Roentgenol. 2006;186:1342–8. https://doi.org/10.2214/AJR.05.0936.
20. Abe H, Schmidt RA, Kulkarni K, Sennett CA, Mueller JS, Newstead GM. Axillary lymph nodes suspicious for breast cancer metastasis: sampling with US-guided 14-gauge core-Needle biopsy—clinical experience in 100 patients. Radiology. 2009;250(1):41–9. https://doi.org/10.1148/radiol.2493071483.
21. Ecanow JS, Hiroyuki A, Newstead GM, Ecanow DB, Jeske JM. Axillary staging of breast cancer: what the radiologist should know. Radiographics. 2013;33:1589–612. https://doi.org/10.1148/rg.336125060.
22. Lee JYM, Dershaw DD. Chapter 5: the axilla. In: Morris EA, Liberman L, editors. Breast MRI: diagnosis and intervention. Springer; 2005. p. 45–50.
23. Baltzer PAT, Matthias D, Burmeister HP, et al. AJR Am J Roentgenol. 2011;196(5):W641–7. https://doi.org/10.2214/AJR.10.4889.
24. Korteweg ME, Zwanenburg JJM, Hoogdium JM, et al. Dissected sentinel lymph nodes of breast cancer patients: characterization with high-spatial-resolution 7-T MR imaging. Radiology. 2011;261(1):127–35.
25. Chesebro AL, Chikarmane SA, Ritner JA, Birdwell RL, Giess C. Troubleshooting to overcome technical challenges in image-guided breast biopsy. Radiographics. 2017;37:705–18. https://doi.org/10.1148/rg.2017160117.

26. Vijayaraghavan GP, Vedantham S, Kataoka M, DeBenedectis C, Quinlan R. The relevance of ultrasound imaging of suspicious axillary lymph nodes and fine-needle aspiration biopsy in the post ACOSOG Z11 era in early breast cancer. Acad Radiol. 2017;24(3):308–15. https://doi.org/10.1016/j.acra.2016.10.005.
27. Mainiero MB, Cinelli CM, Koelliker SL, Graves TA, Chung MA. Axillary ultrasound and fine-needle aspiration in the preoperative evaluation of the breast cancer patient: an algorithm based on tumor size and lymph node appearance. AJR Am J Roentgenol. 2010;195:1261–7. https://doi.org/10.2214/AJR.10.4414.
28. Rao R, Lilley L, Andrews V, Radford L, Ulissey M. Axillary staging by percutaneous biopsy: sensitivity of fine-needle aspiration versus core needle biopsy. Ann Surg Oncol. 2009;16:1170–5. https://doi.org/10.1245/s10434-009-0421-9.
29. Donker M, van Tienhoven G, Straver ME, et al. Radiotherapy or surgery of the axilla after a positive sentinel node in breast cancer (EORTC 10981-22023 AMAROS): a randomised, multicentre, open-label, phase 3 non-inferiority trial. Lancet Oncol. 2014;15(12):1303–10.
30. Giuliano AE, Ballman K, McCall L, et al. Locoregional recurrence after sentinel lymph node dissection with or without axillary dissection in patients with sentinel lymph node metastases: long-term follow-up from the American College of Surgeons Oncology Group (Alliance) ACOSOG Z0011 randomized trial. Ann Surg. 2016;264(3):413–20.
31. Giuliano AE, Ballman KV, McCall L, et al. Effect of axillary dissection vs no axillary dissection on 10-year overall survival among women with invasive breast cancer and sentinel node metastasis: the ACOSOG Z0011 (Alliance) randomized clinical trial. JAMA. 2017;318(10):918–26.
32. Kuehn T, Bauerfeind I, Fehm T, et al. Sentinel-lymph-node biopsy in patients with breast cancer before and after neoadjuvant chemotherapy (SENTINA): a prospective, multicentre cohort study. Lancet Oncol. 2013;14(7):609–18.
33. Boileau JF, Poirier B, Basik M, Holloway CM, Gaboury L, Sideris L, Meterissian S, Arnaout A, Brackstone M, McCready DR, Karp SE, Trop I, Lisbona A, Wright FC, Younan RJ, Provencher L, Patocskai E, Omeroglu A, Robidoux A. Sentinel node biopsy after neoadjuvant chemotherapy in biopsy-proven node-positive breast cancer: the SN FNAC study. J Clin Oncol. 2015;33(3):258–64. https://doi.org/10.1200/JCO.2014.55.7827.
34. Boughey JC, Suman VJ, Mittendorf EA, et al. Sentinel lymph node surgery after neoadjuvant chemotherapy in patients with node-positive breast cancer: the ACOSOG Z1071 (Alliance) Clinical Trial. JAMA. 2013;310(14):1455–61. https://doi.org/10.1001/jama.2013.278932.
35. Boughey JC, Ballman KV, Le-Petross HT, et al. Identification and resection of clipped node decreases the false-negative rate of sentinel lymph node surgery in patients presenting with node-positive breast cancer (T0–T4, N1–N2) who receive neoadjuvant chemotherapy: results from ACOSOG Z1071 (Alliance). Ann Surg. 2016;263(4):802–7. https://doi.org/10.1097/SLA.0000000000001375.
36. Caudle AS, Yang WT, Krishnamurthy S, et al. Improved axillary evaluation following neoadjuvant therapy for patients with node-positive breast cancer using selective evaluation of clipped nodes: implementation of targeted axillary dissection. J Clin Oncol. 2016;34(10):1072–8. https://doi.org/10.1200/JCO.2015.64.0094.
37. Diego EJ, McAuliffe PF, Soran A, et al. Axillary staging after neoadjuvant chemotherapy for breast cancer: a pilot study combining sentinel lymph node biopsy with radioactive seed localization of pre-treatment positive axillary lymph nodes. Ann Surg Oncol. 2016;23(5):1549–53. https://doi.org/10.1245/s10434-015-5052-8.
38. Chang JM, Leung JWT, Moy L, Ha SM, Moon WK. Axillary nodal evaluation in breast cancer: state of the art. Radiology. 2020;295(3):500–15. https://doi.org/10.1148/radiol.2020192534.
39. Hall FM, Kopans DB, Sadowsky NL, Homer MJ. Development of wire localization for occult breast lesions: Boston remembrances. Radiology. 2013;268:622–7. https://doi.org/10.1148/radiol.13121943.
40. Cheang E, Ha R, Thornton CM, Mango VL. Innovations in image-guided preoperative breast lesion localization. Br J Radiol. 2018;91(1085):20170740. https://doi.org/10.1259/bjr.20170740.

41. Pavlicek W, Walton HA, Karstaedt PJ, Gray RJ. Radiation safety with use of I-125 seeds for localization of nonpalpable breast lesions. Acad Radiol. 2006;13:909–15. https://doi.org/10.1016/j.acra.2006.03.017.
42. Jakub JW, Gray RJ, Degnim AC, Boughey JC, Gardner M, Cox CE. Current status of radioactive seed for localization of nonpalpable breast lesions. Am J Surg. 2010;199:522–8. https://doi.org/10.1016/j.amjsurg.2009.05.019.
43. Cox CE, Garcia-Henriquez N, Glancy MJ, Whitworth P, Cox JM, Themar-Geck M, et al. Pilot study of a new nonradioactive surgical guidance technology for locating nonpalpable breast lesions. Ann Surg Oncol. 2016;23:1824–30. https://doi.org/10.1245/s10434-015-5079-x.
44. Mango V, Ha R, Gomberawalla A, Wynn R, Feldman S. Evaluation of the SAVI SCOUT surgical guidance system for localization and excision of nonpalpable breast lesions: a feasibility study. Am J Roentgenol. 2016;15:W69–72. https://doi.org/10.2214/AJR.15.15962.
45. Harvey JR, Lim Y, Murphy J, et al. Safety and feasibility of breast lesion localization using magnetic seeds (Magseed): a multi-centre, open-label cohort study. Breast Cancer Res Treat. 2018;169(3):531–6. https://doi.org/10.1007/s10549-018-4709-y.
46. Nguyen TT, Hieken TJ, Glazebrook KN, Boughey JC. Localizing the clipped node in patients with node-positive breast cancer treated with neoadjuvant chemotherapy: early learning experience and challenges. Ann Surg Oncol. 2017;24(10):3011–6. https://doi.org/10.1245/s10434-017-6023-z.
47. Park S, Koo JS, Kim GM, et al. Feasibility of charcoal tattooing of cytology-proven metastatic axillary lymph node at diagnosis and sentinel lymph node biopsy after neoadjuvant chemotherapy in breast cancer patients. Cancer Res Treat. 2018;50(3):801–12. https://doi.org/10.4143/crt.2017.210.
48. Kim HW, Kim HJ, Jung JH, et al. Ultrasound-guided restaging and localization of axillary lymph nodes after neoadjuvant chemotherapy for guidance of axillary surgery in breast cancer patients: experience with activated charcoal. Ann Surg Oncol. 2018;25:494–500. https://doi.org/10.1245/s10434-017-6250-3.
49. Choy N, Lipson J, Porter C, et al. Initial results with preoperative tattooing of biopsied axillary lymph nodes and correlation to sentinel lymph nodes in breast cancer patients. Ann Surg Oncol. 2015;22:377–82. https://doi.org/10.1245/s10434-014-4034-6.
50. Allweis TM, Menes T, Rotbart N, et al. Ultrasound guided tattooing of axillary lymph nodes in breast cancer patients prior to neoadjuvant therapy, and identification of tattooed nodes at the time of surgery. Eur J Surg Oncol. 2020;46(6):1041–5. https://doi.org/10.1016/j.ejso.2019.11.501.

Chapter 5
Guidelines for Imaging During Neoadjuvant Systemic Therapy

Uzma Waheed and John W. Hall IV

Introduction

Neoadjuvant systemic therapy (NST) is frequently utilized in the management of breast malignancies. Presurgical cytotoxic therapy for locally advanced breast cancer and/or based on tumor subtype may allow for breast conserving or less invasive surgery upon completion. Specifically, HER2-positive and triple-negative (TN) malignancies often benefit from neoadjuvant treatment in the short and long term, while luminal B cancers show less benefit [1]. Attainment of pathologic complete response (pCR) is more frequent in HER2-positive and TN malignancies and is associated with an improved long-term survival [2]. An additional benefit is potential axillary downstaging to reduce axillary surgical extent. Imaging is superior to clinical exam alone and an important adjunct for assessing response for surgical planning following NST [3, 4].

Mammography

Digital mammography (DM) is the standard of care in initial screening and diagnostic evaluation to ascertain the extent of breast carcinoma prior to the initiation of neoadjuvant systemic therapy. More recently, with the advent of digital breast

U. Waheed (✉)
Breast Imaging Division, Department of Radiology, Stanford University, Palo Alto, CA, USA
e-mail: uzmaw@stanford.edu

J. W. Hall IV
UPMC Department of Radiology, Pittsburgh, PA, USA
e-mail: Halljw2@upmc.edu

A. Soran, F. Nakhlis (eds.), *Management of the Breast and Axilla in the Neoadjuvant Setting*, https://doi.org/10.1007/978-3-030-88020-0_5

tomosynthesis (DBT), the ability to assess tumoral characteristics pre- and post-treatment has improved. Still, mammography is often combined with ultrasonography and magnetic resonance imaging (MRI) to improve the accuracy of evaluation of tumor size and extent [3]. The extent to which DM should be utilized for assessment of NST response should consider the initial characteristics of the tumor and be combined with other imaging modalities to improve accuracy of residual disease assessment.

The goals of pre-treatment imaging assessment of the affected breast include initial assessment of tumor size, extent, and to evaluate for axillary involvement. Conventional diagnostic mammography includes full-field craniocaudal (CC) and mediolateral oblique (MLO) views ideally with digital breast tomosynthesis (DBT) when available [5]. DBT aids detection of potential malignancy from overlapping normal fibroglandular tissue. It is technically similar in acquisition to DM with negligible additional radiation exposure that falls within Mammography Quality Standards Act (MQSA) dose limits. Mammography has been shown to be more accurate in the evaluation of invasive ductal carcinoma and low-grade malignancies (sensitivity of 81% for IDC), likely relating to their preponderance to manifest as more discrete masses which can be bidirectionally measured (case 2, Fig. 5.7). Mammographic accuracy for the evaluation of invasive lobular carcinomas and higher-grade malignancies is substantially lower (sensitivity 34% for ILC), related to the more frequent absence of a discrete mass and the infiltrative nature of lobular malignancies [3, 6] (case 3, Fig. 5.12 and case 5, Fig. 5.25). Mammographic sensitivity for detection of tumor and extent prior to systemic neoadjuvant therapy also significantly decreases with increasing breast density, reported to be as low as 45% in extremely dense breasts [6].

Following initial assessment, tissue sampling with core needle biopsy (CNB) is performed with biopsy marker (clip) localization. Mammography is the preferred imaging modality to assess biopsy marker positioning before initiating NST and may also be appropriate surgical localization following NST (case 6, Fig. 5.36). This is a helpful pre-treatment consideration as tumor size and characteristics may significantly change throughout the course of neoadjuvant systemic therapy [5]. Rarely, it may be appropriate to repeat biopsy clip placement within malignancy during therapy as tumor size decreases and if breast-conserving surgery is planned.

The timing of imaging utilization to assess response NST varies between institutions and may require tailoring to specific molecular subtype [5]. Initial pre treatment clinical and image guided staging and final staging following completion of NST are standard. Ongoing clinical exam features help guide the frequency of imaging evaluation to assess therapeutic response. Clinically occult malignancy and those patients with dense or complicated tissue patterns may require more frequent imaging follow-up. Imaging following completion of NST will guide surgical management.

Following the completion of neoadjuvant systemic therapy, the same imaging modalities and protocols should be performed to assess treatment response and adequately compare to initial disease extent (case 6, Fig. 5.34). The ability of conventional digital mammography to accurately assess changes in tumor size and extent is variable and dependent on the initial mammographic appearance. However, limitations exist secondary to the presence of necrosis and treatment related fibrosis, which make it challenging to distinguish residual tumor from post-treatment change [3] (case 1). In fact, this accounts for the wide range of variability in the accuracy of mammography to predict residual tumor size within 1 cm of the pathologic tumor size, ranging from accuracy 32–70% [7, 8]. There is also variability in the ability of mammography to predict a pathologic complete response with sensitivity, specificity, PPV, and NPV of 54.2, 86.3, 54.2, and 86.3, respectively [8]. Nonetheless, mammography has been shown to be more sensitive than clinical examination for the detection of residual carcinoma (79% vs. 49%, respectively) [4, 9]. As previously noted, pre-treatment mammography more accurately predicts residual tumor size and extent when assessing breast carcinomas that initially presented as masses (defined as at least 50% of the tumor margin visible) as opposed to ill-defined regions of architectural distortion or calcification [10]. The addition of digital breast tomosynthesis (DBT) has improved detection rates of breast malignancy on mammogram, specifically when the malignancy presents as a region of architectural distortion [11].

The presence of malignant calcifications can be a misleading feature on mammography when attempting to define tumoral extent upon completion of NST. Multiple studies have shown that new or residual calcifications are not accurate predictors of therapeutic response [12, 13]. Indeed, the presence of new or changing calcifications on mammography has been shown to result in overestimation of residual disease in up to 40% of screened patients [3]. Therefore, the presence, abscence, or change in calcifications should not be used to assess response.

Ductal carcinoma in situ (DCIS) presents a particular challenge for follow-up imaging. Most commonly presenting as calcifications (infrequently architectural distortion, mass, or asymmetry), the response of DCIS to neoadjuvant systemic therapy is inadequately assessed by mammography, with sensitivity reported at 55% [6]. Patient with DCIS, alone or concurrent with invasive carcinoma, should be followed with more advanced imaging, specifically MRI. Calcifications associated with DCIS upon completion of NST should be excised to assess residual disease that may be occult on imaging, including MRI. Given the inadequacy of current imaging, including MRI, to distinguish residual from treated disease in the setting of malignant calcifications, excision of residual calcifications remains important (case 6, Figs. 5.31 and 5.34). This further avoids confusion and potentially unnecessary biopsies at the time of future post-treatment imaging follow-up where these calcifications would be suspicious [13].

Ultrasonography

Sonographic evaluation of breast carcinomas is a frequent addition to initial mammographic imaging evaluation prior to, during, and following completion of NST. In the pre-treatment setting, it allows for better tissue characterization than conventional mammography and often yields the presence of a discrete mass that is more accurately sized [8] (case 1, Fig. 5.3 and case 2, Fig. 5.8). However, in the post-treatment setting, the ability of ultrasonography to accurately predict residual tumor size within 1 cm of the pathologic tumor size remains suboptimal (correlation coefficient 0.42, accuracy 75%). Over- or underestimating pathologic tumor size seems to be equally as likely, probably related to the variable post-treatment appearance of the tumor [3, 7, 8]. Similar to mammography, fibrosis and necrosis can confound assessment of a residual mass(es) (case 3, Fig. 5.15 and case 6, Figs. 5.35 and 5.36) . But studies have demonstrated that residual tumor size is more accurately assessed with ultrasound than by conventional mammography, though still lower than the accuracy of MRI (accuracy of 79% for ultrasound) [3, 5] (Table 5.1). There is also variability in the accuracy of ultrasound in predicting pathologic complete response (pCR) with sensitivity, specificity, positive predictive value (PPV), and negative predictive value (NPV) of 45.8, 93.8, 68.8, and 85.2, respectively [8]. Therefore, ultrasonography is often combined with mammography and/or MRI to increase the accuracy of evaluation of both the initial and residual tumor size/extent [3] (Table 5.2).

Ultrasound evaluation of biopsy-proven DCIS is often challenging and of limited utility. This results from poor sonographic visualization of calcifications, the most common imaging manifestation of DCIS. Discrete masses with increased vascularity, more often seen with invasive breast carcinomas, or ductal dilation are infrequent in the setting of DCIS. Solitary DCIS would not routinely require staging or neoadjuvant treatment.

Ultrasound plays a crucial role in the evaluation of lymph nodes in the axilla. In clinically lymph node-negative patients, axillary ultrasound better assesses lymph node morphology to identify locally advanced disease (case 4, Fig. 5.19) Interrogation with core needle biopsy has been shown to have a higher sensitivity (88%) versus fine needle aspiration (74%) to assess for axillary involvement; however, specificity for both ranges from 99% to 100% [3, 14, 15]. Following the completion of neoadjuvant systemic therapy, US has only been shown to be 70% sensitive for the detection of residual nodal disease [3]. Although ultrasound has been shown to be highly sensitive for the detection of metastatic axillary lymph

Table 5.1 Modality comparison for evaluation of residual disease following NST [3, 4, 8, 59]

	Mammography	Ultrasonography	DCE-MRI	Clinical breast exam
Sensitivity	79%	89–90%	86–92%	49%
Specificity	77%	30–33%	60–89%	92%
Accuracy	32–70%	60% (80% when combined with mammography)	76–90%	54%

Table 5.2 Modality comparison for evaluation of complete pathologic response [3, 4, 8, 59]

	Mammography	Ultrasonography	DCE-MRI
Sensitivity	54%	46%	76–86%
Specificity	86%	94%	45–49%
Accuracy	---	---	74%

nodes, false-negative FNA/CNB rates are up to 20% for sampling by both FNA and CNB [3, 6, 16–18]. Therefore, surgical staging with sentinel lymph node biopsy (SLNB) or targeted SLNB remains the standard of care.

Studies are ongoing regarding the necessity for axillary dissection in patients with biopsy-proven metastatic adenopathy who respond to neoadjuvant treatment. The ACOSOG Z1071 trial found a FNR of 12.6% when two or more sentinel nodes were identified at the time of surgery. However, utilization of targeted SLNB (when a biopsy marker/clip has been placed in a metastatic lymph node at the time of initial FNA or CNB and localized prior to surgery) reduced the FNR to 6.8% (when the marked lymph node was found to be one of the sentinel lymph nodes) [19].

Functional Imaging

Dynamic Contrast-Enhanced Magnetic Resonance Imaging (DCE-MRI/MRI)

MRI provides morphologic and cross-sectional distribution information as well as secondary physiologic information by way of tumor angiogenesis and enhancement kinetic characteristics. In contrast to mammography, MRI sensitivity is not limited by breast tissue density [3] (case 5, Figs. 5.27, 5.28, and 5.29). It is the most robust modality in evaluation of breast carcinomas prior to, during, and following the completion of neoadjuvant systemic therapy and, therefore, the recommended imaging examination in the pre- and post-neoadjuvant systemic therapy setting according to the revised RECIST guidelines [20]. MRI may also be advantageous by showing the type of response, homogeneous or heterogenous. In the case of a heterogenous response to NST, noncontiguous areas of residual disease seen on MRI that may be occult on other modalities potentially altering surgical management (case 5, Fig. 5.30). Correlation of treatment response with MRI at pathology is more accurate than mammography, ultrasound, and clinical exam (Table 5.2). A common criticism of MRI is the high false-positive rate which can result in additional biopsies prior to initiation of neoadjuvant treatment and/or overestimation of disease at the completion of the neoadjuvant chemotherapy. This may be mitigated by greater experience in MRI interpretation and image quality as well as patient factors such as reduced background parenchymal enhancement (BPE).

Standard imaging protocols with 1.5 T or 3 T magnets, dedicated breast coils, and gadolinium-based contrast include axial T1 pre-contrast fat-saturated images and axial dynamic post-contrast-enhanced T1 fat-saturated sequences, with enhancement as an evaluation of tumor angiogenesis [6]. Fluid-sensitive sequences such as T2 and STIR aid interpretation in the pre- and post-treatment settings for necrosis and treatment-related fibrosis and improve specificity (case 3, Fig. 5.16). Sagittal imaging may aid lesion localization and is commonly performed in the delayed post-contrast phase (case 1, Fig. 5.5). Enhancement kinetics, or the manner in which lesions take up the contrast agent, are evaluated on post-processing software and should be used as an adjunct to morphology and imaging characteristics rather than the primary method of evaluation. Washout enhancement defined as initial rapid uptake of contrast and early washout is most suspicious but can also be seen with benign entities such as lymph nodes. Historically, imaging is recommended in the follicular phase of the menstrual cycle to minimize background parenchymal enhancement (BPE); however, this is frequently forgone in the setting of staging malignancy to avoid delays in care. In most cases, MRI should be interpreted with a recent mammogram for correlation.

A crucial first step for utilization of MRI to assess for tumor response in the neoadjuvant setting is to obtain an initial, pre-treatment examination. This estimates tumor size and assesses for additional sites of disease, multifocal or multicentric carcinoma. MRI is also the best tool for assessment of the pectoralis muscle or chest wall invasion and internal mammary lymphadenopathy due to the larger field of view (case 2, Fig. 5.10). The extent of axillary lymphadenopathy can also be established by MRI in both the pre- and post-treatment settings. The non-affected breast is also screened with an incidence of concurrent contralateral breast carcinomas in up to 3–4% of women [3, 21, 22]. Several studies have also shown that in up to 11% of cases, mammographically occult multicentric disease is found on MRI which may alter surgical management in the pre-treatment setting, potentially requiring additional biopsies [21, 22] (case 5, Fig. 5.28).

Utilizing MRI for evaluating pre-treatment extent of disease has been shown to have high sensitivity, variable specificity, and high accuracy (90–96%, 50–97%, and 89%, respectively) [3, 21, 23]. One recent meta-analysis across 14 retrospective studies showed MRI sensitivity and specificity of 84% and 83%, respectively [24]. The variable specificity is a point of concern especially at the initial exam when additional indeterminant or suspicious findings may be identified necessitating further evaluation with percutaneous biopsy, delaying initiation of NST. However, PPV is particularly high in the setting of invasive lobular carcinomas, where MRI has been shown to be more accurate than ultrasonography and mammography in determining disease extent (accuracy 83–85%) [3, 25].

Following the completion of NST, MRI is superior for assessment of residual tumor compared to mammography and ultrasonography, with sensitivity, specificity, and accuracy ranging from 86–92%, 60–89%, and 76–90%, respectively [3] (Table 5.2). Variability in the sensitivity, specificity, and accuracy of MRI in determining residual tumor is highly dependent on the pre-treatment tumor characteristics and tumor subtypes. Discrepancy between imaging assessment of residual disease and pathologic extent is highest for estrogen receptor (ER)-positive breast cancers, cancers of low nuclear grade, and those presenting with diffuse non-mass enhancement [4, 23, 26]. In contrast, MRI is highly accurate in estimating residual tumor size – within 0.1 cm of pathologic size – in triple-negative and HER2-positive subtypes [27]. Further, HER2-positive subtypes, regardless of the hormone receptor status, show the best correlation of post-NST MRI with surgical pathology results (Table 5.3). Recent trials have shown better correlation between tumor size on DCE-MRI compared to pathologic tumor size when volumetric

Table 5.3 MRI for predicting complete pathologic response following NST based on tumor subtype [59]

	Sensitivity	Specificity	Accuracy
HR+/HER2−	86%	45%	80%
HR−/HER2+	83%	47%	69%
HR+/HER2+	77%	49%	70%
TN	81%	49%	69%

measurements are utilized (as opposed to uni- or bidirectional measurements) [28–30]. Another study showed measurement of longest tumor dimension by MRI was more accurate than mammogram and clinical exam in assessing residual tumor size [31].

There are no current recommendations for imaging following an excisional biopsy or lumpectomy with positive margins. However, there have been studies demonstrating the efficacy of DCE-MRI in assessing residual disease with sensitivity of up to 79.9% and specificity between 75% and 90.5% [32]. The higher specificities were achieved approximately 30 days following excisional biopsy/lumpectomy to allow post-surgical changes that may mimic residual carcinoma to subside [33]. Nonetheless, the variable appearance of the post-surgical breast limits the accuracy of MRI to evaluate residual disease extent in the setting of positive surgical margins.

Evaluation of the axilla, both pre- and post-treatment, utilizing MRI delineates the extent of axillary nodal disease including levels I, II, and potentially level III lymph nodes. However, detection of residual nodal disease following completion of neoadjuvant systemic therapy has shown a sensitivity range of 51–61% with a NPV of 83%. In contrast, ultrasonography has shown slightly greater sensitivity of 69.8% for detection of residual nodal disease [3, 4, 34, 35]. Therefore, US evaluation and US-guided axillary CNB/FNA remain useful. And Surgical interrogation of the axilla should not be omitted because of a negative ultrasound or MRI examination.

DCIS presents a challenge in both the pre- and post-treatment settings on MRI. DCE-MRI has been shown to be more sensitive than both ultrasonography and mammography for the initial detection of DCIS (sensitivity 89%) [6, 36]. While MRI is sensitive for the detection of residual DCIS following completion of neoadjuvant systemic therapy, the specificity remains low (sensitivity 93%, specificity 35%) [37]. This especially creates a challenge when invasive cancers coexist with DCIS. DCIS can present with regions of persistent enhancement, above the normal background enhancement of the glandular tissue, which can yield an overestimation of true residual invasive tumor size [6, 31, 37]. But, residual DCIS may be present without abnormal enhancement on MRI, as previously discussed [13] (case 6, Fig. 5.34).

Final considerations include contraindications and relative contraindications to MRI most commonly including renal failure/insufficiency, severe gadolinium contrast allergy, pacemakers, claustrophobia, and pregnancy. Non-severe gadolinium contrast allergies are a relative contradiction with premedication protocols that should be based on institutional and American College of Radiology (ACR) guidelines. As always, there should be a risk-benefit assessment in such patients, including those who are pregnant. While no controlled studies have been performed in pregnant women, no known adverse effects have been reported in clinical settings of gadolinium administration in pregnant women. The risk of breakthrough reactions in patients premedicated for non-severe contrast reactions are rare. Contrast should never be administered in patients who have experienced severe allergic reactions, including anaphylaxis.

Contrast-Enhanced Digital Mammography (CEM/CEDM)

Contrast-enhanced digital mammography (CEM/CEDM) is an FDA-approved, promising emerging technology that rivals MRI in sensitivity and specificity. Like MRI, CEM utilizes a neovascular approach to the detection of malignant angiogenesis. The examination is a dual energy technique performed following administration of iodinated contrast media (same as that used for computed tomography) with standard craniocaudal (CC) and mediolateral oblique (MLO) of both breasts subsequently obtained in two separate acquisitions above ("high energy") and below ("low energy") the k-edge of iodine. "Low-energy" mammogram or mammogram with tomosynethsis is identical to a routine mammogram view. The high energy images are not interpretated but rater used to create recombined or subtraction images used for interpretation. CEM Intrepretation includes assessment of BPE, as with MRI. For the patient, the exam acquisition is similar to a screening mammogram except for iodinated contrast administration and negligible additional radiation as a result of the dual energy technique with two x-ray exposures. Currently, no BI-RADS® lexicon exists for this modality though use of a hybrid mammography and MRI lexicons has been validated [38, 39].

Practically, CEM may be advantageous compared to MRI due to the lower cost in implementation and performance. It can be performed by trained mammography technologists following a vendor-specific upgrade to mammography units and therefore more accessible across practice settings and in rural communities. CEM may also be of benefit for patients when MRI is contraindicated (renal disease, pacemaker, metallic implants) or poorly tolerated (inability to lie prone, claustrophobia). The primary disadvantages compared to MRI are the use of ionizing radiation, limited field of view in imaging the chest wall, internal mammary chain, and axilla, as well as the lack of a widely available CEM-guided biopsy technique. Also in distinction from MRI, enhancement kinetics are not available for CEM because imaging is performed only at a single time point for each view.

Multiple studies have shown CEM efficacy is similar to MRI in tumor detection, tumor extent and size, and detection of additional lesions in the preoperative setting [40–42]. Sensitivity ranged between 96–100% and 96–98% for CEM and MRI, respectively, with fewer false positives as compared with MRI and correlation with postoperative tumor size [40, 41]. Assessment of residual disease following NST is also comparable to MRI and within 1 cm of tumor size by pathology [43–45]. In the setting of assessing response to NST, sensitivity and specificity ranges include 76–84% and 87.5–100% for CEM and 87–92% and 60–75% for MRI with similar

PPV [44, 45]. These highlight the higher specificity of CEM, another potential benefit over MRI which is often critiqued due to variable specificity. However, ongoing study is needed. Though CEM biopsy technology is not yet available, two industry leaders have received premarket FDA 510 k clearance, suggesting wide release in the United States is forthcoming.

Molecular Imaging

Molecular imaging may be utilized prior to the initiation of neoadjuvant systemic therapy in staging for distant metastasis. According to the National Comprehensive Cancer Network (NCCN) guidelines, molecular imaging for evaluation of distant metastases should be considered in patients with signs or symptoms concerning for metastatic disease (i.e., bone pain, elevated alkaline phosphatase, abnormal liver functions tests, or abdominal symptoms) [46].

The most common molecular imaging technique is fluorine-18 fluorodeoxyglucose positron emission tomography (18F-FDG PET), which capitalizes on tumor hypermetabolism of glucose and is performed in conjunction with CT for anatomic detail (case 4, Fig. 5.22). The degree of increased metabolism is quantified by a standard uptake value (SUV), with higher values corresponding to increased metabolic activity. The primary benefit of molecular imaging with 18F-FDG PET is in evaluation of distant metastatic disease. Although recent studies have suggested that decreases in the standardized uptake value (SUV) of invasive breast cancers correlate with pathologic response following the completion of neoadjuvant systemic therapy (sensitivity 84%, specificity 66%, PPV 50%, NPV 91%), the role of molecular imaging for evaluation of residual breast carcinoma remains inadequate [47–49]. This is due to the technical limitation of 18F-FDG PET imaging to detect sub -centimeter lesions with lower spatial resolution as compared to other modalities such as MRI. This also holds true for evaluation of the axilla following neoadjuvant therapy, where 18F-FDG PET has only been shown to be 63.2% sensitive for the detection of residual nodal disease (compared to 69.8% with ultrasonography) [3]. However, 18F-FDG PET shows very high sensitivity and specificity for detection of distant metastases (100% and 96%, respectively) [48, 49].

The current NCCN guidelines recommend evaluation with molecular imaging when clinical signs and/or symptoms raise concern for metastatic disease. A few examples provided include bone pain, elevated alkaline phosphatase, elevated liver functions tests, or abdominal pain. Their current recommendations include the use of computed tomography of the chest, abdomen, and pelvis (CT CAP) along with whole body Tc-99m bone scintigraphy to evaluate for both visceral and bony metastases [46, 50] (case 6, Fig. 5.33). Specifically in the case of bony metastases, the sensitivities of these range from 71–100%, 96%, and 62–100%, respectively [50, 51]. The NCCN guidelines state that 18F-FDG PET is optional in evaluation for distant metastases and could be considered for equivocal results seen on either CT CAP or bone scintigraphy [46]. 18F FDG-PET has been shown in multiple studies to have a higher specificity for bony metastases than bone scintigraphy alone (96–100% vs. 78–100%) [51].

In the neoadjuvant setting, NCCN guidelines recommend the use of CT CAP or bone scintigraphy; however, the frequency of monitoring is not defined and the flare phenomenon (temporarily increased metabolic activity in treated metastases) may confound interpretation. Again, NCCN guidelines list 18F-FDG PET as an optional imaging examination to evaluate treatment response citing the lack of reproducibility in determining standards for disease response [46].

Positron emission mammography (PEM) received FDA approval in 2003 combining the ability to detect hypermetabolic foci within the breast utilizing 18F-FDG, with overall increased spatial resolution when compared to conventional, whole-body 18F-FDG PET. Although not in routine clinical use, PEM has been shown to be more specific than MRI for the detection of pathologic disease extent (80% with PEM vs. 66% with MRI) but with a lower sensitivity (41% with PEM vs. 53% with MRI) [52].

Molecular breast imaging (MBI) and breast-specific gamma imaging (BGSI) are usually performed after IV injection of 99mTc-sestamibi. Imaging is performed with the patient seated and acquisition time is approximately 10 minutes per view, for a total of 40 minutes to complete routine craniocaudal (CC) and mediolateral oblique (MLO) views of both breasts. Like CEM and MRI, normal background parenchymal uptake is characterized. Breast cancer detection with BSGI varies between 69 and 96% with a specificity range of 71–80% [53–55]. Detection of malignancy with MBI is similar to MRI and CEM [56]. However MRI is more sensitive than BGSI for detection of DCIS with and without calcifications [54]. At least one study shows specificity in determining a complete treatment response was greater with BGSI than with MRI (90% vs. 60%) [57]. As with MRI and CEM and in contrast to mammography, sensitivity of MBI/BGSI is not influenced by breast tissue density. However, sensitivity does decrease with decreasing lesion size, particularly when size is smaller than 1 cm. MBI and BGSI are not routinely recommended for detection of breast carcinoma or evaluation for residual tumor following neoadjuvant therapy. This is due to the lower sensitivity when compared with MRI for the diagnosis of sub-centimeter cancers (sensitivity 84%) [58]. However, it may be considered in patients for whom MRI is contraindicated, such as those with a severe gadolinium contrast allergy or MR unsafe implantable devices.

Conclusion

Determination of the appropriate imaging modalities to assess extent of disease and monitor response to neoadjuvant systemic therapy should be based on tumor size, subtype, and the patient's clinical history with multidisciplinary consideration. Accurate assessment of residual tumor with imaging aids selection of the best surgical approach to avoid positive margins, re-excisions, or unnecessary total mastectomy. While standard imaging with tomosynthesis mammogram and ultrasound are necessary, they may underestimate disease extent or overestimate residual disease, especially in patients with dense breasts and those with lobular subtypes. There is strong, consistent evidence to support the routine use of MRI to characterize disease extent, evaluate for contralateral breast disease, and assess therapeutic response following completion of NST. The degree of therapeutic response as characterized by imaging with MRI versus pCR varies by tumor subtype and is most reliable with TN and HER2-positive subtypes. However, lack of MRI enhancement in the setting of DCIS should not preclude excision of malignant calcifications due to insufficient evidence to accurately predict the presence or absence of residual disease.

Molecular imaging with 18F-FDG PET or CT combined with bone scan may be used to evaluate for distant disease when clinically indicated. PET/CT is not recommended as the primary modality to assess response to NST in patients with primary breast carcinoma due to the lower spatial resolution as compared to MRI. While several modalities (CEM/MBI) show sensitivity and specificity comparable to MRI in disease detection and assessment of response, more research is needed and widespread utilization remains limited for a variety of reasons including access, time, and lack of concurrent biopsy technology. However, these modalities may prove to be reasonable alternative in patient for whom MRI is contraindicated.

Axillary staging with ultrasound and ultrasound-guided FNA/CNB is sensitive and specific for the detection of metastatic lymphadenopathy. MRI and cross-sectional imaging better demonstrate the extent of axillary nodal disease including levels I-III and subsequent extent of nodal response to NST. However, sentinel lymph node sampling remains the gold standard due to the insufficiently high false-negative biopsy rates on FNA/CNB.

Case 1

This is a 66-year-old woman with a round and irregular masses and suspicious calcifications in the right breast identified on screening mammography (Figs. 5.1 and 5.2). Ultrasound (US) and US-guided core needle biopsy (CNB) revealed two sites of triple-positive invasive ductal carcinoma (IDC), 8:00 and 9:00 with high Ki-67, between 75 and 90% (Fig. 5.3). Axillary ultrasound revealed an abnormal round level 1 lymph node, CNB-proven metastatic (Fig. 5.4). MRI better delineates the extent of in-breast including non-mass enhancement between the sites of US CNB-proven malignancy and axillary nodal disease including level 2 lymphadenopathy (Figs. 5.5 and 5.6). She completed HER2-based chemotherapy.

Case 2

This is a 47-year-old woman with screen-detected right breast triple-negative (TN) IDC, Ki-67 75% (Fig. 5.7). US better delineates the irregular margins of the mass (Fig. 5.8), and MRI showed abnormal internal mammary chain and intramammary lymphadenopathy (Figs. 5.9 and 5.10) She underwent NST with four cycles of A/C followed by platinum and Taxol with an incomplete response (Fig. 5.11). Breast conservation therapy (BCT) revealed 1.2 cm residual mass within 2.5 cm fibrous tumor bed. One of four lymph nodes were positive for metastatic carcinoma on sentinel lymph node biopsy (SLNB), and one lymph node showed focal therapy changes. She received adjuvant radiation (XRT) and Xeloda.

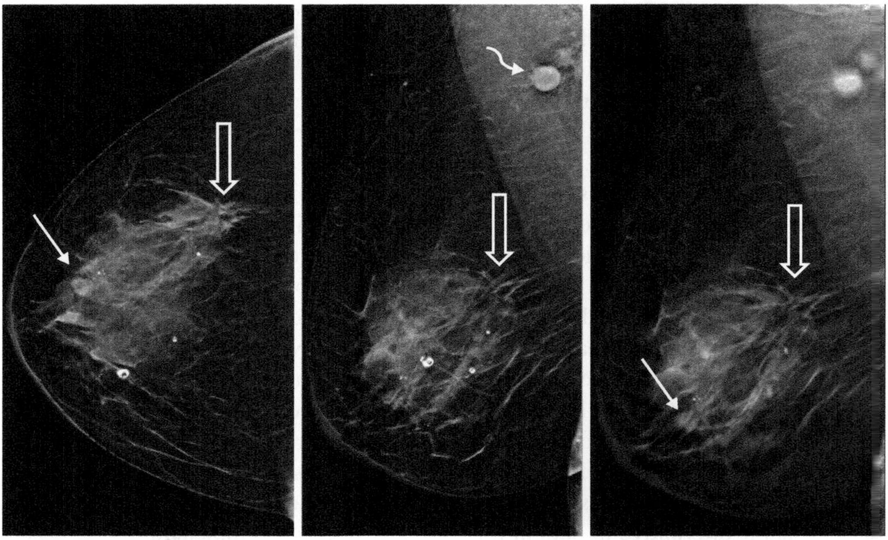

Fig. 5.1 Craniocaudal (CC, left) and mediolateral oblique (MLO, center), and 1 mm tomosynthesis slice MLO (right) views of the right breast. Heterogeneously dense breast tissue. Round (arrow) and irregular (open arrow) masses in the right breast identified on screening mammography. Tomosynthesis better demonstrates the indistinct and irregular margins of the respective masses. Abnormal axillary lymph node with round morphology (curved arrow)

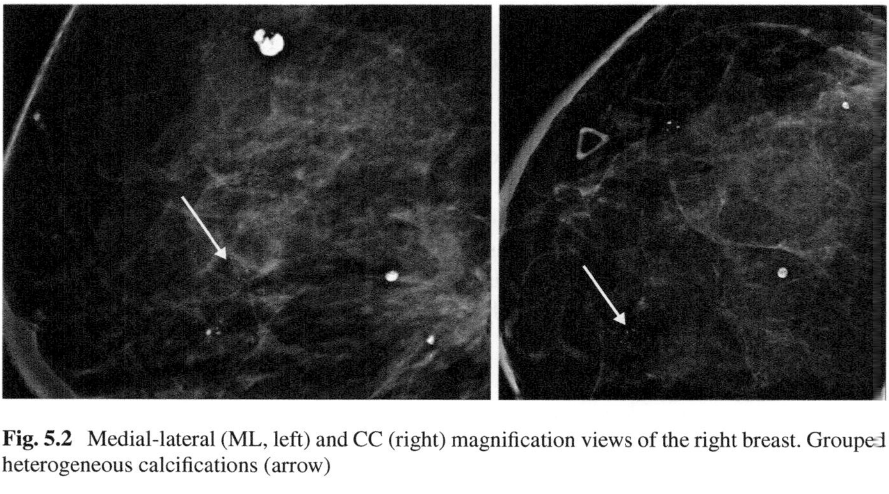

Fig. 5.2 Medial-lateral (ML, left) and CC (right) magnification views of the right breast. Grouped heterogeneous calcifications (arrow)

Case 3

This is a 49-year-old woman with self-detected invasive lobular cancer (ILC) and lobular carcinoma in situ (LCIS) ER/PR-positive, HER2-negative, Ki-67 10%. NST with ACT (Adriamycin, Cytoxan, followed by Taxol). DM revealed a heterogeneously dense breast tissue with a spiculated mass in the upper outer quadrant of the

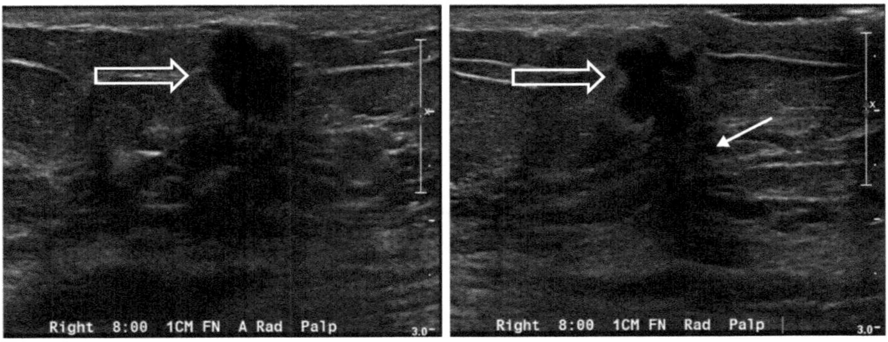

Fig. 5.3 Grayscale ultrasound (US). Irregular hypoechoic mass with an echogenic rim (open arrow) and partial posterior acoustic shadowing (arrow). US CNB revealed triple-positive IDC, Ki-67 90%

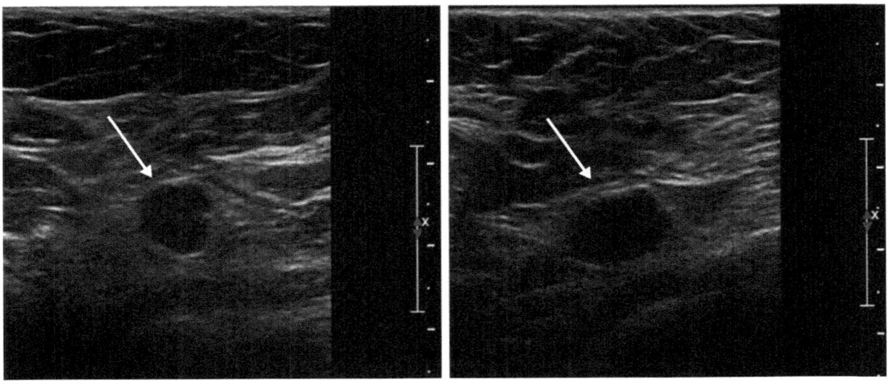

Fig. 5.4 Grayscale US. Abnormal right axillary lymph node (arrow) including a round morphology and absent central fatty hilum

left breast (Fig. 5.12). Ultrasound showed a hypoechoic mass with poorly defined margins (Fig. 5.13). MRI revealed a much larger area of contiguous non mass enhancement and extent of disease spanning at least 7 cm (Fig. 5.14). Following NST, focal residual disease was identified on MRI (Fig. 5.15) though not definitive on US (Fig. 5.16). Segmental mastectomy (SM) showed residual ILC NG II, present as single tumor cells (up to 1 mm) over 3.6 cm area of fibrotic (treated) tissue. She underwent total mastectomy (TM) due to multiple positive margins which showed 5 mm of classic type ILC as well as classic type LCIS and atypical lobular hyperplasia (ALH). 1/3 positive nodes on sentinel lymph node biopsy (SLNB) without extracapsular extension (9.5 mm focus.) RCB (residual cancer burden) II.

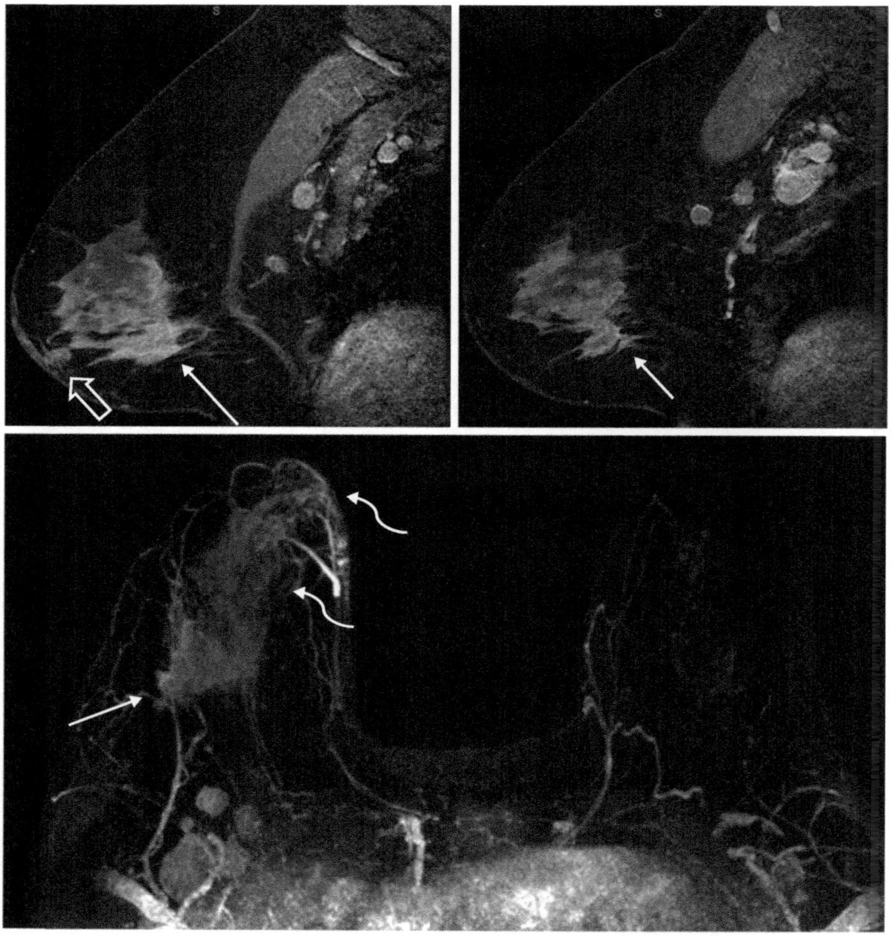

Fig. 5.5 Sagittal T1 delayed post-contrast fat saturation (FS) images (top right and left) and axial maximum intensity projection (MIP, bottom). Irregular enhancing mass (arrow) and round enhancing mass (open arrow) with intervening contiguous non-mass enhancement (NME) extending to the nipple (curved arrows)

Case 4

This is a 39-year-old woman self-detected TN IDC in the right breast, Ki-67 45%. DM showed an irregular mass with calcifications corresponding to the area of concern (Fig. 5.17). US showed a poorly defined hypoechoic shadowing mass (Fig. 5.18), while MRI showed extensive disease involving the upper outer and upper inner breast (Figs. 5.19 and 5.20). US CNB of an abnormal right axillary lymph node was positive for metastatic carcinoma (Fig. 5.21). PET/CT confirmed locally advanced malignancy without distant metastatic disease (Fig. 5.22). Genetic testing revealed a pathogenic BRCA1 mutation. The patient completed AC × 4 and

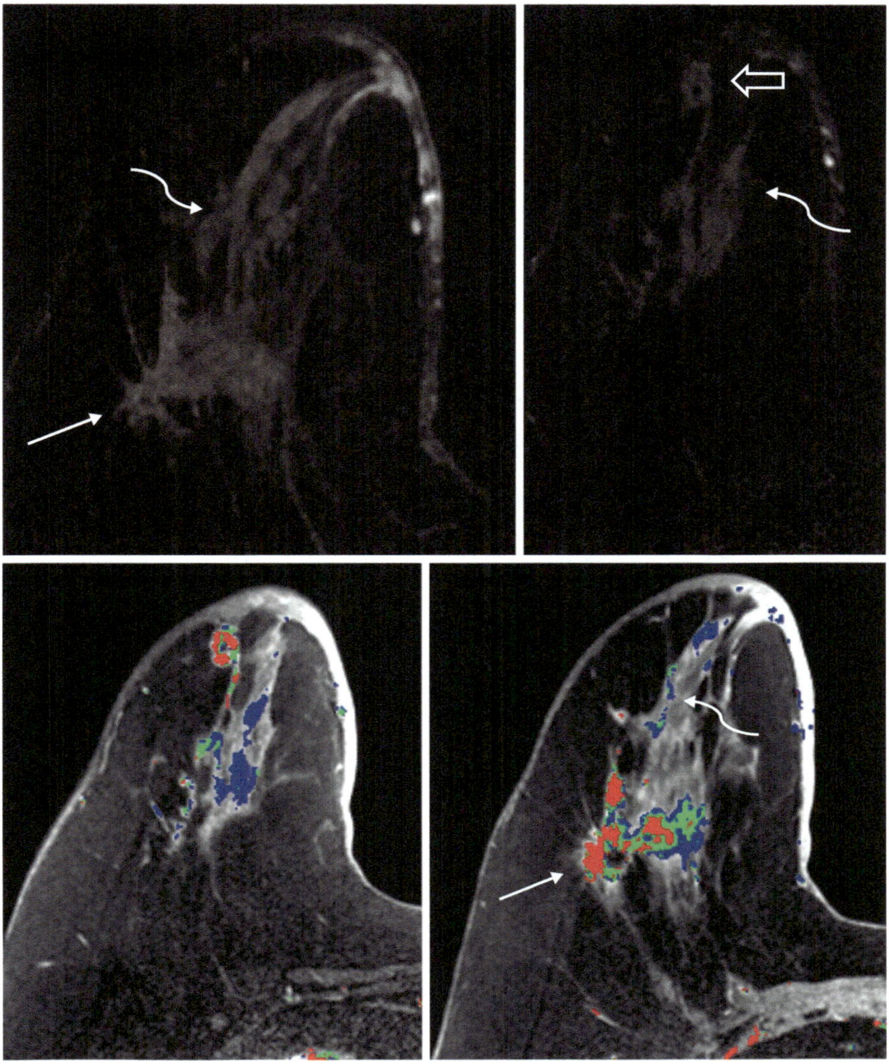

Fig. 5.6 Axial T1 fat saturation (top) and axial post-contrast kinetic overlay images (bottom). Irregular (arrow) and round enhancing (open arrow) masses with washout kinetics (red) and intervening abnormal NME with mixed kinetics (curved arrow)

Taxol and carboplatin NST with a complete imaging response on MRI (Fig. 5.23). Axillary ultrasound showed treatment response within the proven metastatic lymph node (Fig. 5.24). Due to the pathogenic BRCA1 mutation, she underwent skin-sparing total mastectomy (TM). Right breast TM showed residual IDC, few single cells, and clusters of tumors, <0.1 cm in one portion of fibrotic bed. DCIS NG 3, solid type. Lymphovascular invasion (LVI) was identified. 2/3 positive nodes on

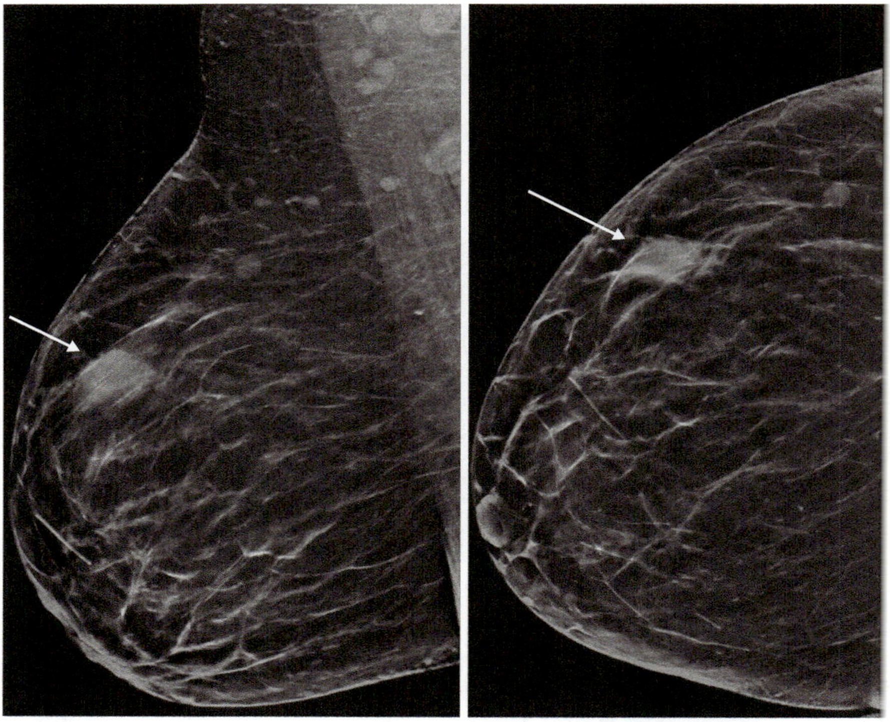

Fig. 5.7 MLO (left) and CC (right) views of the right breast. Scattered fibroglandular breast tissue density. Irregular mass with indistinct margins (arrow) in the upper outer right breast

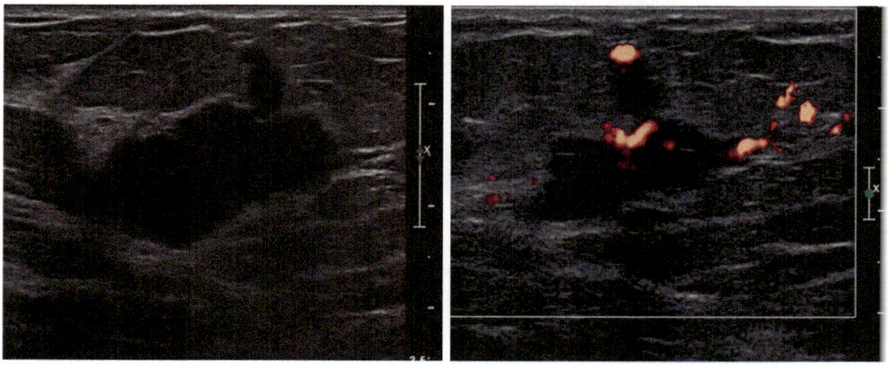

Fig. 5.8 Grayscale US, same patient. Irregular hypoechoic mass with associated vascularity corresponding to the irregular mammographic mass

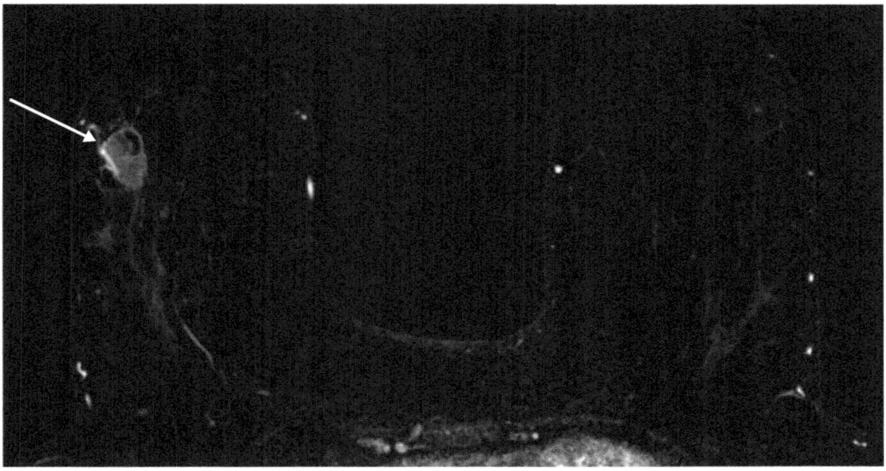

Fig. 5.9 Axial T1 post-contrast subtraction. Irregular enhancing mass corresponding to proven malignancy (arrow)

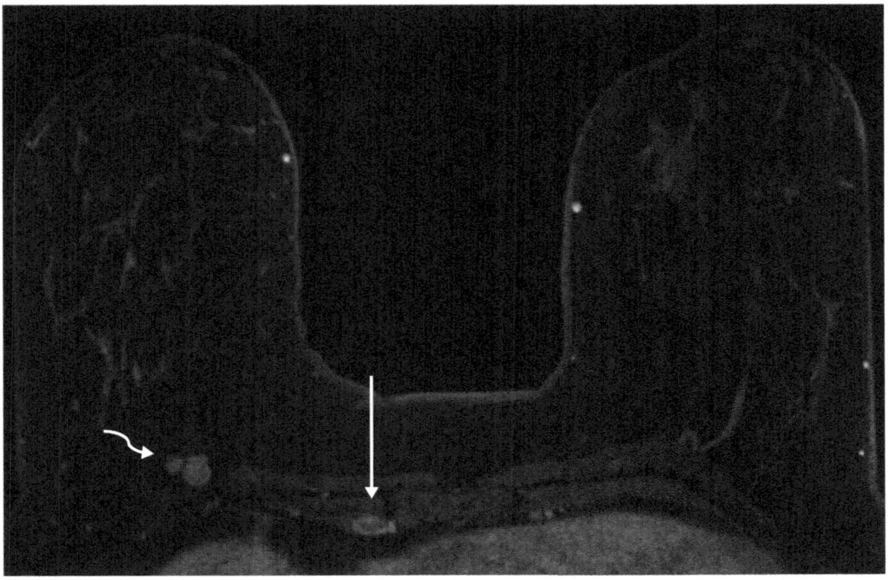

Fig. 5.10 Axial T1 post-contrast fat saturation MRI. Abnormally enlarged right internal mammary chain lymph node (arrow) in the same patient with TN right breast IDC in the upper outer quadrant. Abnormal intramammary lymph nodes are also present (curved arrow)

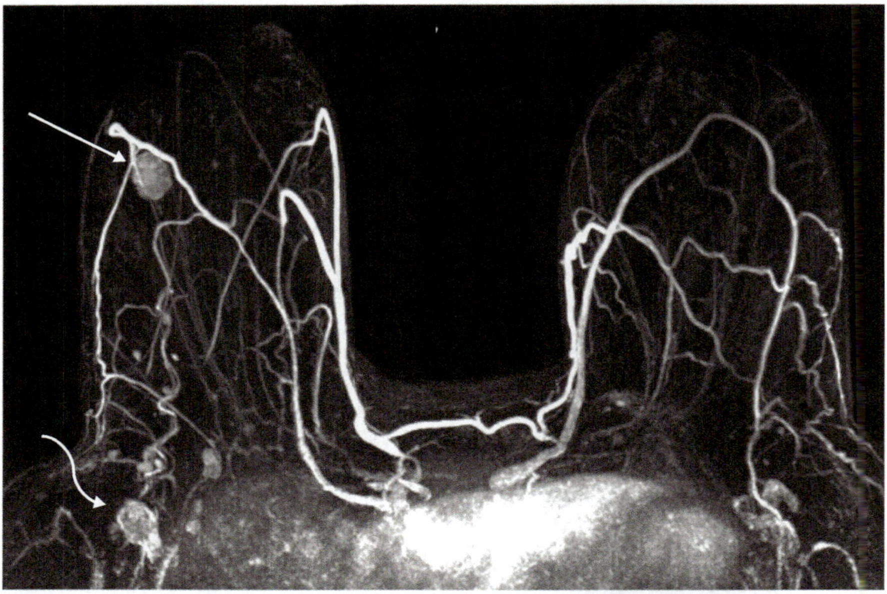

Fig. 5.11 Post-NST MRI axial MIP image shows incomplete response to NST with a smaller residual oval enhancing mass (arrow) and abnormal level 1 axillary lymph node (curved arrow)

SLNB and she underwent axillary dissection (AD) with 7/10 positive lymph node with therapy changes; the largest metastatic lymph node focus was 6 mm. RCB II.

Case 5

This is a 51-year-old woman with right breast 9:00 ILC, ER positive, PR negative, HER2+ Ki-67 5%. At the time of her screening mammogram, she underwent screening US as part of a research study. DM with tomosynthesis failed to demonstrate a discrete abnormality (Fig. 5.25), while US showed a vague hypoechoic area of shadowing (Fig. 5.26) which underwent US CNB. MRI demonstrates a 5 cm extent of asymmetric NME (Fig. 5.27) corresponding to disease extent. Even in retrospect, a mammographic abnormality was not identified corresponding to the US or MRI findings. At the time of initial MRI, bilateral axillary lymphadenopathy and an enhancing mass with contiguous NME were identified in the contralateral left breast at the 6:00 position (Fig. 5.28); MRI-guided CNB revealed classic type ILC, ER positive, PR weakly positive, HER2 amplified by FISH, and nuclear grade 2 DCIS. US CNB of bilateral axillary lymph nodes both proved positive for metastatic carcinoma (Fig. 5.29).

She completed NST with Abraxane/Herceptin. MRI following NST shows near complete response with small residual enhancing foci (Fig. 5.30). Right TM revealed rare minute areas of residual ILC up to 1 mm within a 5.8 cm fibrotic area. Left TM revealed complete pathologic response to NST. One right and two left axillary LNs were partially fibrotic indicating treatment response. Right T1cN1, Left T1bN1.

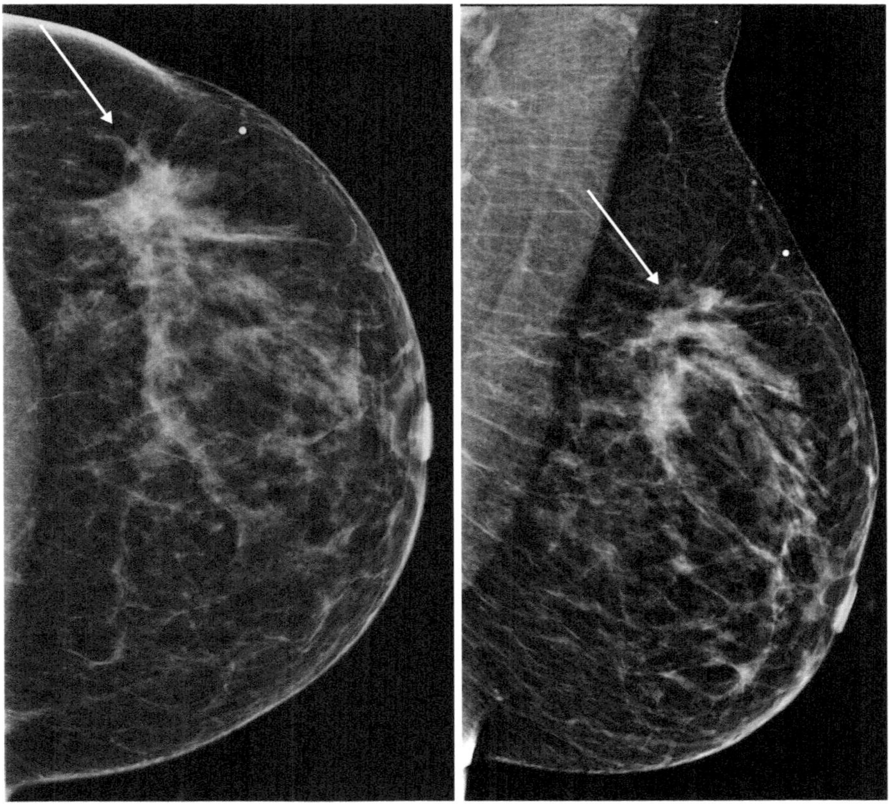

Fig. 5.12 CC (left) and MLO (right) views of the left breast. Irregular spiculated mass in the upper outer left breast (arrow)

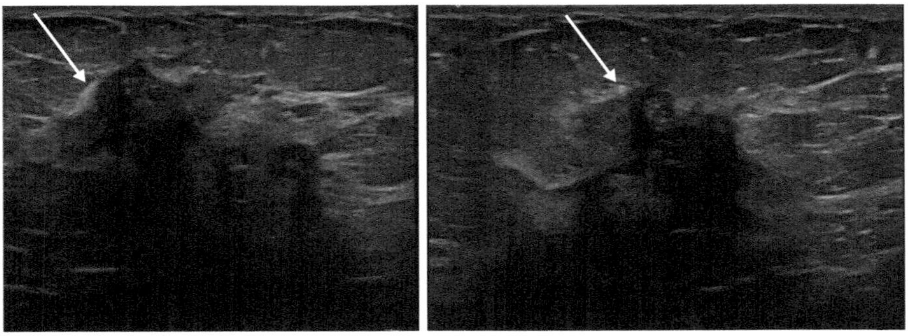

Fig. 5.13 Grayscale ultrasound. Irregular poorly delineated hypoechoic mass with posterior acoustic shadowing

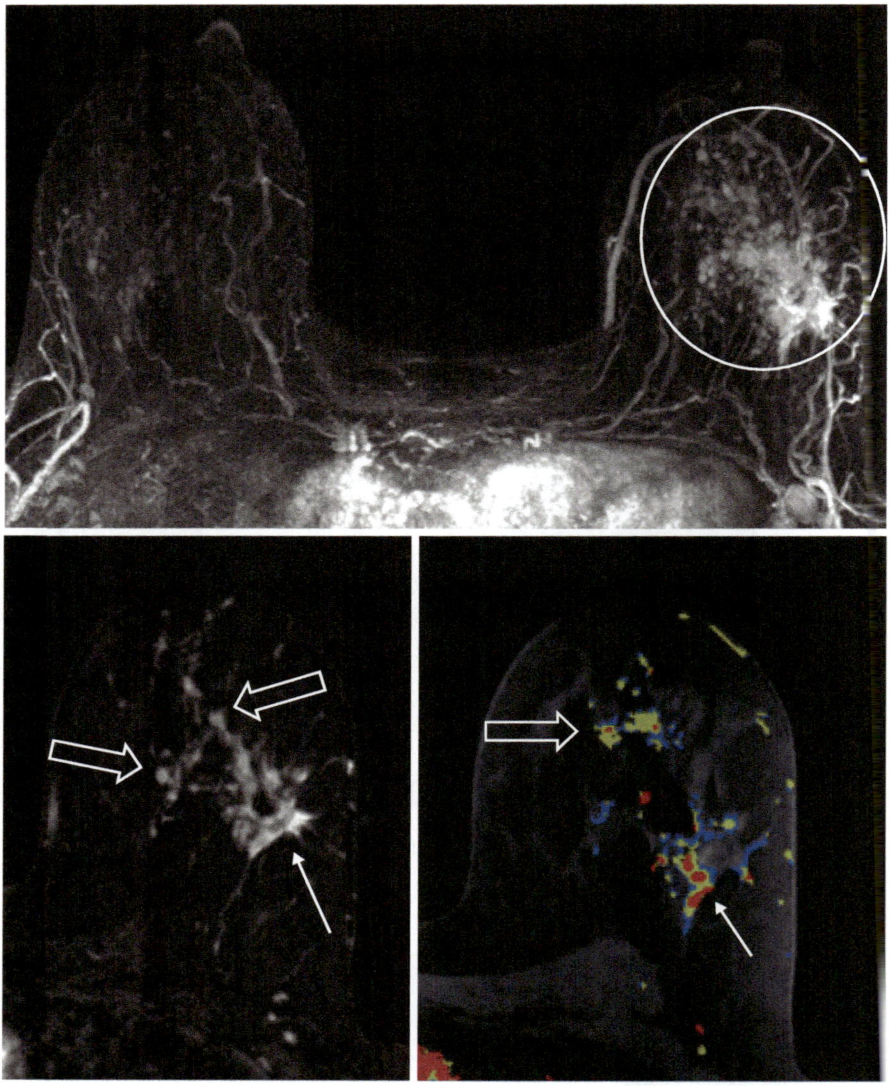

Fig. 5.14 MIP (top), post-contrast subtraction (bottom left), and kinetic color map (bottom right) MRI. The index heterogeneously enhancing mass with distortion (arrow) shows mixed enhancement with washout kinetics (red, arrow). Anterior clumped non-mass enhancement (NME, open arrow) is contiguous with the irregular mass and spans 7.2 cm in greatest AP dimension. Left axillary node biopsy (NS) positive for metastatic carcinoma

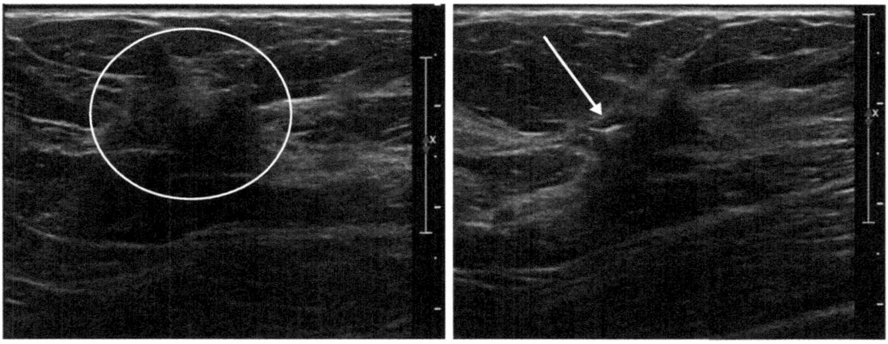

Fig. 5.15 Grayscale US images post-NST. An irregular hypoechoic mass-like area with architectural distortion remains at the site of proven malignancy as demonstrated by the echogenic biopsy clip (arrow). It is frequently difficult to delineate residual disease extent from treatment-related fibrosis on post-NST ultrasound

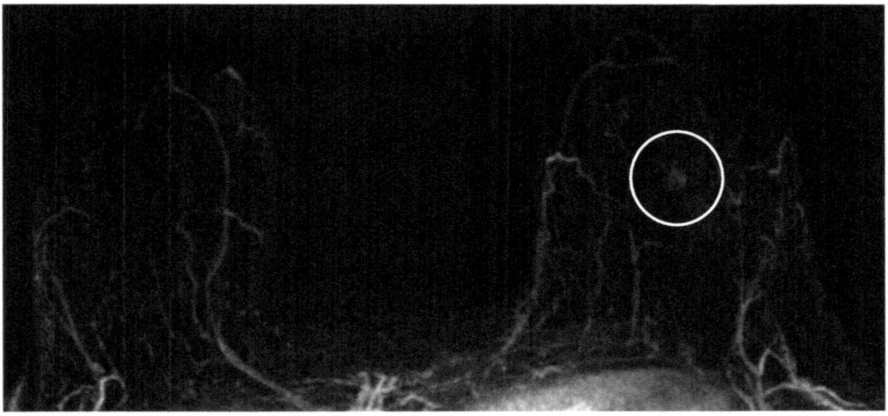

Fig. 5.16 Post-NST MIP MRI. Small residual enhancing mass in the upper outer left breast measuring 0.7 cm (circle). Following NST there was resolution of pre-treatment NME extent. Biopsy-proven malignant axillary disease also improved, not shown (NS)

Case 6

This 39-year-old woman presented with a palpable area in the left breast and thickening of the left nipple. Mammography demonstrated heterogeneously dense breast tissue with linear and segmental pleomorphic left breast calcifications spanning greater than 5 cm (Fig. 5.31). Skin thickening of the nipple and peri-areolar skin were also present (Fig. 5.31). US (NS) showed poorly delineated hypoechoic area

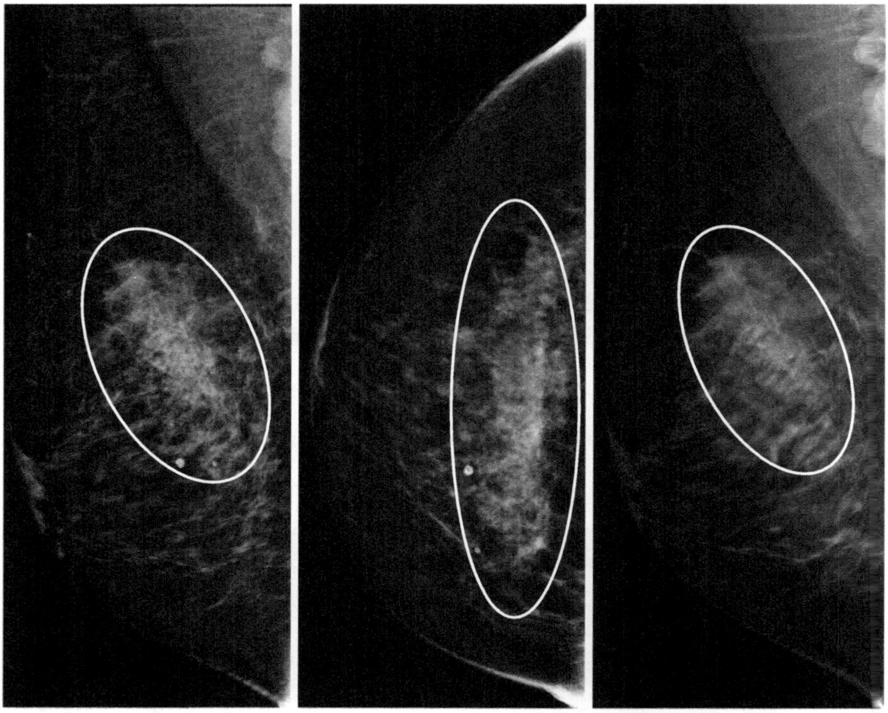

Fig. 5.17 MLO (left), CC (center), and single slice tomosynthesis MLO (right) images of the right breast demonstrating an irregular mass with calcifications in the upper outer and upper medial right breast (circle)

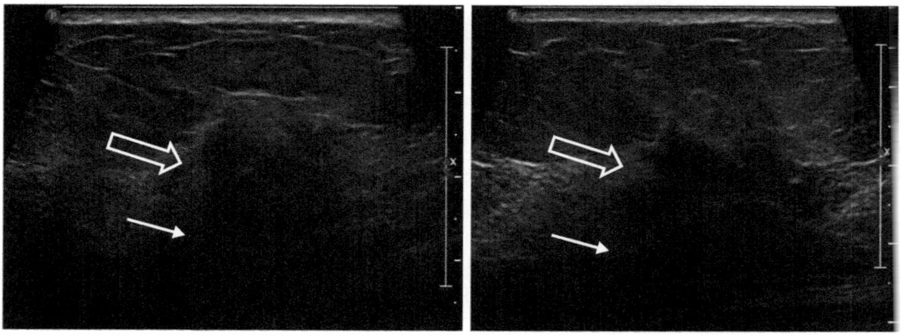

Fig. 5.18 Grayscale ultrasound images of the right breast at the 10:00 (left) and 12:00 (right) positions. Irregular hypoechoic masses (open arrows) with marked posterior shadowing (arrow), making the posterior extent of disease difficult to delineate

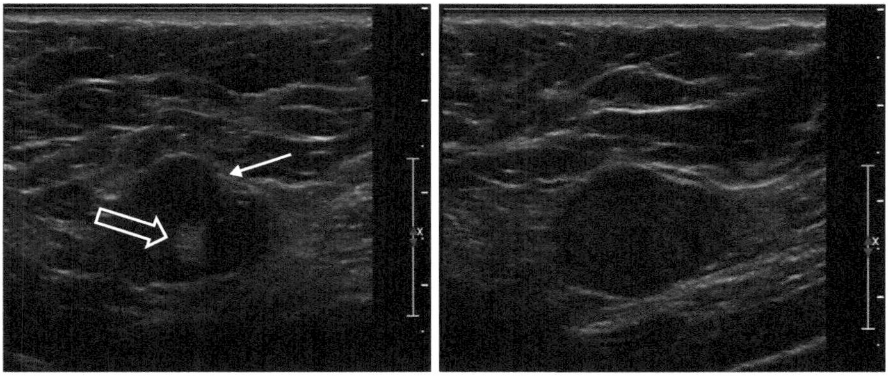

Fig. 5.19 Abnormal level 1 right axillary lymph node with eccentric nodular cortical thickening (arrow) and partially effaced central hilum. US CNB was positive for metastatic carcinoma

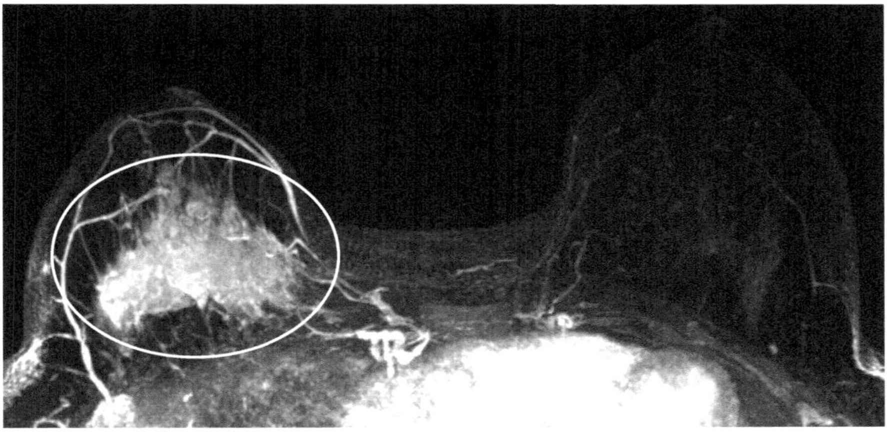

Fig. 5.20 Axial MIP MRI shows "shrunken" right breast compared to the left breast with diffuse irregular right breast enhancement breast spanning upper medial and upper lateral quadrants (circle)

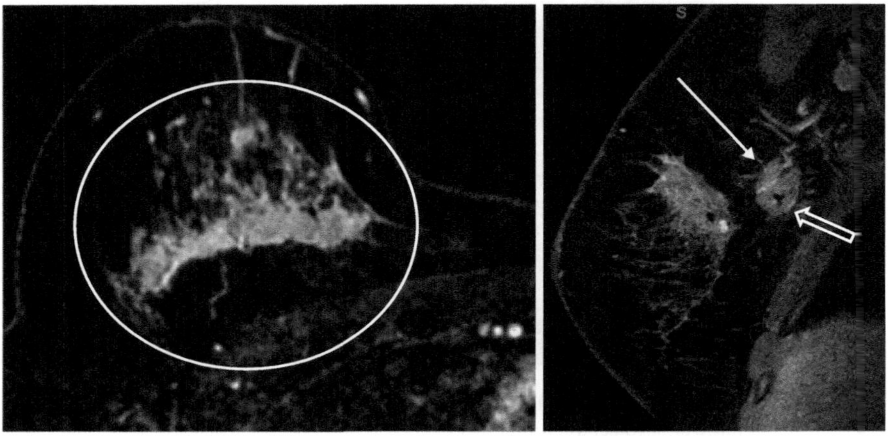

Fig. 5.21 Axial T1 post-contrast subtraction (left) and sagittal T1 delayed post-contrast fat saturation(right) images. Irregular enhancing mass and NME encompass the superior right breast, including upper medial and upper lateral quadrants (circle). Kinetic color map (NS) showed predominant washout kinetics. Biopsy-proven metastatic lymph node (arrow) with central clip artifact (open arrow)

in the retroareolar left breast without a discrete mass. A small hypoechoic mass was identified left breast 2:00 (Fig. 5.32), and US CNB revealed IDC (ER/PR positive, HER2 negative Ki-67 15%). Stereotactic biopsy of left breast calcifications 4:00 (Fig. 5.31) revealed IDC and ductal carcinoma in situ (DCIS). An abnormal level 1 left axillary node underwent US CNB and was positive for metastatic carcinoma (NS). MRI revealed NME spanning 9.5 cm in the lateral left breast (Fig. 5.34). Staging CT showed lytic lesions in at least two lumbar vertebral bodies consistent with metastases in this young patient (Fig. 5.33). Genetic testing was negative for pathogenic mutations. The patient underwent NST with ACT. Despite post-NST US and MRI findings consistent with a complete imaging response (Figs. 5.34, 5.35, and 5.36), residual disease was identified following two site radioactive seed localized (RSL) segmental mastectomy (SM) (Fig. 5.37). Due to this and the extent of residual calcifications, TM was ultimately performed. This case illustrates the challenge in interpreting the significance of residual calcifications following NST. The lack of MRI enhancement was a false negative in this case as surgical pathology showed residual disease, ultimately requiring TM.

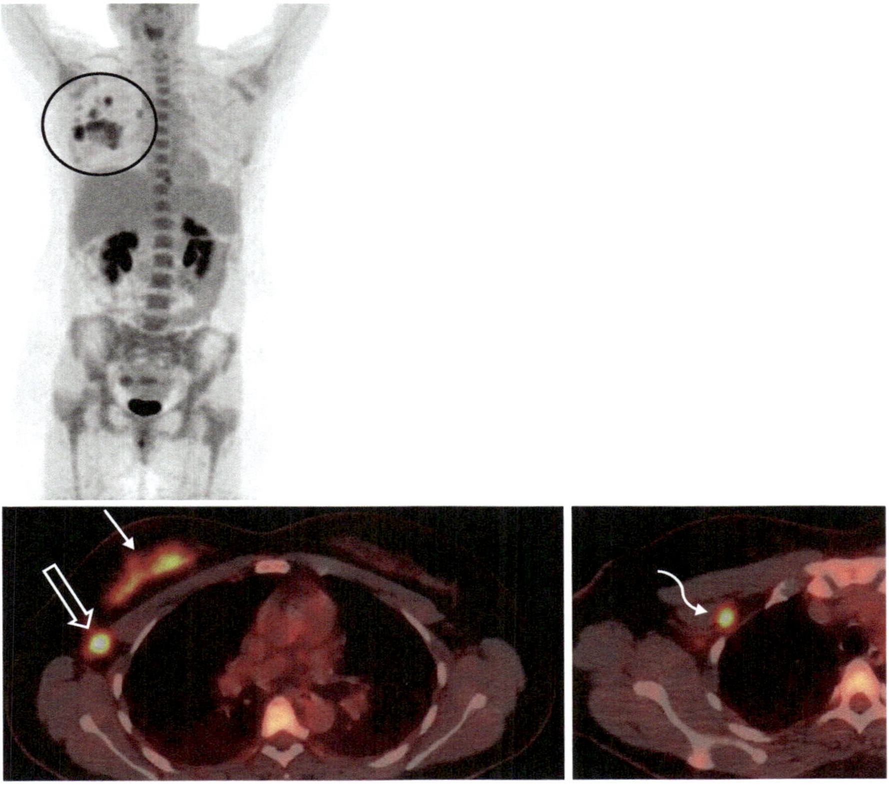

Fig. 5.22 Coronal MIP (top) and axial fused PET/CT images (bottom right and left). Increased FDG radiotracer update corresponding to right breast malignancy (arrow, max SUV 6.6) and multiple abnormal right axillary level 1 (open arrow) and level 2 (curved arrow) lymph nodes (max SUV 7.3). No distant disease was identified

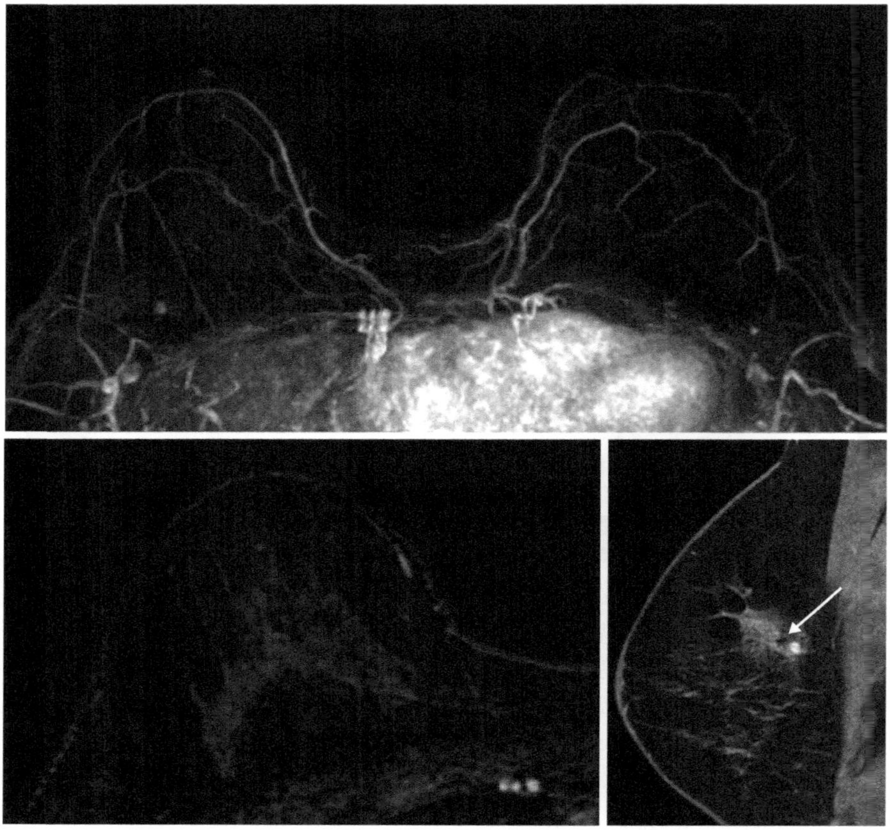

Fig. 5.23 MRI following NST demonstrates a complete imaging response on axial MIP (top) and axial T1 post-contrast subtraction (bottom left) and sagittal T1 post-contrast fat saturation images (bottom, right). Biopsy clip susceptibility artifact (arrow) is again noted

Fig. 5.24 Grayscale US images of biopsy-proven right axillary LN following NST show decrease in size, consistent with therapeutic response (arrow). Central echogenic biopsy clip is noted (open arrow)

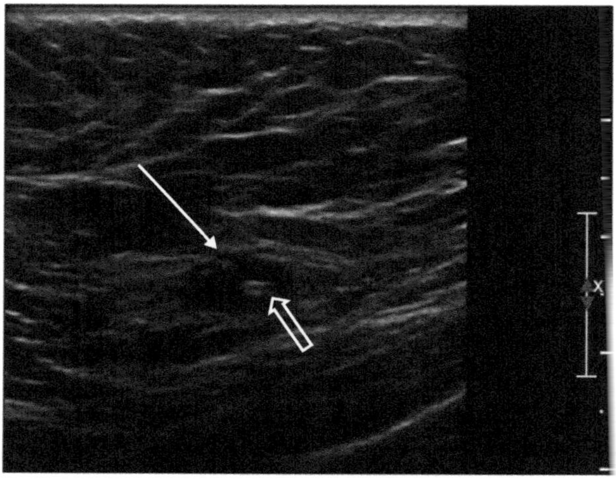

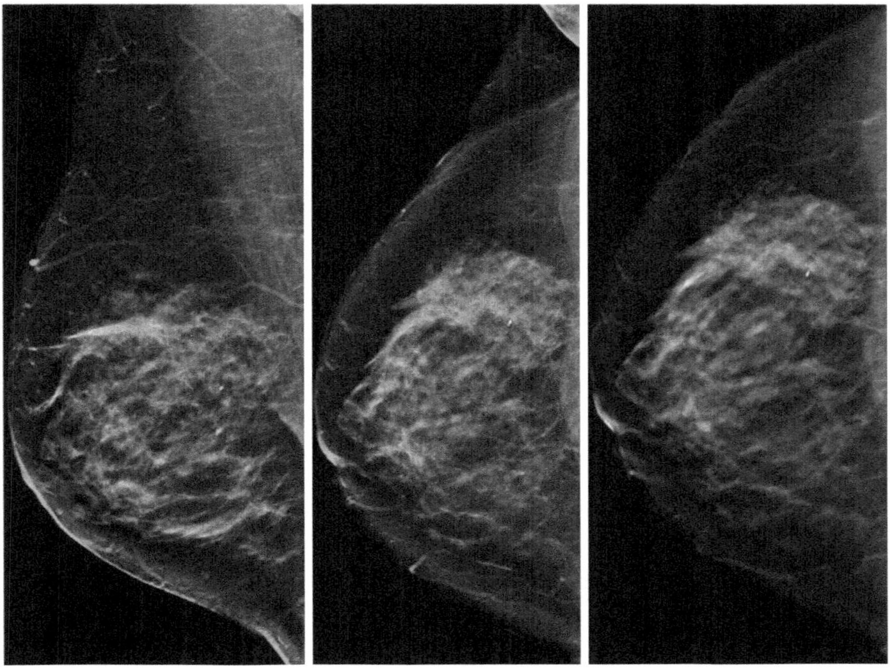

Fig. 5.25 MLO (left), CC (center), and tomosynthesis CC (right) views of the right breast. Heterogeneously dense breast tissue without a discrete abnormality

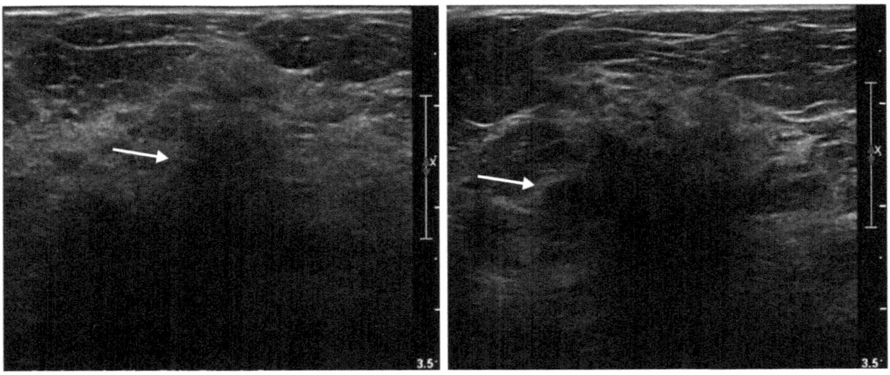

Fig. 5.26 Screening ultrasound performed as part of a research study and subsequent diagnostic ultrasound images show an ill-defined hypoechoic area (arrow) with shadowing. US CNB revealed ILC

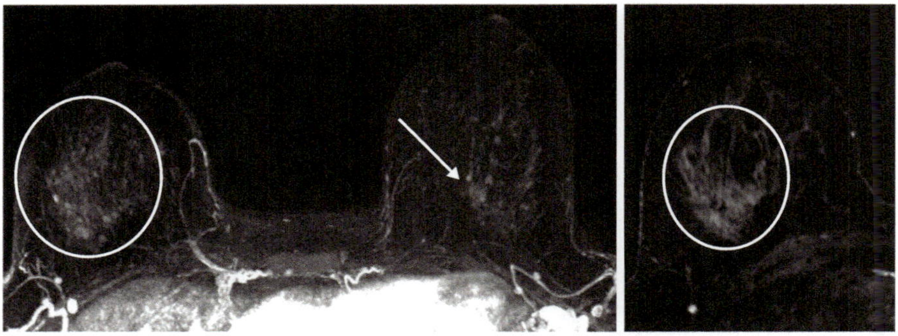

Fig. 5.27 Axial MIP (left) and axial post-contrast subtraction (right) MRI shows extensive disease in the right breast with asymmetric clumped NME in the upper outer right breast spanning 5 cm (circles), mammographically occult, and greater than the sonographic extent which was poorly defined. In the *left breast*, there is an enhancing mass and clumped NME (arrow), MRI guided core biopsy proven ILC

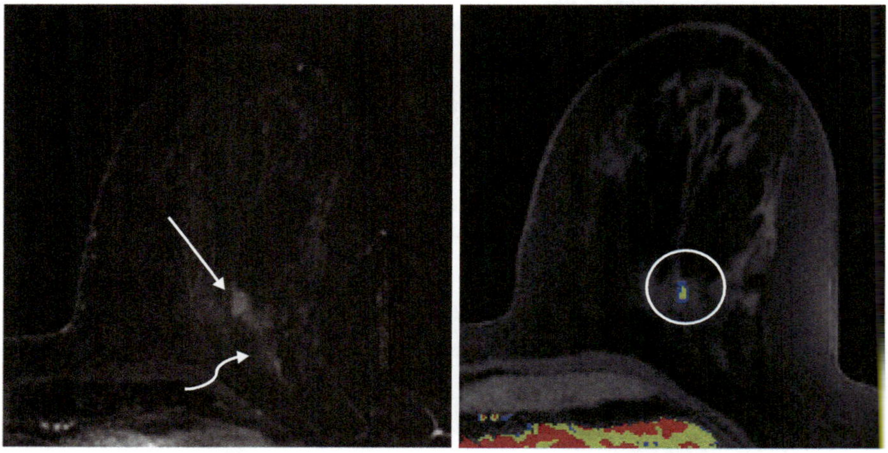

Fig. 5.28 Same patient. Axial T1 post-contrast subtraction (left) and axial T1 FS color overlay (right) of the *left breast*. Enhancing mass (arrow) with posterior clumped NME (curved arrow) demonstrating mixed persistent and plateau enhancement kinetics (circle). MRI-guided core biopsy revealed ILC (ER positive, PR weakly positive, HER2 equivocal, amplified by FISH) and DCIS)

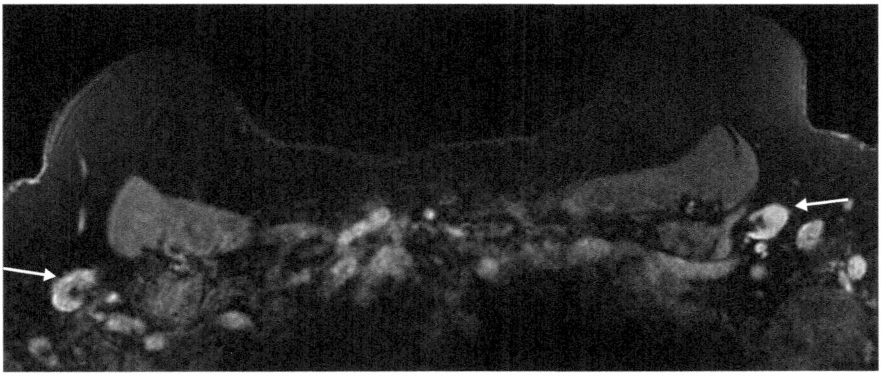

Fig. 5.29 Axial T1 FS post-contrast image. Bilateral level 1 axillary lymphadenopathy with cortical thickening (arrows). Subsequent bilateral axillary US and bilateral core biopsies revealed bilateral metastatic carcinoma

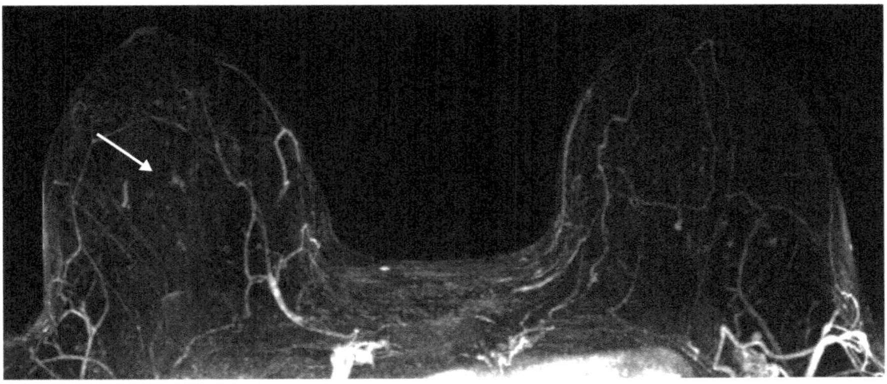

Fig. 5.30 Post-NST MIP MRI shows near complete resolution of abnormal enhancement in both breasts. Small residual enhancing focus in the right breast (arrow)

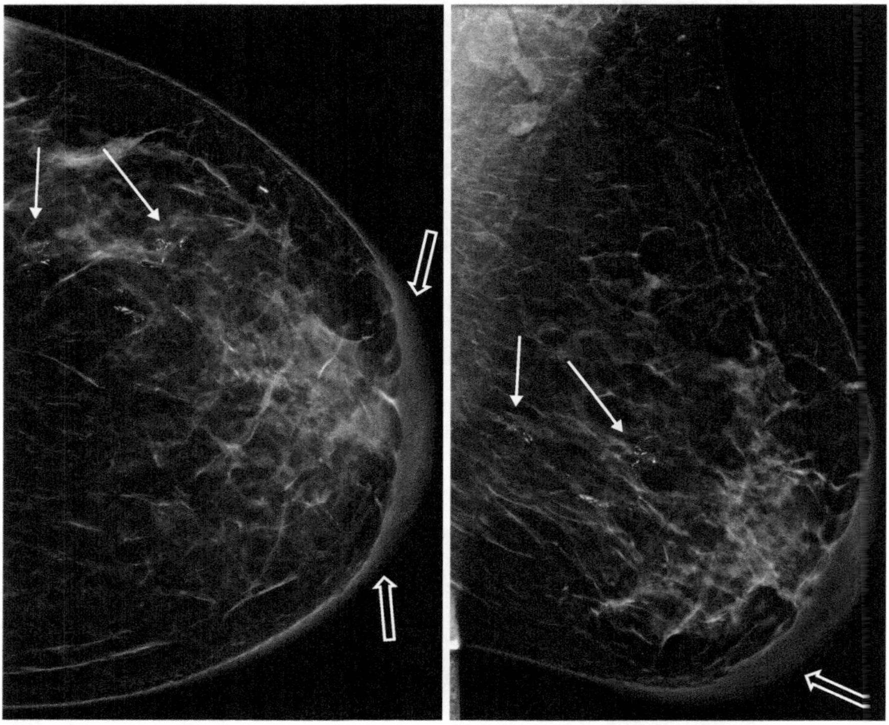

Fig. 5.31 CC (left) and MLO (right) mammographic views of the left breast. Heterogeneously dense breast tissue. Skin thickening (open arrow) and pleomorphic linear and segmental calcifications (arrows). Stereotactic biopsy of calcifications showed nuclear grade 2 IDC and nuclear grade 2 DCIS

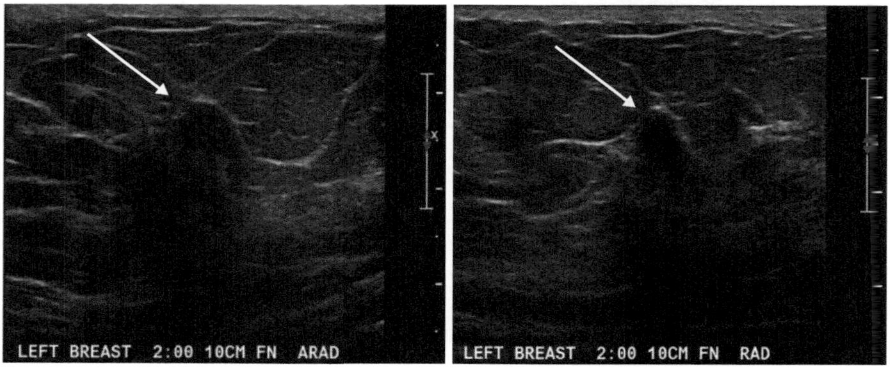

Fig. 5.32 Grayscale US. Round hypoechoic mass with indistinct margins (arrow) and posterior shadowing. US CNB revealed nuclear grade 2 IDC, ER/PR positive, HER2 negative

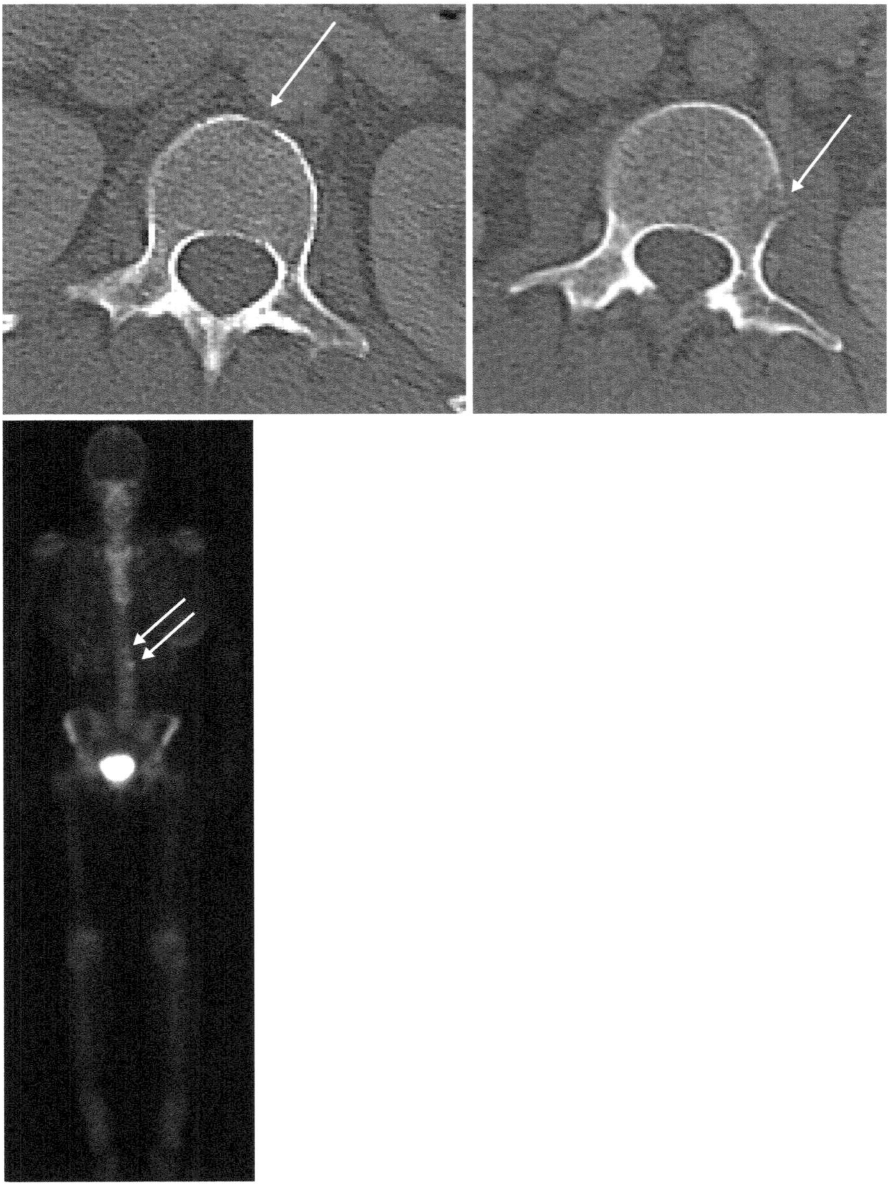

Fig. 5.33 Axial computed tomography (CT) images on bone window (top right and left) and 99-technetium-labeled methyl diphosphate (MDP) bone scan (bottom). CT demonstrates a lytic lesion in the anterior L1 and left lateral L2 vertebral bodies (arrows) with cortical disruption most consistent with metastases in this young patient. Bone scan confirms a corresponding focal abnormal radiotracer uptake at the L2 vertebral body (curved arrow)

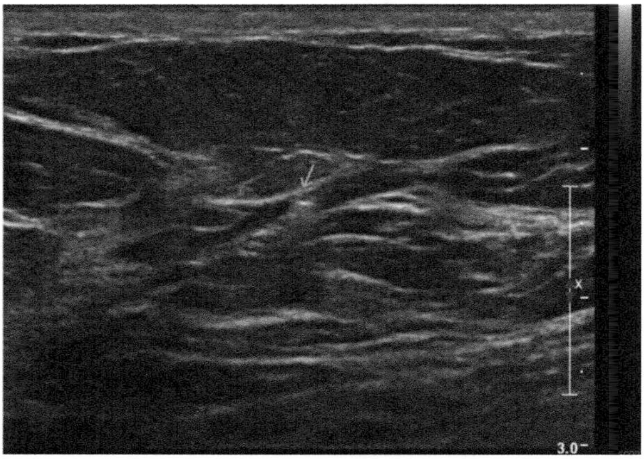

Fig. 5.34 Grayscale US following NST. Branching duct with internal heterogeneity and a central echogenic biopsy clip (arrow) corresponding to the site of proven IDC and ductal carcinoma in situ (DCIS)

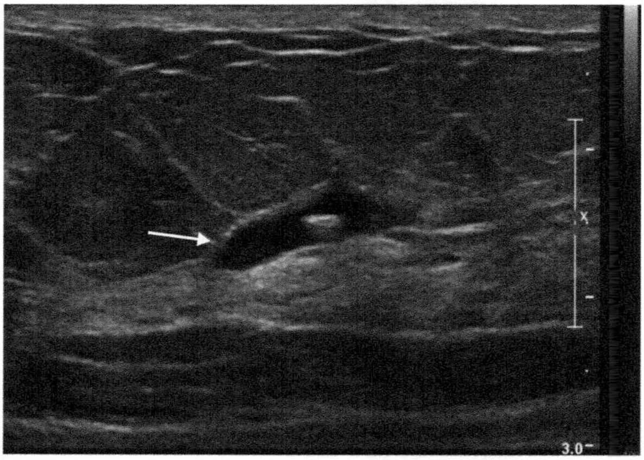

Fig. 5.35 Grayscale US following NST. Anechoic hydrophilic biopsy clip (arrow) without a residual mass identified at the site of proven IDC

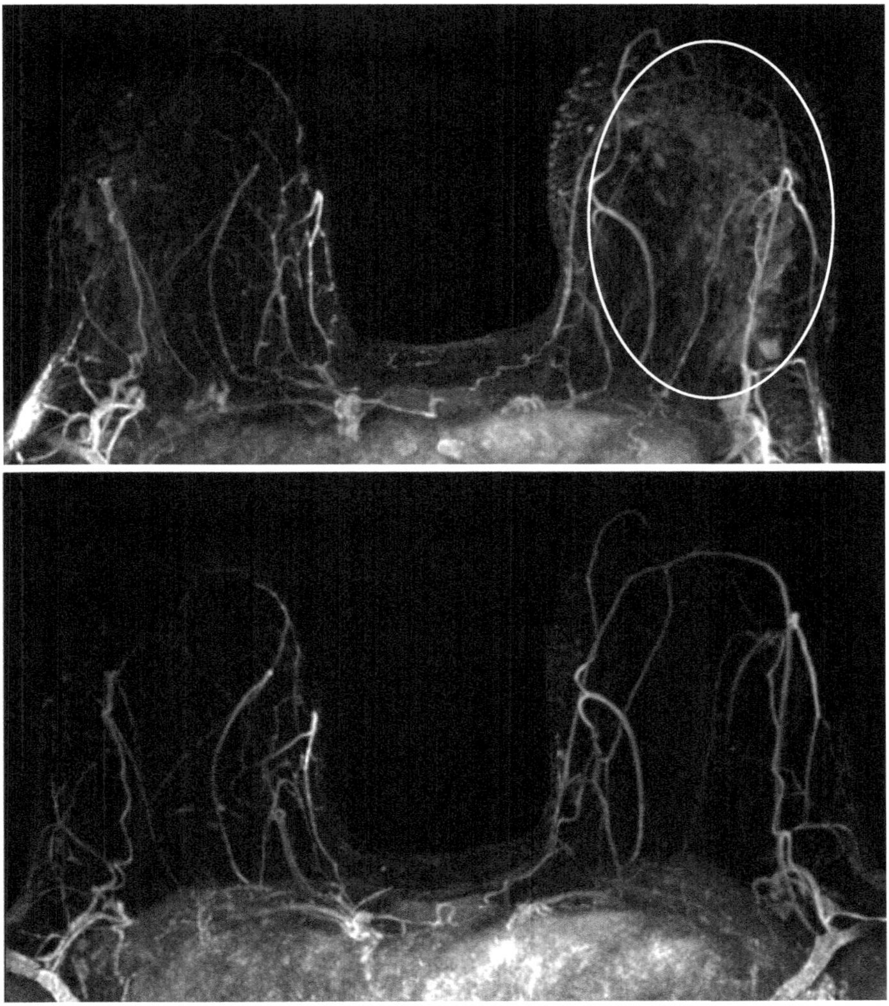

Fig. 5.36 Pre-NST (top) and post-NST (bottom) MRI axial MIP images. The pre-treatment MRI demonstrates extensive abnormal non-mass enhancement in the lateral left breast spanning up to 9.5 cm (circle). The post-treatment MRI demonstrates a complete imaging response. However, SM demonstrated residual IDC present as small clusters of tumor cells and residual DCIS. The patient ultimately underwent total mastectomy and delayed reconstruction

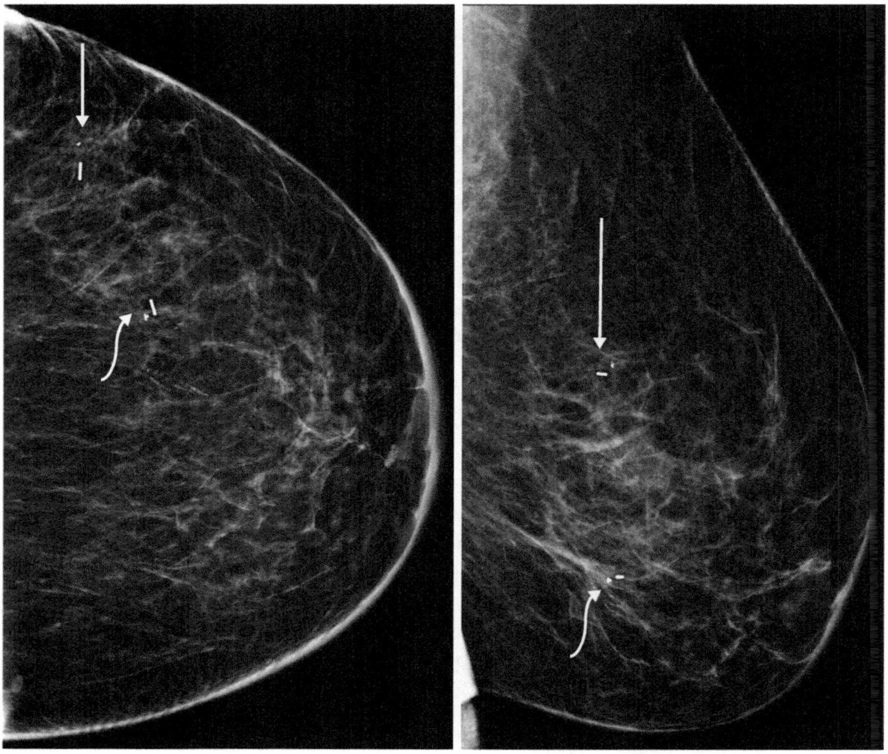

Fig. 5.37 Surgical localization. CC (left) and MLO (right) views following NST. Biopsy clips show corresponding placement of radioactive seeds in the upper outer (arrow) and lower outer (curved arrow) left breast at sites of proven malignancy for surgical guidance at the time of initial SM. Of note, left breast skin thickening has improved

References

1. Haque W, Verma V, Hatch S, Suzanne Klimberg V, Brian Butler E, Teh BS. Response rates and pathologic complete response by breast cancer molecular subtype following neoadjuvant chemotherapy. Breast Cancer Res Treat. 2018;170:559–67.
2. Cortazar P, Zhang L, Untch M, et al. Pathological complete response and long-term clinical benefit in breast cancer: the CTNeoBC pooled analysis. Lancet Lond Engl. 2014;384:164–72.
3. Slanetz PJ, Moy L, Baron P, et al. ACR appropriateness criteria ® monitoring response to neoadjuvant systemic therapy for breast cancer. J Am Coll Radiol. 2017;14:S462–75.
4. Dialani V, Chadashvili T, Slanetz PJ. Role of imaging in neoadjuvant therapy for breast cancer. Ann Surg Oncol. 2015;22:1416–24.
5. Fowler AM, Mankoff DA, Joe BN. Imaging neoadjuvant therapy response in breast cancer. Radiology. 2017;285:358–75.
6. Berg WA, Gutierrez L, NessAiver MS, Carter WB, Bhargavan M, Lewis RS, Ioffe OB. Diagnostic accuracy of mammography, clinical examination, US, and MR imaging in preoperative assessment of breast cancer. Radiology. 2004;233:830–49.

7. Chagpar AB, Middleton LP, Sahin AA, et al. Accuracy of physical examination, ultrasonography, and mammography in predicting residual pathologic tumor size in patients treated with neoadjuvant chemotherapy. Ann Surg. 2006;243:257–64.
8. Keune JD, Jeffe DB, Schootman M, Hoffman A, Gillanders WE, Aft RL. Accuracy of ultrasonography and mammography in predicting pathologic response after neoadjuvant chemotherapy for breast cancer. Am J Surg. 2010;199:477–84.
9. Helvie MA, Joynt LK, Cody RL, Pierce LJ, Adler DD, Merajver SD. Locally advanced breast carcinoma: accuracy of mammography versus clinical examination in the prediction of residual disease after chemotherapy. Radiology. 1996;198:327–32.
10. Huber S, Wagner M, Zuna I, Medl M, Czembirek H, Delorme S. Locally advanced breast carcinoma: evaluation of mammography in the prediction of residual disease after induction chemotherapy. Anticancer Res. 2000;20:553–8.
11. Skaane P, Bandos AI, Niklason LT, Sebuødegård S, Østerås BH, Gullien R, Gur D, Hofvind S. Digital mammography versus digital mammography plus Tomosynthesis in breast cancer screening: the Oslo Tomosynthesis Screening Trial. Radiology. 2019;291:23–30.
12. Weiss A, Lee KC, Romero Y, Ward E, Kim Y, Ojeda-Fournier H, Einck J, Blair SL. Calcifications on mammogram do not correlate with tumor size after neoadjuvant chemotherapy. Ann Surg Oncol. 2014;21:3310–6.
13. Felicano Y, Mamtani A, Morrow M, Stempel MM, Patil S, Jochelson MS. Do calcifications on mammography after neoadjuvant chemotherapy for breast cancer always need to be excised? Ann Surg Oncol. 2017;24:1492–8.
14. Henry-Tillman R, Glover-Collins K, Preston M, Gallagher K, Tummel E, Robertson YV, Ochoa D, Korourian S, Westbrook K, Klimberg VS. The SAVE review: sonographic analysis versus excision for axillary staging in breast cancer. J Am Coll Surg. 2015;220:560–7.
15. Balasubramanian I, Fleming CA, Corrigan MA, Redmond HP, Kerin MJ, Lowery AJ. Meta-analysis of the diagnostic accuracy of ultrasound-guided fine-needle aspiration and core needle biopsy in diagnosing axillary lymph node metastasis. BJS: Br J Surg. 2018;105:1244–53.
16. Khan A, Sabel MS, Nees A, Diehl KM, Cimmino VM, Kleer CG, Schott AF, Hayes DF, Chang AE, Newman LA. Comprehensive axillary evaluation in neoadjuvant chemotherapy patients with ultrasonography and sentinel lymph node biopsy. Ann Surg Oncol. 2005;12:697–704.
17. Bedrosian I, Bedi D, Kuerer HM, et al. Impact of clinicopathological factors on sensitivity of axillary ultrasonography in the detection of axillary nodal metastases in patients with breast cancer. Ann Surg Oncol. 2003;10:1025–30.
18. Moorman AM, Bourez RLJH, de Leeuw DM, Kouwenhoven EA. Pre-operative ultrasonographic evaluation of axillary lymph nodes in breast cancer patients: for which group still of additional value and in which group cause for special attention? Ultrasound Med Biol. 2015;41:2842–8.
19. Boughey JC, Ballman KV, Le-Petross HT, McCall LM, Mittendorf EA, Ahrendt GM, Wilke LG, Taback B, Feliberti EC, Hunt KK. Identification and resection of the clipped node decreases the false negative rate of sentinel lymph node surgery in patients presenting with node positive breast cancer (T0-T4, N1-2) who receive neoadjuvant chemotherapy – results from ACOSOG Z1071 (Alliance). Ann Surg. 2016;263:802–7.
20. Eisenhauer EA, Therasse P, Bogaerts J, et al. New response evaluation criteria in solid tumours: revised RECIST guideline (version 1.1). Eur J Cancer Oxf Engl 1990. 2009;45:228–47.
21. Hollingsworth AB, Stough RG, O'Dell CA, Brekke CE. Breast magnetic resonance imaging for preoperative locoregional staging. Am J Surg. 2008;196:389–97.
22. Lehman CD, Gatsonis C, Kuhl CK, et al. MRI evaluation of the contralateral breast in women with recently diagnosed breast cancer. N Engl J Med. 2007;356:1295–303.
23. Ko ES, Han B-K, Kim RB, et al. Analysis of factors that influence the accuracy of magnetic resonance imaging for predicting response after neoadjuvant chemotherapy in locally advanced breast cancer. Ann Surg Oncol. 2013;20:2562–8.
24. Jun W, Cong W, Xianxin X, Daqing J. Meta-analysis of quantitative dynamic contrast-enhanced MRI for the assessment of neoadjuvant chemotherapy in breast cancer. Am Surg. 2019;85:645–53.

25. Yeh ED, Slanetz PJ, Edmister WB, Talele A, Monticciolo D, Kopans DB. Invasive lobular carcinoma: spectrum of enhancement and morphology on magnetic resonance imaging. Breast J. 2003;9:13–8.
26. Bouzón A, Acea B, Soler R, Iglesias Á, Santiago P, Mosquera J, Calvo L, Seoane-Pillado T, García A. Diagnostic accuracy of MRI to evaluate tumour response and residual tumour size after neoadjuvant chemotherapy in breast cancer patients. Radiol Oncol. 2016;50:73–9.
27. McGuire KP, Toro-Burguete J, Dang H, Young J, Soran A, Zuley M, Bhargava R, Bonaventura M, Johnson R, Ahrendt G. MRI staging after neoadjuvant chemotherapy for breast cancer: does tumor biology affect accuracy? Ann Surg Oncol. 2011;18:3149–54.
28. Henderson SA, Muhammad Gowdh N, Purdie CA, Jordan LB, Evans A, Brunton T, Thompson AM, Vinnicombe S. Breast cancer: influence of tumour volume estimation method at MRI on prediction of pathological response to neoadjuvant chemotherapy. Br J Radiol. 2018; https://doi.org/10.1259/bjr.20180123.
29. Hylton NM, Blume JD, Bernreuter WK, et al. Locally advanced breast cancer: MR imaging for prediction of response to neoadjuvant chemotherapy—results from ACRIN 6657/I-SPY trial. Radiology. 2012;263:663–72.
30. Partridge SC, Gibbs JE, Lu Y, Esserman LJ, Tripathy D, Wolverton DS, Rugo HS, Hwang ES, Ewing CA, Hylton NM. MRI measurements of breast tumor volume predict response to neoadjuvant chemotherapy and recurrence-free survival. Am J Roentgenol. 2005;184:1774–81.
31. Scheel JR, Kim E, Partridge SC, et al. MRI, clinical examination, and mammography for preoperative assessment of residual disease and pathologic complete response after neoadjuvant chemotherapy for breast cancer: ACRIN 6657 trial. Am J Roentgenol. 2018;210:1376–85.
32. Chae EY, Cha JH, Kim HH, Shin HJ, Kim H, Lee J, Cheung JY. Evaluation of residual disease using breast MRI after excisional biopsy for breast cancer. Am J Roentgenol. 2013;200:1167–73.
33. Frei KA, Kinkel K, Bonel HM, Lu Y, Esserman LJ, Hylton NM. MR imaging of the breast in patients with positive margins after lumpectomy. Am J Roentgenol. 2000;175:1577–84.
34. Giuliano AE, Ballman KV, McCall L, et al. Effect of axillary dissection vs no axillary dissection on 10-year overall survival among women with invasive breast cancer and sentinel node metastasis: the ACOSOG Z0011 (Alliance) randomized clinical trial. JAMA. 2017;318:918.
35. Hyun SJ, Kim E-K, Moon HJ, Yoon JH, Kim MJ. Preoperative axillary lymph node evaluation in breast cancer patients by breast magnetic resonance imaging (MRI): can breast MRI exclude advanced nodal disease? Eur Radiol. 2016;26:3865–73.
36. Greenwood HI, Wilmes LJ, Kelil T, Joe BN. Role of breast MRI in the evaluation and detection of DCIS: opportunities and challenges. J Magn Reson Imaging: JMRI. 2020;52:697–709.
37. Kim HJ, Im Y-H, Kim HJ, et al. Accuracy of MRI for estimating residual tumor size after neoadjuvant chemotherapy in locally advanced breast cancer: relation to response patterns on MRI. Acta Oncol. 2007;46:996–1003.
38. Kamal RM, Helal MH, Mansour SM, Haggag MA, Nada OM, Farahat IG, Alieldin NH. Can we apply the MRI BI-RADS lexicon morphology descriptors on contrast-enhanced spectral mammography? Br J Radiol. 2016;89:20160157.
39. Travieso-Aja MM, Maldonado-Saluzzi D, Naranjo-Santana P, Fernández-Ruiz C, Severino-Rondón W, Rodríguez Rodríguez M, Luzardo OP. Evaluation of the applicability of BI-RADS® MRI for the interpretation of contrast-enhanced digital mammography. Radiol Engl Ed. 2019;61:477–88.
40. Contrast-enhanced spectral mammography versus MRI: initial results in the detection of breast cancer and assessment of tumour size | SpringerLink. https://link.springer.com/article/10.1007%2Fs00330-013-3007-7. Accessed 19 Dec 2020.
41. Jochelson MS, Dershaw DD, Sung JS, Heerdt AS, Thornton C, Moskowitz CS, Ferrara J, Morris EA. Bilateral contrast-enhanced dual-energy digital mammography: feasibility and comparison with conventional digital mammography and MR imaging in women with known breast carcinoma. Radiology. 2013;266:743–51.
42. Chou C-P, Lewin JM, Chiang C-L, Hung B-H, Yang T-L, Huang J-S, Liao J-B, Pan H-B. Clinical evaluation of contrast-enhanced digital mammography and contrast enhanced tomosynthesis—comparison to contrast-enhanced breast MRI. Eur J Radiol. 2015;84:2501–8.

43. Patel BK, Hilal T, Covington M, Zhang N, Kosiorek HE, Lobbes M, Northfelt DW, Pockaj BA. Contrast-enhanced spectral mammography is comparable to MRI in the assessment of residual breast cancer following neoadjuvant systemic therapy. Ann Surg Oncol. 2018;25:1350–6.
44. Iotti V, Ravaioli S, Vacondio R, et al. Contrast-enhanced spectral mammography in neoadjuvant chemotherapy monitoring: a comparison with breast magnetic resonance imaging. Breast Cancer Res: BCR. 2017;19:106.
45. Barra FR, Sobrinho AB, Barra RR, Magalhães MT, Aguiar LR, de Albuquerque GFL, Costa RP, Farage L, Pratesi R. Contrast-enhanced mammography (CEM) for detecting residual disease after neoadjuvant chemotherapy: a comparison with breast magnetic resonance imaging (MRI). Biomed Res Int. 2018;2018:8531916.
46. NCCN imaging appropriate use criteria. https://www.nccn.org/professionals/imaging/default.aspx. Accessed 21 Dec 2020.
47. Groheux D, Espié M, Giacchetti S, Hindié E. Performance of FDG PET/CT in the clinical management of breast cancer. Radiology. 2013;266:388–405.
48. Koolen BB, Vrancken Peeters M-JTFD, Aukema TS, et al. 18F-FDG PET/CT as a staging procedure in primary stage II and III breast cancer: comparison with conventional imaging techniques. Breast Cancer Res Treat. 2012;131:117–26.
49. Wang Y, Zhang C, Liu J, Huang G. Is 18F-FDG PET accurate to predict neoadjuvant therapy response in breast cancer? A meta-analysis. Breast Cancer Res Treat. 2012;131:357–69.
50. Broos WAM, van der Zant FM, Wondergem M, Knol RJJ. Accuracy of 18F-NaF PET/CT in bone metastasis detection and its effect on patient management in patients with breast carcinoma. Nucl Med Commun. 2018;39:325–33.
51. Hamaoka T, Madewell JE, Podoloff DA, Hortobagyi GN, Ueno NT. Bone imaging in metastatic breast cancer. J Clin Oncol. 2004;22:2942–53.
52. Berg WA, Madsen KS, Schilling K, Tartar M, Pisano ED, Larsen LH, Narayanan D, Ozonoff A, Miller JP, Kalinyak JE. Breast cancer: comparative effectiveness of positron emission mammography and MR imaging in presurgical planning for the ipsilateral breast. Radiology. 2011;258:59–72.
53. Brem RF, Petrovitch I, Rapelyea JA, Young H, Teal C, Kelly T. Breast-specific gamma imaging with 99mTc-Sestamibi and magnetic resonance imaging in the diagnosis of breast cancer--a comparative study. Breast J. 2007;13:465–9.
54. Kim JS, Lee SM, Cha ES. The diagnostic sensitivity of dynamic contrast-enhanced magnetic resonance imaging and breast-specific gamma imaging in women with calcified and non-calcified DCIS. Acta Radiol Stockh Swed 1987. 2014;55:668–75.
55. Zhou M, Johnson N, Gruner S, Ecklund GW, Meunier P, Bryn S, Glissmeyer M, Steinbock K. Clinical utility of breast-specific gamma imaging for evaluating disease extent in the newly diagnosed breast cancer patient. Am J Surg. 2009;197:159–63.
56. Sumkin JH, Berg WA, Carter GJ, et al. Diagnostic performance of MRI, molecular breast imaging, and contrast-enhanced mammography in women with newly diagnosed breast cancer. Radiology. 2019;293:531–40.
57. Kim S, Plemmons J, Hoang K, Chaudhuri D, Kelley A, Cunningham T, Hoefer R. Breast-specific gamma imaging versus MRI: comparing the diagnostic performance in assessing treatment response after neoadjuvant chemotherapy in patients with breast cancer. Am J Roentgenol. 2019;212:696–705.
58. Urbano N, Scimeca M, Tancredi V, Bonanno E, Schillaci O. 99mTC-sestamibi breast imaging: current status, new ideas and future perspectives. Semin Cancer Biol. 2020; https://doi.org/10.1016/j.semcancer.2020.01.007.
59. Santos JFDL, Cantor A, Amos KD, et al. Magnetic resonance imaging as a predictor of pathologic response in patients treated with neoadjuvant systemic treatment for operable breast cancer. Cancer. 2013;119:1776–83.

Part III
Neoadjuvant Systemic Therapy

Chapter 6
Neoadjuvant Systemic Therapy for Breast Cancer Based on Underlying Tumor Biology

William M. Sikov

Introduction

Neoadjuvant therapy is defined as systemic therapy administered to patients with non-metastatic cancer prior to definitive surgical therapy. In the treatment of breast cancer, this has typically been chemotherapy, though other types of treatment, including endocrine therapies in patients with hormone receptor-positive/HER2-negative breast cancer (HR+/HER2-BC) and HER2-targeted therapies, in patients with HER2-positive breast cancer (HER2+BC), are also employed in this setting, and there is ongoing interest in assessing other types of treatment, including molecularly targeted agents and immunotherapy, in this setting. While rapidly evolving, this chapter will review current "Neoadjuvant systemic therapy for breast cancer based on underlying tumor biology."

While neoadjuvant therapy was originally administered only to patients with locally advanced cancers who were not candidates for primary surgery, the effectiveness of this treatment at inducing both clinical and pathologic responses, particularly in patients with more aggressive breast cancers, led to it being investigated in patients with less extensive disease, and its role has expanded rapidly over the past 20 years. Current indications for consideration of neoadjuvant therapy include the following:

- Patients with locally advanced/unresectable cancers, including inflammatory carcinomas (T4d).
- Patients who desire breast-conserving surgery (BCS) but are not candidates for this at diagnosis or are likely to have a suboptimal cosmetic outcome due to the size and/or location of the breast mass.

W. M. Sikov (✉)
Breast Health Center, Program in Women's Oncology, Women and Infants Hospital of Rhode Island and Warren Alpert Medical School of Brown University, Providence, RI, USA
e-mail: wsikov@wihri.org

A. Soran, F. Nakhlis (eds.), *Management of the Breast and Axilla in the Neoadjuvant Setting*, https://doi.org/10.1007/978-3-030-88020-0_6

- Patients with limited axillary lymph node involvement (clinical N1, cN1) in whom axillary lymph node dissection (ALND) would be the standard of care if they underwent primary surgery but might be candidates for more limited axillary sampling such as sentinel lymph node biopsy (SLNB) if they become clinically (ycN0) and pathologically (ypN0) node-negative following neoadjuvant therapy.
- Patients in whom surgery must be delayed for any reason, such as resolution of an intercurrent medical condition, including pregnancy.
- Patients with triple-negative breast cancer (TNBC) or HER2+BC in whom response to neoadjuvant therapy would impact the decision as to whether to administer adjuvant capecitabine (in TNBC) or ado-trastuzumab emtansine (in HER2+BC).
- Another potential role for neoadjuvant therapy is to identify patients in whom adjuvant treatment can be deescalated following documentation of response. Examples of this include patients with HR+/HER2-BC who receive neoadjuvant endocrine therapy in whom adjuvant chemotherapy might be omitted based on their response to that treatment and the recently initiated CompassHER-pCR trial (EA1181) on which patients with clinical stage II–III HER2+BC who achieve a pathologic complete response (pCR) with weekly paclitaxel, trastuzumab, and pertuzumab avoid more aggressive chemotherapy.

The primary goal of systemic therapy in patients with non-metastatic breast cancer, whether administered prior to or after surgery, is to reduce the risk of distant recurrence and death caused by their cancer. Initially, there were concerns that delaying surgery to administer neoadjuvant therapy might allow the cancer to spread. Conversely, some argued that starting systemic therapy without the delay necessitated by surgery could reduce the risk of distant recurrence and death. However, several randomized studies, including NSABP B-18, demonstrated equivalent rates of distant recurrence and death whether the same chemotherapy was administered before or after surgery [1–5]. A meta-analysis of ten trials involving 4756 patients that compared pre- vs. postoperative chemotherapy demonstrated no significant differences in risks of distant recurrence and breast cancer mortality between neoadjuvant and adjuvant chemotherapy [6]. Patients receiving neoadjuvant chemotherapy (NACT) were more likely to undergo BCS (65% vs. 49%), and while this was associated with a higher rate of local recurrences at 15 years (2_% vs. 16%), it did not adversely impact the risk of distant recurrence or death.

Not only does neoadjuvant therapy have clinical utility in a variety of settings, but it is also increasingly employed in clinical trials to assess the efficacy of novel agents and regimens. In 2014 the US Food and Drug Administration (FDA) issued guidance that encouraged the pharmaceutical industry to apply for accelerated approval of a new drug if its use was associated with a significant increase in pCRs (usually defined as the absence of residual invasive disease in the breast and any sampled ipsilateral axillary lymph nodes, but permitting the presence of residual ductal carcinoma in situ, which does not appear to increase the risk of distant disease recurrence, designated ypT0/isN0), especially in HER2+BC or TNBC, with full approval contingent upon subsequent demonstration of improvement in long-term outcomes, such as disease-free survival (DFS) and/or overall survival (OS). This was based in part on a meta-analysis performed at their request which confirmed the correlation between achievement of pCR and substantial reductions in the risks of distant disease recurrence and breast cancer mortality, particularly in those more aggressive breast cancer subtypes [7]. The hope was that this guidance would encourage the more rapid development and approval of life-saving treatments than possible with adjuvant trials, which typically require much larger numbers of patients and longer follow-up to demonstrate superiority of an investigational approach over the control regimen. In addition, administering treatment in the neoadjuvant setting allows researchers to monitor clinical response on serial physical examinations and imaging studies and to obtain tumor tissue and blood samples before, during, and, in patients who do not achieve pCR, after treatment, to try to identify biologic markers of response or resistance.

Neoadjuvant Treatment Options

As neoadjuvant treatment options differ by breast cancer subtype, treatment in HR+/HER2-BC, HER2+BC, and TNBC will be addressed separately.

Neoadjuvant Therapy in Hormone Receptor-Positive/HER2-Negative Breast Cancer (HR+/HER2-BC)

About 2/3 of breast cancers diagnosed in the United States are hormone receptor-positive and HER2-negative, but the biology of these cancers varies greatly, dictating a variety of approaches to treatment in the neoadjuvant, as well as the adjuvant, setting. Many HR+/HER2-BC are relatively indolent, with a low fraction of actively dividing cells, making them much less sensitive to cytotoxic therapies. In the meta-analysis conducted by Cortazar and colleagues, only 7.5% of patients with low- or intermediate-grade HR+/HER2-BC achieved a pCR with NACT, and while patients who achieved a pCR had a very good prognosis, it was not significantly better than for patients in this subgroup found to have residual disease at surgery [7]. In comparison, patients with high-grade HR+/HER2-BC had a slightly higher pCR rate with NACT (16.2%), and in these patients achievement of pCR was associated with a highly significant reduction in risk of recurrence.

For lower-risk HR+/HER2-BC patients, an alternative to NACT may be neoadjuvant endocrine therapy (NET). While NET is no more likely than NACT to induce a pCR in the breast or clear axillary nodes, in appropriately selected patients it appears to be as likely to induce a clinical response and improve the patient's chances of successful BCS, and it is associated with many fewer side effects than chemotherapy [8]. Selecting appropriate patients for NET involves determining whether their tumor biology suggests a potential benefit from this treatment, but basing this assessment on factors such as receptor status and tumor grade is inaccurate, especially given the frequency of disagreement on tumor grade between pathologists. A preferable approach is to submit the patient's diagnostic biopsy for gene expression analysis, such as the Oncotype Dx assay. Not only are patients with low and intermediate Oncotype Dx Recurrence Scores unlikely to demonstrate a major clinical or pathologic response to NACT [9–11], randomized trials in the adjuvant setting fail to demonstrate improvements in invasive recurrence-free survival with the addition of chemotherapy to endocrine therapy in node-negative (TAILORx) [12] or limited (1–3) node-positive (RxPONDER) [13] patients. Thus, NACT should be administered to patients with locally advanced (clinical T4 or N2) cancers or those with less extensive disease but a high-risk Oncotype score (>26) who would typically receive adjuvant chemotherapy following primary surgery.

When selecting a NACT regimen for appropriate HR+/HER2-BC patients, it is appropriate to administer treatment similar to what the patient would receive in the adjuvant setting. In patients with more extensive disease, this typically involves sequential administration of an anthracycline-based regimen, usually four cycles of doxorubicin or epirubicin with cyclophosphamide (AC/EC), given either every 2 or 3 weeks (as the superiority of "dose-dense" or every 2-week treatments has been demonstrated only for more aggressive breast cancer subtypes [14], the treatment schedule can be chosen based on balancing a reduction in the overall duration of treatment versus giving the patient more time to recover between treatments) and a taxane, either weekly (×twelve cycles) or every 2-week (×four cycles) paclitaxel or every 3-week (×four cycles) docetaxel. While data suggest slightly higher response rates and fewer subsequent chemotherapy dose reductions when the taxane component is administered first, presumably due to less hematopoietic stem cell toxicity with the taxane than with the anthracycline/alkylating agent combination, either sequence is acceptable. In patients with clinically negative nodes or limited (≤3) nodal involvement, but in whom chemotherapy is indicated by gene expression analysis, the combination of docetaxel and cyclophosphamide (every 3 weeks × four to six cycles) should be considered, given that addition of an anthracycline failed to demonstrate significant improvement in DFS in the adjuvant setting in these subsets of HR+/HER2-BC patients in the Anthracyclines in Early Breast Cancer (ABC) combined analysis [15].

In postmenopausal patients for whom NET is appropriate, studies have demonstrated higher response rate for aromatase inhibitors than for tamoxifen [8, 16]. To achieve this same advantage, premenopausal patients should receive an aromatase inhibitor concurrent with ovarian function suppression, typically with a long-acting LHRH analog such as goserelin or leuprolide. A study comparing the available aromatase inhibitors – anastrozole, letrozole, and exemestane – failed to demonstrate any differences in clinical or pathologic response rates between these agents [17]. In the absence of evidence of disease progression on NET, which is rare in appropriately selected patients, this treatment should continue for at least 6 months, as both clinical and pathologic response improve with longer durations of treatment [18], and longer treatment in the preoperative setting will be offset by a shorter duration of this treatment after surgery. Assessing the tumor cell proliferative (Ki-67) rate on biopsies obtained after 2–4 weeks on NET has been studied [17, 19]; while failure of NET to suppress proliferation may identify patients less likely to respond to this treatment, the clinical utility of such measurements (i.e., improved responses with alternative treatment such as chemotherapy) has not been demonstrated, and thus this remains a research tool and not routinely performed outside of a clinical trial.

At this point in time, there is no evidence that administering agents other than an aromatase inhibitor (along with ovarian function suppression in premenopausal women) significantly enhances response to NET. These include using fulvestrant in place of or in combination with anastrozole [20], adding tamoxifen to anastrozole [21], or adding a targeted agent, such as gefitinib or everolimus [8]. Given their activity in combination with endocrine therapies in the metastatic setting, ongoing trials evaluate the addition of cdk 4/6 inhibitors and PIK3CA inhibitors to NET.

Given the rarity of achievement of a pCR with NET, evaluation of a patient's response to this treatment, and the implications of this response on subsequent treatment, may be important. To address this, Ellis and colleagues developed the Preoperative Endocrine Prognostic Index (PEPI), which combines assessment of residual disease in the breast and axillary nodes (ypTN) with estrogen receptor expression after exposure to NET and measurement of tumor cell proliferation (Ki-67) in the surgical specimen [22, 23]. Their analysis suggests that patients with PEPI scores of 0 have an excellent prognosis without subsequent chemotherapy, while patients with higher scores (PEPI >0) might benefit from receiving adjuvant chemotherapy. While this may be a useful adjunct to assessing response to NET, it is also reasonable to make decisions about adjuvant chemotherapy based on more established criteria, including stage and, in N0-1 patients, Oncotype Dx Recurrence Score performed on their pretreatment tumor sample.

Neoadjuvant Therapy in HER2-Positive Breast Cancer (HER2+BC)

While the role of the human epidermal growth factor receptor 2 (HER2) in normal human physiology has yet to be determined, it has been demonstrated that activation of the intracellular tyrosine kinase domain of the receptor initiates a signal transduction cascade that results in enhanced transcription of genes that increase cell proliferation, invasiveness, angiogenesis, and resistance to apoptotic signals. In 15–20% of breast cancers, amplification and/or overexpression of the HER2-*neu* gene on chromosome 17 leads to an overabundance of this transmembrane receptor. The etiology of this somatic mutation is unknown, but the excess of HER2 promotes formation of HER2 homodimers that induce constitutive activation of those pathways, which is reflected in the aggressive biology of these cancers. Blocking activation of these pathways not only reduces tumor cell proliferation, but also restores sensitivity to agents that induce apoptosis, such as chemotherapy drugs. Hormone receptor-negative/HER2+ cancers (HR-/HER2+BC, which account for 40–45% of HER2+BC) exhibit, on average, higher levels of HER2 overexpression, higher rates of proliferation, and greater sensitivity to treatments that disrupt HER2-activated signaling than in hormone receptor-positive/HER2+ cancers (HR+/HER2+BC). After demonstrating synergistic cytotoxicity in HER2+BC cell lines between a variety of chemotherapeutic agents and trastuzumab, a monoclonal antibody that binds to an extracellular epitope on HER2 and blocks the conformational change induced by HER2 homodimerization which activates the receptor's tyrosine kinase moiety, randomized trials demonstrated that the addition of trastuzumab to chemotherapy enhances response and improves survival in patients with metastatic HER2+BC and markedly reduces the risk of distant recurrence and improves survival in patient with early-stage HER2+BC [24, 25].

In the neoadjuvant setting, the addition of trastuzumab to NACT markedly increases achievement of pCR in HER2+BC and, since HER2+BC patients who achieve pCR are much less likely to recur, significantly improves DFS and OS [7, 26–28]. In a 2016 meta-analysis of 36 neoadjuvant trials that enrolled nearly 5800 HER2+BC patients, those achieving pCR (ypT0/isN0) had a 63% reduction in events and a 66% reduction in deaths from any cause compared to patients with residual invasive disease, with an even greater reduction in events (71%) seen in the HR-/HER2+BC subgroup [29]. In patients who fail to achieve a pCR, the extent of residual invasive disease, as measured by Residual Cancer Burden (RCB), which was developed by Symmans and colleagues at the MD Anderson Cancer Center, which stratifies patients by the extent of residual disease in the breast and axillary nodes, has been shown to be predictive of 5- and 10-year relapse-free survival [30]. This may be particularly useful in deciding which patients might benefit from administration of adjuvant ado-trastuzumab emtansine (T-DM1) based on results from the KATHERINE trial [31] (discussed below).

While some HER2+BC patients can achieve pCR with HER2-targeted therapy (with the addition of endocrine therapy in those with HR+/HER2+BC cancers) alone (discussed below), in patients who have no contraindication to receiving NACT, the current standard of care is administration of a combination of NACT and HER2-targeted therapy. Efforts to increase pCR rates and/or reduce toxicity associated with NACT plus trastuzumab have focused on enhancing HER2 blockade and exploring alternative chemotherapy regimens. These approaches are discussed below.

HER2-Targeted Therapies

In the phase II NOAH trial, the addition of every 3-week trastuzumab to anthracycline- and taxane-based neoadjuvant chemotherapy significantly increased the pCR rate (38% vs. 19% with chemotherapy alone) and 5-year EFS (58% vs. 43%) [32, 33]. Even among patients who achieved pCR, those who had received trastuzumab had significantly improved EFS compared to those who had not, indicating the superiority of this regimen at eradicating occult metastatic disease as well as overt disease in the breast and axilla [33]. A subsequent meta-analysis confirmed the value of the addition of trastuzumab to NACT on both pCR rates and long-term outcomes, consistent with improvements seen with the addition of trastuzumab to chemotherapy in the adjuvant setting [7].

Lapatinib is a small molecule inhibitor of the tyrosine kinase domain of HER2, and the addition of this agent demonstrated substantial activity in patients with metastatic HER2+BC who had progressed on a trastuzumab-containing regimen, suggesting the appearance or selection of a subclone of malignant cells that exploits alternative pathways to activating the HER2 tyrosine kinase. In several randomized studies, the addition of lapatinib to NACT plus trastuzumab has been shown to increase the pCR rate, while substituting lapatinib for trastuzumab resulted in equivalent or lower pCR rates [34–38]. However, the addition of lapatinib was also associated with a significant increase in side effects, especially diarrhea, rash, and liver function test abnormalities, likely related to off-target inhibition of the tyrosine kinase for HER1, the epidermal growth factor receptor. As consistent improvement in long-term outcomes has not been demonstrated for addition of lapatinib to chemotherapy plus trastuzumab in either the neoadjuvant [39] or adjuvant [40] setting, there is no indication for its routine use in the neoadjuvant setting, and further studies with this agent in that setting are not anticipated. However, the potential benefit of adding a tyrosine kinase inhibitor on pCR rates and long-term outcomes in nonmetastatic HER2+BC is likely to be revisited with the development of tucatinib, a tyrosine kinase inhibitor with much greater specificity for HER2 over HER1, which was recently approved in the metastatic setting.

Pertuzumab is a monoclonal antibody that binds to a different epitope on HER2 than trastuzumab, resulting in inhibition of the formation of HER2/HER3 heterodimers, which has been proposed as both the mechanism of activation of HER2 in normal physiology and a likely mechanism of resistance to trastuzumab. The addition of pertuzumab to trastuzumab induces responses in about half of patients with metastatic HER2+BC who progress on a trastuzumab-containing regimen, suggesting the frequency of the appearance of a subclone of malignant cells that exploit this mechanism. While the existence of such a subclone is likely much less common in patients with early-stage HER2+BC (unfortunately, at present we have no way of prospectively identifying cancers with this alteration), its existence could explain the failure of some patients with HER2+BC to achieve pCR with NACT plus trastuzumab. To explore this, the phase II NeoSphere study randomized 417 patients with stage II–III HER2+BC to four cycles of docetaxel plus trastuzumab (the control arm), docetaxel plus pertuzumab, docetaxel plus both trastuzumab and pertuzumab, or trastuzumab and pertuzumab without docetaxel. All patients received three cycles of fluorouracil, epirubicin, and cyclophosphamide (FEC) after surgery (patients on the dual antibody only arm also received four cycles of docetaxel before starting FEC) and completed a year of trastuzumab. The breast pCR (ypT0/is Nany) rate on the control arm was 29%; the addition of pertuzumab significantly increased it to 46% ($p = 0.0141$), while substitution of pertuzumab for trastuzumab reduced the breast pCR rate to 24%, and with dual antibody therapy alone it was 17% [41]. The addition of pertuzumab to docetaxel and trastuzumab had no appreciable impact on adverse events, including cardiotoxicity. While the study was not large enough for definitive evaluation of the treatment arms on long-term outcomes, 5-year progression-free survival was numerically higher with docetaxel plus trastuzumab and pertuzumab arm compared to the control arm (86% vs. 81%, HR 0.69, 95% CI 0.34–1.40) [42]. The randomized phase II TRYPHAENA study was designed to assess the incidence and severity of cardiotoxicity with anthracycline-containing (FEC followed by docetaxel with trastuzumab and pertuzumab (FEC-THP) and FEC with concurrent trastuzumab and pertuzumab followed by docetaxel with trastuzumab and pertuzumab (FECHP-THP)) regimens vs. an anthracycline-free regimen (every 3-week docetaxel, carboplatin, trastuzumab, and pertuzumab, TCHP); while it was not powered to compare pCR rates between these arms, on all three arms pCR rates were higher (FEC-THP 55%, FECHP-THP 56%, TCHP 64%) than would be expected for non-pertuzumab-containing regimens [43]. The incidence of cardiotoxicity was slightly lower in the TCHP arm, but this regimen was associated with higher rates of hematologic toxicities and diarrhea. Three-year DFS was similar across the three arms (87–90%) [44]. Based on these two studies, the FDA granted accelerated approval for the addition of pertuzumab to NACT and trastuzumab, and, despite the absence of a larger randomized trial or demonstration of significant improvements in long-term outcomes with its addition, this has become the standard of care for stage II–III HER2+BC.

One of the most common toxicities associated with the combination of NACT, trastuzumab, and pertuzumab is diarrhea. The etiology of this toxicity – and its apparent greater frequency and severity when the chemotherapy regimen includes carboplatin, which is not often associated with diarrhea in other settings – is unknown but may reflect the physiologic role of signaling modulated by the HER2/HER3 heterodimer, which is blocked by this treatment. Patients initiating this treatment should be instructed on appropriate management of diarrhea.

Both single-agent trastuzumab and the combination of trastuzumab and pertuzumab are available as subcutaneous (SC) formulations which are FDA approved for use in the neoadjuvant setting in place of the intravenous versions of these agents based on studies which demonstrated similar pCR rates and toxicities, though one study reported a higher rate of adverse events with the SC formulation of trastuzumab, due to more frequent infections [45, 46]. While there are potential cost and convenience advantages to the SC formulations, including at-home administration once the patient has completed chemotherapy and surgery, the uptake of SC therapy varies widely between countries, likely based on differences in medication coverage and reimbursement for treatment.

Over the last few years, several trastuzumab biosimilars have been developed and approved based on phase III studies which have demonstrated equivalent pCR rates to the original formulation when administered with NACT in HER2+BC [47–49]. Their use is usually determined by purchasing managers for individual hospitals, cancer centers, and physician offices, and they should be considered interchangeable with the original formulation.

Ado-trastuzumab emtansine (T-DM1) in an antibody-drug conjugate composed of trastuzumab linked to a potent antimicrotubule agent (emtansine) that is released only after the agent, attached to HER2 by its trastuzumab moiety, is endocytosed by the HER2+ cancer cell and the linker metabolized as part of normal cell "recycling." It has demonstrated impressive single-agent activity in patients with metastatic HER2+BC who had progressed on a trastuzumab-containing regimen and is associated with far fewer serious adverse events than standard chemotherapy plus trastuzumab. It is FDA approved both in the metastatic setting and for patients with residual disease after NACT plus trastuzumab (+/− pertuzumab) (see below). In the West German Study Group's ADAPT/T-DM1 study in patients with HR+/HER2+BC, T-DM1, either as a single agent or concurrent with endocrine therapy, induced much higher pCR rates (41% and 42%, respectively) than trastuzumab plus endocrine therapy (15%) [50], and in the Swedish PREDIX HER2 trial, the pCR rate with single-agent T-DM1 was similar to that seen with docetaxel, trastuzumab, and pertuzumab (44% and 46%, respectively) [51]. However, in the KRISTINE/TRIO-021 study, the pCR rate with T-DM1 plus pertuzumab was significantly lower than with TCHP (44% vs. 56%, $p = 0.016$), and 3-year EFS was also significantly lower (85% vs. 94%) due to a higher incidence of locoregional progression prior to surgery, though postoperative invasive DFS was similar (93% vs. 92%) [52, 53]. Thus, while TCHP is more likely to induce pCR, and T-DM1 is not FDA approved in the neoadjuvant setting, administration of this agent could be considered in patients who are not candidates for standard neoadjuvant therapy, due to age or medical comorbidities, or refuse that treatment.

Another option for patients with comorbidities that preclude the use of NACT could be administration of HER2-targeted therapies alone. As mentioned above, on the NeoSphere study, 17% of patients assigned to trastuzumab and pertuzumab alone achieved pCR, including 27% of HR-/HER2+BC patients but only 6% of HR+/HER2+BC patients [41]. The single-arm TBCRC023 pilot study demonstrated pCR rates as high as 33% in patients with HR+/HER2+BC who received 24 weeks of trastuzumab, lapatinib, and endocrine therapy, compared to 9% after only 12 weeks, while the pCR rate in HR-/HER2+BC was 18% and did not increase with an additional 12 weeks of treatment [54].

It had been hypothesized that the lower pCR rates seen in HR+/HER2+BC (compared to HR-/HER2+BC) might be due to "cross talk" between signaling pathways activated by HER2 and those activated by binding of estrogen to the estrogen receptor. To test this hypothesis, the NSABP B-52 study randomized patients with HR+/HER2+BC to neoadjuvant TCHP with or without an aromatase inhibitor (plus ovarian function suppression in premenopausal women). While estrogen deprivation did not adversely impact the pCR rate, neither did it significantly improve it. The pCR rate with TCHP alone was 41%; with the addition of estrogen deprivation, it rose modestly to 46% ($p = 0.39$) [55]. Thus, while concurrent endocrine therapy with NACT and dual HER2-targeted therapy is not clearly contraindicated, neither is it recommended.

Neoadjuvant Chemotherapy for HER2+BC

A variety of chemotherapeutic agents demonstrate additive or synergistic cytotoxicity with trastuzumab against HER2+BC cell lines in vitro and thus are potential partners for HER2-targeted therapies in the metastatic and neoadjuvant settings. As with the initial trials of the addition of trastuzumab to adjuvant chemotherapy, most early trials of neoadjuvant therapy utilized regimens consisting of an anthracycline-containing combination followed, or preceded, by a taxane plus trastuzumab (due to the high incidence of cardiotoxicity seen in the study that led to the approval of trastuzumab for metastatic HER2+BC; trastuzumab is usually not administered concurrent with the anthracycline, but typically with the taxane). A few examples:

- In the ACOSOG Z1041 study, patients with operable HER2+BC were randomized to four cycles of FEC followed by weekly paclitaxel with trastuzumab or to the alternative sequence. The overall pCR rate was 55% and did not differ between the two arms [56].
- In the NSABP B-41 study, 49% of patients with operable HER2+BC treated with four cycles of AC followed by weekly paclitaxel and trastuzumab achieved pCR, including 43% of clinically node-positive patients [36].
- In the GeparQuinto (GBG) study, patients who received four cycles of EC and trastuzumab followed by four cycles of every 3-week docetaxel and trastuzumab had a pCR rate of 45% [57].

In all of these studies, the pCR rate was higher in HR-/HER2+BC than in HR+/HER2+BC.

Based on results from the BCIRG006 adjuvant trial, in which patients who received the anthracycline-free regimen of every 3-week docetaxel, carboplatin, and trastuzumab (TCH) had similar outcomes to those who received AC followed by docetaxel and trastuzumab (though the study was not designed to directly compare these two arms, both were superior to AC followed by docetaxel without trastuzumab) [58], anthracycline-free chemotherapy regimens have been explored in the neoadjuvant setting, a trend which accelerated with demonstration of the higher pCR rates achieved with dual HER2-targeted therapy. Results from the randomized phase II TRYPHAENA study are discussed above [43, 44]. However, the study that confirmed that an anthracycline-free NACT regimen is as effective as an anthracycline-containing one in HER2+BC was the TRAIN-2 study [59, 60]. This trial, which was conducted by the Dutch Breast Cancer Research Group (BOOG), randomized 438 patients with stage II–III HER2+BC to three cycles of FEC followed by six cycles of paclitaxel days 1 and 8 with carboplatin (AUC 6), trastuzumab, and pertuzumab on day 1 every 3 weeks for six cycles versus the paclitaxel, carboplatin, trastuzumab, and pertuzumab regimen alone for nine cycles. The primary objective of the study was to demonstrate superiority of the anthracycline-containing regimen, but results showed that not only were pCR rates identical between the two arms (67% and 68%, respectively), but 3-year EFS (93%) and OS (98%) were as well. While most acute toxicities were comparable between the two arms, there was a significantly higher incidence of febrile neutropenia on the anthracycline-containing arm (10% vs. 1%, $p < .05$) and non-significantly higher rates of grade >3 diarrhea (17% vs. 12%) and peripheral neuropathy (7% vs. 5%) on the anthracycline-free arm. With anthracycline-containing NACT, cardiotoxicity rates were significantly higher, and two patients (1%) developed acute leukemia during follow-up compared to none on the anthracycline-free arm. Based on these results, an anthracycline-free regimen should be considered the preferred approach in patients with stage II–III HER2+BC who receive neoadjuvant therapy. No study has directly compared every 3-week docetaxel-based TCHP regimen to a weekly paclitaxel-based regimen such as that used in TRAIN-2, so the choice between these regimens is up to the individual oncologist.

GeparSepto compared 12 weeks of weekly nanoparticle albumin-bound (nab)-paclitaxel at 150 mg/m^2 (subsequently reduced to 125 mg/m^2 due to excessive neurotoxicity at the original dose) to standard paclitaxel at 80 mg/m^2 with trastuzumab and pertuzumab, followed by four cycles of EC [61]. While the nab-paclitaxel regimen had numerically higher pCR rates, overall (62% vs. 54%) and in the HR+/HER2+BC and HR-/HER2+BC subpopulations, this did not reach statistical significance. The activity of nab-paclitaxel as part of an anthracycline-free NACT regimen with trastuzumab and pertuzumab has not been studied in a large population of HER2+ patients.

Neoadjuvant Therapy Options in Lower-Risk HER2+BC Patients and Those with Comorbidities

In patients with lower-risk HER2+BC, such as clinical T1cN0, who, for whatever reason, are candidates for neoadjuvant therapy, and in patients with stage II–III disease with medical comorbidities that contraindicate use of the more aggressive regimens described above, less intensive treatment is indicated. Based on results from the APT adjuvant trial [62], a suitable regimen would be the combination of weekly paclitaxel and trastuzumab × 12 weeks; while there is no evidence that adding pertuzumab to this regimen will improve long-term outcomes, it would likely increase the pCR rate and thus including it is a reasonable option.

A slightly more intensive but still relatively brief regimen and well-tolerated regimen worth considering in patients with clinical stage IIA disease, such as T2N0, with T <3.5 cm in greatest dimension (since the APT trial included few patients with tumors >2 cm in size), is four cycles of every 3-week docetaxel, cyclophosphamide, and trastuzumab (again, with or without pertuzumab), based on its efficacy and tolerability in the adjuvant setting [63].

Neoadjuvant Therapy for Triple-Negative Breast Cancer (TNBC)

While there is heterogeneity within the entity referred to as triple-negative breast cancer (TNBC), including small numbers of patients with biologically less aggressive variants that express neither hormone receptors nor HER2, most of these cancers are high-grade and thus responsive to cytotoxic agents. Patients with TNBC who achieve a pCR with NACT have an excellent prognosis; in a recent meta-analysis, TNBC patients who achieved pCR had a 5-year event-free survival (EFS) rate of 90%, compared to 57% for patients with residual disease at surgery [26]. How pCR is achieved does not appear to affect the excellent prognosis associated with it. However, in randomized multicenter studies, less than 1/3 of TNBC patients achieve pCR with "standard" NACT, such as a sequence of weekly or every 2-week paclitaxel followed by or following an anthracycline-based regimen such as AC (Table 6.1). As a result, several clinical trials have investigated additions or alternatives to that regimen, most often the antiangiogenic monoclonal antibody bevacizumab, the chemotherapeutic agent carboplatin, or an immune checkpoint inhibitor.

The addition of bevacizumab to NACT chemotherapy in TNBC has been evaluated by four large, randomized studies [64–67]. Of these three – GeparQuinto, ARTemis, and CALGB 40603 – reported significant increases in the pCR rate (NSABP B-40 did not). Despite this, and despite the expected association between pCR and improved long-term outcomes, in none of the studies did the addition of bevacizumab significantly improve DFS or OS in TNBC [68–71]. Exploratory analyses suggest that there may be a weaker correlation between pCRs achieved with the addition of bevacizumab and long-term outcomes than pCRs achieved with NACT alone. For example, in GeparQuinto, patients with TNBC who achieved pCR with the addition of bevacizumab were twice as likely to suffer a DFS event compared to pCRs achieved without this agent [68]. In ARTemis, while only 2% of TNBC patients who achieved pCR with NACT alone suffered a DFS event, these occurred in 19% of pCRs achieved with the addition of bevacizumab, and achievement of a pCR with bevacizumab did not improve DFS or OS compared to patients with residual disease [69]. These findings led the ARTemis investigators to hypothesize that while the addition of bevacizumab to NACT may enhance response in an angiogenesis-driven breast tumor, it may not have a similar effect at sites of occult micrometastatic disease that may be less reliant on neoangiogenesis. This might also explain the failure of the addition of bevacizumab to improve DFS or OS in TNBC in large adjuvant trials, such as E5103 and BEATRICE [72, 73], or to improve OS in metastatic TNBC despite higher response rates and improved time to progression [74]. Given our reliance on the prognostic value of pCR in TNBC, particularly to determine which patients might benefit from receiving subsequent adjuvant therapy (see below), if achievement of pCR with bevacizumab is not a reliable predictor of improved long-term outcomes, that would be a compelling reason to avoid its use in the neoadjuvant setting.

Table 6.1 Neoadjuvant chemotherapy for TNBC: pathologic complete response (pCR) rates without and with carboplatin

	Control (no carboplatin) regimen			Carboplatin-containing regimen		
Study	*N*	Regimen	pCR	*N*	Regimen	pCR
CALGB 40603 [66]	107	wP → ddAC	39%	111	wPq3Cb → ddAC	49%
	105	(wP → ddAC) + Bev	43%	110	(wPq3Cb → ddAC) + Bev	60%
BrighTNess [76]	158	wP → AC	31%	160	wPq3Cb → AC	58%
				316	wPq3CbVel → AC	53%
GeparSepto [61]	137	wP → EC	26%	NA		
GeparSixto [75, 77]	157	wPwnpLDBev	43%	158	wPwCbwnpLDBev	53%
KEYNOTE-522 [81]	NA			84	wPq3Cb → AC/EC	56%
				116	wPwCb → AC/EC	48%
				165	(wPq3Cb → AC/EC) + Pembro	64%
				231	(wPwCb → AC/EC) + Pembro	67%
				466	10–12 doses of wPCb (−/+ Pembro)	55%/70%
				132	<10 doses of wPCb (−/+ Pembro)	36%/51%
GeparX [80]	NA			159	wnPxCb → EC	60%
				158	nPCb d 1,8 q21d → EC	50%
NeoSTOP [82]	NA			52	Txq3Cb × 6	52%
				48	wPq3Cb → ddAC	55%

wP weekly paclitaxel, *nP* nab-paclitaxel, *AC* doxorubicin and cyclophosphamide, *dd* dose-dense (every 2 weeks), *Bev* bevacizumab, *q3Cb* every 3-week carboplatin, *wCb* weekly carboplatin, *Vel* veliparib, *EC* epirubicin and cyclophosphamide, *wnpLD* weekly non-pegylated liposomal doxorubicin, *Pembro* pembrolizumab, *Tx* docetaxel, *NA* not applicable

Three large randomized studies – GeparSixto, CALGB 40603, and BrighTNess – have demonstrated significant increases in pCR rates with the addition of carboplatin to taxane- and anthracycline-based neoadjuvant chemotherapy in TNBC [66, 75, 76]; these results are supported by results from other multicenter studies utilizing similar neoadjuvant regimens (Table 6.1). While none of the randomized studies was powered to definitively determine whether the addition of carboplatin improves long-term outcomes, results from GeparSixto are encouraging. In 315 TNBC patients, the addition of weekly carboplatin (initially AUC 2, reduced to AUC 1.5 due to excessive hematologic toxicities) to a control regimen of weekly paclitaxel, weekly non-pegylated liposomal doxorubicin, and every 3-week bevacizumab significantly improved DFS (HR 0.456; 95% CI 0.25–0.83, $p = .008$) [77, 78]. OS was also improved, though this did not achieve statistical significance (HR 0.55; 95% CI

0.27–1.14, $p = .104$). In contrast, improvement in EFS and OS was not seen in the intention-to-treat population with addition of carboplatin to a more standard neoadjuvant regimen consisting of weekly paclitaxel followed by dose-dense AC (with half of the patients in each group also receiving bevacizumab) in CALGB 40603 [79]. However, results from this study are skewed by a subset of patients assigned to carboplatin who missed multiple doses of treatment during weekly paclitaxel (35% compared to 15% of patients not assigned to carboplatin) due to increased hematologic toxicity and the study's dose modification guidelines, which mandated that treatment with weekly paclitaxel (+/− carboplatin) be omitted, rather than just delayed pending recovery, for low blood counts or other toxicities [46]. These patients had a significantly lower pCR rate (41% vs. 61%) and inferior 5-year EFS (58% vs. 79%) compared to patients assigned to carboplatin who received treatment as planned. If these patients are excluded, the addition of carboplatin improved 5-year EFS from 72% to 79%, which trends toward significance (HR 0.72, $p = .016$) [79]. We await long-term outcomes from the BrighTNess trial, which utilized an identical treatment regimen to CALGB 40603, but permitted treatment delays, resulting in a much higher percentage of patients on the carboplatin arm receiving treatment as planned [76]. Given the magnitude of the pCR increase with carboplatin in that study (an absolute increase of 27% compared to 13% in CALGB 40603), we have reason to be optimistic that it will demonstrate substantial improvements in long-term outcomes as well. The BrighTNess study also included a third arm, on which patients received both carboplatin and the PARP inhibitor veliparib during weekly paclitaxel, which failed to demonstrate an increase in the pCR rate over that achieved with carboplatin alone [76]. Results from the GeparX study support the importance of paclitaxel/carboplatin dose delivery on achievement of pCR in TNBC [80]; on that study, TNBC patients randomized to receive nab-paclitaxel 125 mg/m^2 and carboplatin AUC 2 weekly for 12 weeks had a significantly higher pCR rate than patients who received the same treatment days 1 and 8 only every 21 days for four cycles (thus, a maximum of eight doses of paclitaxel), both followed by four cycles of EC (60.4% vs. 50.0%, $p = .056$), despite patients assigned to uninterrupted weekly treatment being more likely to discontinue this phase of treatment early.

While long-term outcome data are limited, the substantially higher pCR rates reported from multiple studies support the routine addition of carboplatin to taxane- and anthracycline-based NACT in TNBC, utilizing dosing guidelines (like those from BrighTNess) designed to avoid missed treatment doses which appears to compromise outcomes. In terms of the optimal treatment schedule (weekly versus every 3 weeks) and dose (AUC 1.5–2 for weekly, 5–6 for every 3 weeks) for carboplatin when administered with weekly paclitaxel, there have been no randomized studies comparing the two. The KEYNOTE-522 study (discussed under Immunotherapy below) allowed treating physicians to choose between weekly and every 3-week carboplatin, with the majority (58%) selecting the weekly regimen [81]. There is also reason to believe that inclusion of carboplatin might allow us to eliminate anthracyclines from the NACT regimen in many patients with TNBC. In a randomized phase II study, six cycles of docetaxel and carboplatin achieved a pCR rate (52%) similar to that seen with weekly paclitaxel and every 3-week carboplatin followed by four cycles of dose-dense AC (55%) [82]. In addition, in a recently published phase III adjuvant trial of 647 TNBC patients, those assigned to six cycles of weekly paclitaxel and carboplatin had significantly improved 5-year DFS compared to a control regimen of three cycles of cyclophosphamide, epirubicin, and fluorouracil followed by three cycles of docetaxel (CEF-T) (86.5% vs 80.3%, HR = 0.65; 95% CI, 0.44–0.96, $p = 0.03$) [83].

Immunotherapy for TNBC in the Neoadjuvant Setting

One of the mysteries in the development and progression of breast cancer is why these abnormal cells are not recognized as such and destroyed by the immune system. On histologic examination there is evidence that, in some cases at least, the immune system has identified the cancer as "foreign" and recruited immune effector cells, as evidenced by the presence of tumor-infiltrating lymphocytes (TILs), which are more prevalent and numerous in aggressive breast cancer subtypes, such as HER2+BC and TNBC. The presence of TILs is both prognostic, in terms of risk of distant recurrence and death, and predictive of response to NACT [84]. So, if TILs are present, what prevents the immune system from attacking the cancer? Over recent years a variety of substances have been identified that may be produced by cancer cells which interact with receptors on immune effector cells and suppress their activation, and agents have been developed to block this interaction. These agents, often referred to as immune checkpoint inhibitors (ICIs), are typically monoclonal antibodies (mAbs) that target either the programmed cell death protein 1 (PD-1), an inhibitory molecule expressed by T lymphocytes, especially T effector cells such as killer T cells, or its ligand (PD-L1) and have demonstrated antitumor efficacy in an increasing number of malignancies, including in metastatic TNBC that expresses PD-L1, leading to their approval by the FDA [85]. Several studies have investigated the impact of the addition of ICIs to neoadjuvant chemotherapy on pCR rates in HER2-negative breast cancer, especially TNBC. The hope is that the addition of such agents will not only increase the pCR rate but also enhance eradication of occult metastatic disease. Trials assessing the addition of an ICI to neoadjuvant chemotherapy for TNBC in chemotherapy that have reported results are listed in Table 6.2:

- The phase III KEYNOTE-522 study demonstrated that the addition of pembrolizumab (a PD-1-targeted mAb) to NACT consisting of weekly paclitaxel and carboplatin (the latter administered either weekly or every 3 weeks at the discretion of the treating physician) followed by AC or EC raised the overall pCR rate from 51% to 65% [81]. While patients with PD-L1-expressing (PD-L1+) cancers had higher pCR rates whether they received pembrolizumab or not, the addition of pembrolizumab increased pCR rates in both PD-L1+ and PD-L1-negative (PD-L1−) cancers. Preliminary data suggest that the addition of pembrolizumab may

Table 6.2 Impact of addition of immune checkpoint inhibitors to neoadjuvant chemotherapy in triple-negative breast cancer

Study (reference)	Chemo regimen	Subgroup	N	pCR[a] (%)	N	pCR[a] (%)	EFS results (IT vs Control)
			Immunotherapy agent (target)		Control		
			Pembrolizumab (PD-1)		Placebo		
KEYNOTE-522 [81]	Weekly paclitaxel with carboplatin (weekly or every 3 weeks) × 12 weeks followed by doxorubicin or epirubicin and cyclophosphamide × four cycles	All	784	65	390	51	At 18 months – 91 versus 85% HR 0.63; 95% CI 0.43–0.97)
		PD-L1+	656	69	317	55	
		PD-L1−	127	45	69	30	
			Atezolizumab (PD-L1)		Placebo		
Impassion031 [86]	Weekly nab-paclitaxel × 12 followed by doxorubicin and cyclophosphamide × four cycles	All	165	58	168	41	HR 0.76 (95% CI 0.4–1.44)
		PD-L1+	77	69	75	49	
		PD-L1−	88	48	93	34	
			Atezolizumab		None		
NeoTRIPaPDL1 [87]	Nab-paclitaxel and carboplatin days 1 and 8 every 21 days × eight cycles	All	138	44	142	41	Not reported
		PD-L1+	79	52	77	48	
		PD-L1−	59	32	65	32	
			(PD-L1)		Placebo		
GeparNUEVO [88]	Weekly nab-paclitaxel × 12 followed epirubicin and cyclophosphamide × four cycles	All	88	53	86	44	Not reported
		PD-L1+	69	58	69	51	
		PD-L1−	11	44	9	18	
		Window[b]	59	61	58	41	

[a]pCR – ypT0/isN0

[b]The first 117 patients treated on GeparNeuvo received a single dose of either durvalumab or placebo 2 weeks before starting neoadjuvant chemotherapy with the same agent; this was omitted after the study's Independent Data Monitoring Committee expressed concern about the delay in the start of chemotherapy; another 57 patients were subsequently treated without this "window" treatment

also improve EFS, but in February 2021 the FDA deferred a decision on approval of this agent in the neoadjuvant setting pending longer follow-up.

- The phase III Impassion031 demonstrated that the addition of the PD-L1-targeted mAb atezolizumab to NACT, consisting of weekly nab-paclitaxel followed by AC, increased the overall pCR rate from 41% to 58% [86]. As in the KEYNOTE-522 study, an increase in pCR was seen in both PD-L1+ and PD-L1− patients. While early EFS results are promising, this study was not powered to definitively address this endpoint.
- In contrast, the NeoTRIPaPDL1 study did not demonstrate a significant increase in pCR rates with the addition of atezolizumab to NACT consisting of nab-paclitaxel and carboplatin administered days 1 and 8 every 21 days for eight cycles, overall or in either the PD-L1+ or PD-L1− subsets [87].
- In the German Breast Group's phase II GeparNuevo study, while the addition of the PD-L1-targeted mAb durvalumab to NACT, consisting of weekly nab-paclitaxel followed by EC, increased pCR rates in all patients, including those with PD-L1+ or PD-L1− cancers, these increases did not reach statistical significance [88]. However, among 117 patients who received "window" treatment with a single dose of their assigned study drug 2 weeks before starting nab-paclitaxel, those who received durvalumab had a significantly higher pCR rate, suggesting a potential benefit for this type of "immune priming."

While results from some of these studies are encouraging in regard the impact of adding an ICI to NACT on pCR rates (and possibly EFS) in TNBC, many questions remain. These include whether the choice of agent (PD-1- versus PD-L1-targeted) is important, the optimal timing and duration of treatment, selection of the accompanying NACT regimen, the appropriate target population (especially whether to include PD-L1− cancers), as well as the impact of immunotherapy on long-term outcomes such as EFS and OS. Until we have answers to at least some of the questions, routine inclusion of an ICI in neoadjuvant therapy for TNBC will likely not be accepted as the standard of care.

Post-neoadjuvant Systemic Therapy

Patients who achieve a pCR with neoadjuvant therapy have a very good prognosis. Despite this, most receive adjuvant systemic therapy determined by their tumor subtype. Patients with HR+/HER-BC typically receive adjuvant endocrine therapy for at least 5 years, with either tamoxifen, an aromatase inhibitor, or a sequence of the two, depending on their menopausal status and tolerance of this treatment. The benefit of extended (>5 years) adjuvant endocrine therapy to reduce the risk of late distant recurrence has not been studied in this group of patients but is likely small given their good prognosis. Similarly, in premenopausal women who received ovarian function suppression with a long-acting LHRH analog during either NACT (to protect ovarian function) or as part of their NET, the benefit of continuing ovarian function suppression in the postoperative setting has not been studied, but the possible benefit of this treatment should be weighed against its short- and long-term side effects. In patients with HER2+BC who achieve a pCR with neoadjuvant therapy, the standard of care is to complete a year of trastuzumab, as in patients treated in the adjuvant setting, though the benefit of this treatment has not been studied, with the addition of adjuvant endocrine therapy if HR+. Resumption of pertuzumab (in addition to trastuzumab) after surgery in patients who achieve pCR with NACT and dual HER2-targeted therapy is controversial; this has not been studied, is not without toxicity and costs, and is unlikely to impact long-term outcomes given the marginal benefit of adding pertuzumab to adjuvant chemotherapy and trastuzumab in the APHINITY trial [89]. In patients with TNBC who achieve pCR, there is no standard postoperative systemic treatment.

Until recently, there were no recommended treatments for patients with a suboptimal response to NACT. Patients with HR+ cancers typically received adjuvant endocrine therapy and those with HER2+BC received adjuvant trastuzumab. Patients with TNBC were sometimes offered adjuvant chemotherapy, despite the lack of evidence that it would reduce the risk of disease recurrence. Then, in 2015, Masuda and colleagues presented the results of the CREATE-X trial, on which 910 patients with HER2-BC with residual invasive disease in the breast or axillary nodes after NACT were randomly assigned to a 6-month course of adjuvant capecitabine or observation [90]. The study demonstrated significant improvements in both 5-year DFS (74.1% vs. 67.6%, HR 0.70, 95% CI 0.53–0.92; $p = 0.01$) and OS (89.2% vs. 83.6%, HR 0.59, 95% CI 0.39–0.90: $p = 0.01$) with capecitabine. When stratified by hormone receptor status, significant benefits were seen only in patients with TNBC, with 42% and 48% improvements in DFS and OS, respectively, while outcomes in patients with HR+HER2-BC did not significantly improve. Another interesting observation was that patients with the poorest histologic response to neoadjuvant chemotherapy (grade 0, 1a, or 1b by Japanese Breast Cancer Society response criteria) received the greatest benefit from adjuvant capecitabine, while DFS improvement was not statistically significant in patients with a moderate or marked response to their prior treatment (grades 2 and 3), which raises questions about the heterogeneous biology of TNBC and its response to short-term intensive intravenous chemotherapy versus extended duration oral chemotherapy.

As mentioned above, in patients with HER2+ breast cancer, standard adjuvant therapy was trastuzumab, despite persistence of disease in the breast or axilla on this agent as part of their neoadjuvant regimen. Given its activity in metastatic HER2+BC that had progressed on trastuzumab and its favorable toxicity profile, the KATHERINE trial assessed substituting ado-trastuzumab emtansine (T-DM1) for standard trastuzumab in 1486 patients with residual disease after NACT and trastuzumab [31]. Treatment with T-DM1 significantly improved invasive DFS. Estimated percentages of patients who would be free of invasive disease at 3 years were 88.3% in the T-DM1 group compared to 77.0% in the trastuzumab group (HR, 0.50; 95% CI 0.39 to 0.64; $p < 0.001$), and while treatment with T-DM1 was associated with more frequent side effects than trastuzumab, it was well tolerated overall, with more than 70% of patients completing the planned 14 cycles of treatment.

These two studies not only changed the standard of care for patients with TNBC and HER2+BC who fail to achieve pCR but also established the value of using the "post-neoadjuvant" setting to test the benefit of treatments in patients identified at increased risk for distant recurrence by their failure to achieve pCR. Several ongoing and proposed studies in various breast cancer subtypes have adopted this approach.

In patients with HR+/HER2- breast cancer who received NACT, due to extent of disease at diagnosis or a high-risk Oncotype Dx Recurrence Score (>26) and fail to achieve pCR, standard adjuvant therapy consists of endocrine therapy with tamoxifen, an aromatase inhibitor, or a sequence of the two for up to 10 years. In these higher-risk women, the addition of a 5-year course of ovarian function suppression, if premenopausal, or ovarian ablation (particularly if likely to be within 5 years of natural menopause) is warranted, as is the addition of adjuvant bisphosphonate therapy [91].

Perhaps the patients in whom choice of post-neoadjuvant therapy generates the most controversy are those with HR+/HER2-BC that failed to respond to NET, whether by clinical criteria or PEPI score at surgery. While some argue that this lack of response indicates a poorer prognosis, justifying administration of adjuvant chemotherapy, slow-growing cancers may not achieve a significant response to NET, yet are unlikely to benefit from chemotherapy. A reasonable approach may be to make recommendations about adjuvant chemotherapy based on the same criteria one would employ in the adjuvant setting, by administering chemotherapy to patients with extensive nodal disease (pathologic N2-3, including those with involvement of >4 axillary lymph nodes) or an Oncotype Dx Recurrence Score (performed on the diagnostic biopsy, not the surgical specimen) of at least 26 while relying on endocrine therapy for pathologic N0-1 with an Oncotype of <25.

Conclusion

The role of neoadjuvant therapy is likely to continue to expand, given its impact on surgical management and usefulness to direct postoperative therapy. While tumor subtype as defined by hormone receptor and HER2 expression largely defines neoadjuvant treatment options for individual patients today, as our understanding of the molecular determinants of cancer behavior and response to treatment advances, our interventions will hopefully become more precise and personalized, enhancing efficacy and reducing unnecessary toxicity. Novel approaches to post-neoadjuvant therapy in patients who fail to achieve pCR are also being evaluated, including tucatinib (A011801) and trastuzumab deruxtecan (DESTINY-Breast05) in HER2+BC and pembrolizumab in TNBC (S1418), and the role of NET in HR+/HER2-BC is likely to expand. Table 6.3 summarizes current neoadjuvant treatment recommendations by tumor subtype, but these are certain to change as results from ongoing and planned studies become available.

Table 6.3 Breast cancer subtype and preferred neoadjuvant regimen(s) – 2021

HR+/ HER2-BC	Locally advanced (clinical stage T4 or N2) or high-risk Oncotype (>25)		Sequential AC × 4 -T (either every 3-week docetaxel × 4 or paclitaxel every 2–3 weeks × 4 or weekly × 12) (in either order)	In clinical T1-2N0, every 3-week TC × 4–6 cycles can be considered
	Clinical stage T1-2 N0-1 with low-intermediate risk Oncotype (<25)	Postmenopausal	Aromatase inhibitor for 6 months or longer	
		Premenopausal	Ovarian function suppression with goserelin (SC) or leuprolide (IM) and an aromatase inhibitor for 6 months or longer	
TNBC	Weekly paclitaxel with weekly or every 3-week carboplatin × 12 weeks followed by dose-dense AC × 4		In patients with contraindication to anthracyclines, every 3-week docetaxel and carboplatin × six cycles should be considered	
HER2+BC	Every 3-week docetaxel, carboplatin, trastuzumab, and pertuzumab (TCHP) × 6 or weekly paclitaxel with weekly or every 3-week carboplatin and every 3-week trastuzumab and pertuzumab × 18 weeks		Lower-risk patients in whom neoadjuvant therapy is indicated could receive less intensive therapy, such as weekly paclitaxel and trastuzumab (+/− pertuzumab) × 12 weeks (in clinical T1N0) or every 3-week docetaxel, cyclophosphamide and trastuzumab (+/− pertuzumab) × four cycles (in clinical T2 (<3.5 cm) N0)	

References

1. van der Hage JA, van de Velde CJ, Julien JP, et al. Preoperative chemotherapy in primary operable breast cancer: results from the European Organization for Research and Treatment of Cancer trial 10902. J Clin Oncol. 2001;19:4224–37.
2. Fisher B, Bryant J, Wolmark N, Mamounas E, et al. Effect of preoperative chemotherapy on the outcome of women with operable breast cancer. J Clin Oncol. 1998;16:2672–85.
3. Gianni L, Baselga J, Eiermann W, et al. Feasibility and tolerability of sequential doxorubicin/paclitaxel followed by cyclophosphamide, methotrexate, and fluorouracil and its effects on tumor response as preoperative therapy. Clin Cancer Res. 2005;11:8715–21.
4. Rastogi P, Anderson SJ, Bear HD, et al. Preoperative chemotherapy: updates of National Surgical Adjuvant Breast and Bowel Project Protocols B-18 and B-27. J Clin Oncol. 2008;26:778–85.
5. Mauri D, Pavlidis N, Ioannidis JP. Neoadjuvant versus adjuvant systemic treatment in breast cancer: a meta-analysis. J Natl Cancer Inst. 2005;97:188–94.
6. Early Breast Cancer Trialists' Collaborative Group (EBCTCG). Long-term outcomes for neoadjuvant versus adjuvant chemotherapy in early breast cancer: meta-analysis of individual patient data from ten randomised trials. Lancet Oncol. 2018;19:27–39.
7. Cortazar P, Zhang L, Untch M, et al. Pathological complete response and long-term clinical benefit in breast cancer: the CTNeoBC pooled analysis. Lancet. 2014;384:164–72.

8. Spring LM, Gupta A, Reynolds KL, et al. Neoadjuvant endocrine therapy for estrogen receptor-positive breast cancer: a systemic review and meta-analysis. JAMA Oncol. 2016;2:1477–86.
9. Bear HD, Wan W, Robidoux A, et al. Using the 21-gene assay from core needle biopsies to choose neoadjuvant therapy for breast cancer: a multicenter trial. J Surg Oncol. 2017;115:917–23.
10. Pease AM, Riba LA, Gruner RA, Tung NM, James TA. Oncotype DX Recurrence Score as predictor of response to neoadjuvant chemotherapy. Ann Surg Oncol. 2019;26:366–71.
11. Akashi-Tanaka S, Shimizu C, Ando M, et al. 21-Gene expression profile assay on core needle biopsies predicts responses to neoadjuvant endocrine therapy in breast cancer patients. Breast. 2009;18:171–4.
12. Sparano JA, Gray RJ, Makower DF, et al. Prospective validation of a 21-gene expression assay in breast cancer. N Engl J Med. 2015;373:2005–14.
13. Kalinsky K, Barlow WE, Meric-Bernstam F, Gralow JR, Albain KS. First results from a phase III randomized clinical trial of standard adjuvant endocrine therapy (ET) +/− chemotherapy (CT) in patients (pts) with 1–3 positive nodes, hormone receptor-positive (HR+) and HER2-negative (HER2-) breast cancer (BC) with recurrence score (RS)<25: SWOG S1007(RxPONDER). Presented at SABCS 2020, Abstract GS3-00.
14. Berry DA, Cirrincione C, Henderson IC, et al. Estrogen-receptor status and outcomes of modern chemotherapy for patients with node-positive breast cancer. JAMA. 2006;295:1658–67.
15. Blum JL, Flynn PJ, Yothers G, et al. Anthracyclines in early breast cancer: the ABC trials-USOR 06-090, NSABP B-46-I/USOR 07132, and NSABP B-49 (NRG oncology). J Clin Oncol. 2017;35:2647.2655.
16. Seo JH, Kim YH, Kim JS. Meta-analysis of pre-operative aromatase inhibitor versus tamoxifen in postmenopausal woman with hormone receptor-positive breast cancer. Cancer Chemother Pharmacol. 2009;63:261–6.
17. Ellis MJ, Suman VJ, Hoog J, et al. Randomized phase II neoadjuvant comparison between letrozole, anastrozole, and exemestane for postmenopausal women with estrogen receptor-rich stage 2 to 3 breast cancer: clinical and biomarker outcomes and predictive value of the baseline PAM50-based intrinsic subtype-ACOSOG Z1031. J Clin Oncol. 2011;29:2342–9.
18. Dixon JM, Renshaw L, Macaskill EJ, et al. Increase in response rate by prolonged treatment with neoadjuvant letrozole. Breast Cancer Res Treat. 2009;113:145–51.
19. Dowsett M, Smith IE, Ebbs SR, et al. Prognostic value of Ki67 expression after short-term presurgical endocrine therapy for primary breast cancer. J Natl Cancer Inst. 2007;99:167–70.
20. Ma CX, Suman VJ, Leitch AM, et al. ALTERNATE: neoadjuvant endocrine treatment (NET) approaches for clinical stage II or III estrogen receptor-positive HER2-negative breast cancer (ER+ HER2- BC) in postmenopausal (PM) women: alliance A011106. J Clin Oncol. 2020;38(15 suppl):Abstract 504.
21. Smith IE, Dowsett M, Ebbs SR, et al. Neoadjuvant treatment of postmenopausal breast cancer with anastrozole, tamoxifen, or both in combination: the IMmediate Preoperative Anastrozole, Tamoxifen, or Combined with Tamoxifen (IMPACT) multicenter double-blind randomized trial. J Clin Oncol. 2005;23:5108–16.
22. Ellis MJ, Tao Y, Luo J, et al. Outcome prediction for estrogen receptor-positive breast cancer based on postneoadjuvant endocrine therapy tumor characteristics. J Natl Cancer Inst. 2008;100:1380–8.
23. Ellis MJ, Suman VJ, Hoog J, et al. Ki67 proliferation index as a tool for chemotherapy decisions during and after neoadjuvant aromatase inhibitor treatment of breast cancer: results from the American College of Surgeons Oncology Group Z1031 trial (Alliance). J Clin Oncol. 2017;35:1061–9.
24. Slamon DJ, Leyland-Jones B, Shak S, et al. Use of chemotherapy plus a monoclonal antibody against HER2 for metastatic breast cancer that overexpresses HER2. N Engl J Med. 2001;344:783–92.

25. Romond EH, Perez EA, Bryant J, et al. Trastuzumab plus adjuvant chemotherapy for operable HER2-positive breast cancer. N Engl J Med. 2005;353:1673–84.
26. Spring LM, Fell G, Arfe A, et al. Pathological complete response after neoadjuvant chemotherapy and impact on breast cancer recurrence and survival: a comprehensive meta-analysis. Clin Cancer Res. 2020;26:2838–48.
27. von Minckwitz G, Untch M, Blohmer JU, et al. Definition and impact of pathologic complete response on prognosis after neoadjuvant chemotherapy in various intrinsic breast cancer subtypes. J Clin Oncol. 2012;30:1796–804.
28. Untch M, Fasching PA, Konecny GE, et al. Pathologic complete response after neoadjuvant chemotherapy plus trastuzumab predicts favorable survival in human epidermal growth factor receptor 2-overexpressing breast cancer: results from the TECHNO trial of the AGO and GBG study groups. J Clin Oncol. 2011;29:3351–7.
29. Broglio KR, Quintana M, Foster M, et al. Association of pathologic complete response to neoadjuvant therapy in HER2-positive breast cancer with long-term outcomes: a meta-analysis. JAMA Oncol. 2016;2:751–60.
30. Symmans WF, Wei C, Gould R, et al. Long-term prognostic risk after neoadjuvant chemotherapy associated with residual cancer burden and breast cancer subtype. J Clin Oncol. 2017;35:1049–60.
31. von Minckwitz G, Huang C-S, Mano MS, et al. Trastuzumab emtansine for residual invasive HER2-positive breast cancer. N Engl J Med. 2019;380:617–28.
32. Gianni L, Eiermann W, Semiglazov V, et al. Neoadjuvant chemotherapy with trastuzumab followed by adjuvant trastuzumab versus neoadjuvant chemotherapy alone, in patients with HER2-positive locally advanced breast cancer (the NOAH trial): a randomised controlled superiority trial with a parallel HER2-negative cohort. Lancet. 2010;375:377–84.
33. Gianni L, Eiermann W, Semiglazov V, et al. Neoadjuvant and adjuvant trastuzumab in patients with HER2-positive locally advanced breast cancer (NOAH): follow-up of a randomised controlled superiority trial with a parallel HER2-negative cohort. Lancet Oncol. 2014;15:640–7.
34. Guarneri V, Frassoldati A, Bottini A, et al. Preoperative chemotherapy plus trastuzumab, lapatinib, or both in human epidermal growth factor receptor 2-positive operable breast cancer: results of the randomized phase II CHER-LOB study. J Clin Oncol. 2012;30:1989–95.
35. Baselga J, Bradbury I, Eidtmann H, et al. Lapatinib with trastuzumab for HER2-positive early breast cancer (NeoALTTO): a randomised, open-label, multicentre, phase 3 trial. Lancet. 2012;379:633–40.
36. Robidoux A, Tang G, Rastogi P, et al. Lapatinib as a component of neoadjuvant therapy for HER2-positive operable breast cancer (NSABP protocol B-41): an open-label, randomised phase 3 trial. Lancet Oncol. 2013;14:1183–92.
37. Carey LA, Berry DA, Cirrincione CT, et al. Molecular heterogeneity and response to neoadjuvant human epidermal growth factor receptor 2 targeting in CALGB 40601, a randomized phase III trial of paclitaxel plus trastuzumab with or without lapatinib. J Clin Oncol. 2016;34:542–9.
38. Hicks M, Macrae ER, Abdel-Rasoul M, et al. Neoadjuvant dual HER2-targeted therapy with lapatinib and trastuzumab improves pathologic complete response in patients with early stage HER2-positive breast cancer: a meta-analysis of randomized prospective clinical trials. Oncologist. 2015;20:337–42.
39. Huober J, Holmes E, Baselga J, et al. Survival outcomes of the NeoALTTO study (BIG 1-06): updated results of a randomised multicenter phase III neoadjuvant clinical trial in patients with HER2-positive primary breast cancer. Eur J Cancer. 2019;118:169–77.
40. Piccart-Gebhart M, Holmes E, Baselga J, et al. Adjuvant lapatinib and trastuzumab for early human epidermal growth factor receptor 2-positive breast cancer: results from the randomized phase III Adjuvant Lapatinib and/or Trastuzumab Treatment Optimization trial. J Clin Oncol. 2016;34:1034–42.
41. Gianni L, Pienkowski T, Im YH, et al. Efficacy and safety of neoadjuvant pertuzumab and trastuzumab in women with locally advanced, inflammatory, or early HER2-positive breast

cancer (NeoSphere): a randomised multicentre, open-label, phase 2 trial. Lancet Oncol. 2012;13:25–32.

42. Gianni L, Pienkowski T, Im YH, et al. 5-year analysis of neoadjuvant pertuzumab and trastuzumab in patients with locally advanced, inflammatory, or early-stage HER2-positive breast cancer (NeoSphere): a multicentre, open-label, phase 2 randomised trial. Lancet Oncol. 2016;17:791–800.
43. Schneeweiss A, Chia S, Hickish T, et al. Pertuzumab plus trastuzumab in combination with standard neoadjuvant anthracycline-containing and anthracycline-free chemotherapy regimens in patients with HER2-positive early breast cancer: a randomized phase II cardiac safety study (TRYPHAENA). Ann Oncol. 2013;24:2278–84.
44. Schneeweiss A, Chia S, Hickish T, et al. Long-term efficacy analysis of the randomised, phase II TRYPHAENA cardiac safety study: evaluating pertuzumab and trastuzumab plus standard neoadjuvant anthracycline-containing and anthracycline-free chemotherapy regimens in patients with HER2-positive early breast cancer. Eur J Cancer. 2018;89:27–35.
45. Ismael G, Hegg R, Muehlbauer S, et al. Subcutaneous versus intravenous administration of (neo)adjuvant trastuzumab in patients with HER2-positive, clinical stage I-III breast cancer (HannaH study): a phase 3, open-label, multicentre, randomised trial. Lancet Oncol. 2012;13:869–78.
46. Jackisch C, Hegg R, Stroyakovskiy D, et al. Total pathologic complete response (tpCR) and event-free survival (EFS) with subcutaneous (SC) or intravenous (IV) trastuzumab in HER2-positive early breast cancer (EBC). J Clin Oncol. 2015;33(15 suppl):Abstract 585.
47. Stebbing J, Baranau Y, Baryash V, et al. CT-P6 compared with reference trastuzumab for HER2-positive breast cancer: a randomised, double-blind, active-controlled, phase 3 equivalence trial. Lancet Oncol. 2017;18:917–28.
48. Pivot X, Bondarenko I, Nowecki Z, et al. Phase III, randomized, double-blind study comparing the efficacy, safety, and immunogenicity of SB3 (trastuzumab biosimilar) and reference trastuzumab in patients treated with neoadjuvant therapy for human epidermal growth factor receptor 2-positive early breast cancer. J Clin Oncol. 2018;36:968–74.
49. Pivot X, Bondarenko I, Nowecki Z, et al. A phase III study comparing SB3 (a proposed trastuzumab biosimilar) and trastuzumab reference product in HER2-positive early breast cancer treated with neoadjuvant-adjuvant treatment: final safety, immunogenicity, and survival results. Eur J Cancer. 2018;93:19–27.
50. Harbeck N, Gluz O, Christgen M, et al. De-escalation strategies in human epidermal growth factor receptor 2 (HER2)-positive early breast cancer (BC): final analysis of the West German Study Group Adjuvant Dynamic Marker-Adjusted Personalized Therapy trial optimizing risk assessment and therapy response prediction in early BC HER2- and hormone receptor-positive phase II randomized trial-efficacy, safety, and predictive markers for 12 weeks of neoadjuvant trastuzumab emtansine with or without endocrine therapy (ET) versus trastuzumab plus ET. J Clin Oncol. 2017;35:3046–54.
51. Bergh JCS, Andersson A, Bjohle J, et al. Docetaxel, trastuzumab, pertuzumab versus trastuzumab emtansine as neoadjuvant treatment of HER2-positive breast cancer: Results from the Swedish PREDIX HER2 trial identifying a new potential de-escalation standard? J Clin Oncol. 2019;37(15 suppl):Abstract 501.
52. Hurvitz SA, Martin M, Symmans WF, et al. Neoadjuvant trastuzumab, pertuzumab, and chemotherapy versus trastuzumab emtansine plus pertuzumab in patients with HER2-positive breast cancer (KRISTINE): a randomised, open-label, multicentre, phase 3 trial. Lancet Oncol. 2018;19:115–26.
53. Hurvitz SA, Martin M, Jung KH, et al. Neoadjuvant trastuzumab emtansine and pertuzumab in human epidermal growth factor receptor 2-positive breast cancer: three-year outcomes from the phase III KRISTINE study. J Clin Oncol. 2019;37:2206–16.
54. Rimawi MF, Niravath PA, Wang T, et al. TBCRC023: a randomized phase II neoadjuvant trial of lapatinib plus trastuzumab without chemotherapy for 12 versus 24 weeks in patients with HER2-positive breast cancer. Clin Cancer Res. 2020;26:821–7.

55. Rimawi MF, Cecchini RS, Rastogi P, et al. A phase III trial evaluating pCR in patients with HR+, HER2-positive breast cancer treated with neoadjuvant docetaxel, carboplatin, trastuzumab, and pertuzumab (TCHP) +/− estrogen deprivation: NRG Oncology/NSABP B-52. Cancer Res. 2017;77(4 suppl):Abstract S3-06.
56. Buzdar AU, Suman VJ, Meric-Bernstam F, et al. Fluorouracil, epirubicin, and cyclophosphamide (FEC-75) followed by paclitaxel plus trastuzumab versus paclitaxel plus trastuzumab followed by FEC-75 plus trastuzumab as neoadjuvant treatment for patients with HER2-positive breast cancer (Z1041): a randomised, controlled, phase 3 trial. Lancet Oncol. 2013;14:1317–25.
57. Untch M, Loibl S, Bischoff J, et al. Lapatinib versus trastuzumab in combination with neoadjuvant anthracycline-taxane-based chemotherapy (GeparQuinto, GBG 44): a randomised phase 3 trial. Lancet Oncol. 2012;13:135–44.
58. Slamon D, Eiermann W, Robert N, et al. Adjuvant trastuzumab in HER2-positive breast cancer. N Engl J Med. 2011;365:1273–83.
59. van Ramshorst MS, van der Voort A, van Werkhoven ED, et al. Neoadjuvant chemotherapy with or without anthracyclines in the presence of dual HER2 blockade for HER2-positive breast cancer (TRAIN-2): a multicentre, open-label, randomised, phase 3 trial. Lancet Oncol. 2018;19:1630–40.
60. van der Voort A, van Ramshorst MS, van Werkhoven ED, et al. Three-year follow-up of neoadjuvant chemotherapy with or without anthracyclines in the presence of dual HER2-blockade for HER2-positive breast cancer (TRAIN-2): a randomized phase III trial. J Clin Oncol. 2020;8(15 suppl):Abstract 501.
61. Loibl S, Jackisch C, Schneeweiss A, et al. Dual HER2-blockade with pertuzumab and trastuzumab in HER2-positive early breast cancer: a subanalysis of data from the randomized phase III GeparSepto trial. Ann Oncol. 2017;28:497–504.
62. Tolaney SM, Barry WT, Dang CT, et al. Adjuvant paclitaxel and trastuzumab for node-negative, HER2-positive breast cancer. N Engl J Med. 2015;372:134–41.
63. Jones SE, Collea R, Paul D, et al. Adjuvant docetaxel and cyclophosphamide plus trastuzumab in patients with HER2-amplified early-stage breast cancer: a single-group, open-label, phase 2 study. Lancet Oncol. 2013;14:1121–8.
64. von Minckwitz G, Eidtmann H, Rezai M, et al. Neoadjuvant chemotherapy and bevacizumab for HER2-negative breast cancer. N Engl J Med. 2012;366:299–309.
65. Earl HM, Hiller L, Dunn JA, et al. Efficacy of neoadjuvant bevacizumab added to docetaxel followed by fluorouracil, epirubicin, and cyclophosphamide, for women with HER2-negative early breast cancer (ARTemis): an open-label, randomized, phase 3 trial. Lancet Oncol. 2015;16:656–66.
66. Sikov WM, Berry DA, Perou CP, et al. Impact of the addition of carboplatin and/or bevacizumab to neoadjuvant weekly paclitaxel followed by dose-dense doxorubicin and cyclophosphamide on pathologic complete response rates in stage II-III triple-negative breast cancer: CALGB 40603 (Alliance). J Clin Oncol. 2015;33:13–21.
67. Bear HD, Tang G, Rastogi P, et al. Bevacizumab added to neoadjuvant chemotherapy for breast cancer. N Engl J Med. 2012;366:310–20.
68. von Minckwitz G, Loibl S, Untch M, et al. Survival after neoadjuvant chemotherapy with or without bevacizumab or everolimus for HER2-negative primary breast cancer (GBG-GeparQuinto). Ann Oncol. 2014;25:2363–72.
69. Earl HM, Hiller L, Dunn JA, et al. Disease-free and overall survival at 3.5 years for neoadjuvant bevacizumab added to docetaxel followed by fluorouracil, epirubicin and cyclophosphamide, for women with HER2-negative early breast cancer: ARTemis trial. Ann Oncol. 2017;28:1817–24.
70. Bear HD, Tang G, Rastogi P, Geyer CE Jr, et al. Neoadjuvant plus adjuvant bevacizumab in early breast cancer (NSABP B-40 [NRG Oncology]): secondary outcomes of a phase 3, randomised controlled trial. Lancet Oncol. 2015;16:1037–48.
71. Sikov WM, Berry DA, Perou CM, et al. Event-free and overall survival following neoadjuvant weekly paclitaxel and dose-dense AC +/− carboplatin and/or bevacizumab in triple-

negative breast cancer: Outcomes from CALGB 40603 (Alliance). Cancer Res. 2016;76(4 suppl):Abstract GS2-05.
72. Miller KD, O'Neill AM, Gradishar W, et al. Double-blind phase III trial of adjuvant chemotherapy with and without bevacizumab in patients with lymph node–positive and high-risk lymph node–negative breast cancer (E5103). J Clin Oncol. 2018;36:2621–9.
73. Bell R, Brown J, Parmar M, et al. Final efficacy and updated safety results of the randomized phase III BEATRICE trial evaluating adjuvant bevacizumab-containing therapy in triple-negative early breast cancer. Ann Oncol. 2017;28:754–60.
74. Miller K, Wang M, Gralow J, et al. Paclitaxel plus bevacizumab versus paclitaxel alone for metastatic breast cancer. N Engl J Med. 2007;357:2666–76.
75. von Minckwitz G, Schneeweiss A, Loibl S, et al. Neoadjuvant carboplatin in patients with triple-negative and HER2-positive early breast cancer (GeparSixto; GBG 66): a randomised phase 2 trial. Lancet Oncol. 2014;15:747–56.
76. Loibl S, O'Shaughnessy J, Untch M, et al. Addition of the PARP inhibitor veliparib plus carboplatin or carboplatin alone to standard neoadjuvant chemotherapy in triple-negative breast cancer (BrighTNess): a randomised, phase 3 trial. Lancet Oncol. 2018;19:497–509.
77. Hahnen E, Lederer B, Hauke J, et al. Germline mutation status, pathologic complete response, and disease-free survival in triple-negative breast cancer – secondary analysis of the GeparSixto randomized clinical trial. JAMA Oncol. 2017;2:1378–85.
78. Loibl S, Weber KE, Timms KM, et al. Survival analysis of carboplatin added to an anthracycline/taxane-based neoadjuvant chemotherapy and HRD score as predictor of response-final results from GeparSixto. Ann Oncol. 2018;29:2341–7.
79. Sikov WM, Polley M-Y, Twohy E, et al. CALGB (Alliance) 40603: long-term outcomes (LTOs) after neoadjuvant chemotherapy (NACT) +/− carboplatin (Cb) and bevacizumab (Bev) in triple-negative breast cancer (TNBC). J Clin Oncol. 2019;37(15 suppl):Abstract 591.
80. Blohmer J-U, Link T, Kummel S, et al. Investigating denosumab as an add-on treatment to neoadjuvant chemotherapy and two different nab-paclitaxel schedules in a 2x2 design in primary breast cancer – first results of the GeparX study. Cancer Res. 2019;80(4 suppl):Abstract GS3-01.
81. Schmid P, Cortes J, Pusztai L, et al. Pembrolizumab for early triple-negative breast cancer. N Engl J Med. 2020;382:810–21.
82. Sharma P, Kimler B, O'Dea A, et al. Results of randomized phase II trial of neoadjuvant carboplatin plus docetaxel or carboplatin plus paclitaxel followed by AC in stage I–III triple-negative breast cancer (NCT02413320). J Clin Oncol. 2019;37(15 suppl):Abstract 516.
83. Yu K-D, Ye F-G, He M, et al. Effect of adjuvant paclitaxel and carboplatin on survival in women with triple-negative breast cancer: a phase 3 randomized clinical trial. JAMA Oncol. 2020;6:1390–6.
84. Denkert C, von Minckwitz G, Darb-Esfahani S, et al. Tumour-infiltrating lymphocytes and prognosis in different subtypes of breast cancer: a pooled analysis of 3771 patients treated with neoadjuvant therapy. Lancet Oncol. 2018;19:40–50.
85. Schmid P, Adams S, Rugo HS, et al. Atezolizumab and nab-paclitaxel in advanced triple-negative breast cancer. N Engl J Med. 2018;379:2108–21.
86. Mittendorf EA, Zhang H, Barrios CH, et al. Neoadjuvant atezolizumab in combination with sequential nab-paclitaxel and anthracycline-based chemotherapy versus placebo and chemotherapy in patients with early-stage triple-negative breast cancer (IMpassion031): a randomised, double-blind, phase 3 trial. Lancet. 2020;396:1090–100.
87. Gianni L, Huang CS, Egle D, et al. Pathologic complete response (pCR) to neoadjuvant treatment with and without atezolizumab in triple negative, early high-risk and locally advanced breast cancer. NeoTRIPaPDL1 Michaelangelo randomized trial. Cancer Res. 2019;80(4 suppl):Abstract GS3-04.
88. Loibl S, Untch M, Burchard N, et al. A randomised phase II study investigating durvalumab in addition to an anthracycline taxane-based neoadjuvant therapy in early triple-negative breast cancer: clinical results and biomarker analysis of GeparNuevo study. Ann Oncol. 2020;30:1279–88.

89. Von Minckwitz G, Procter M, de Azambuja E, et al. Adjuvant trastuzumab and pertuzumab in early HER2-positive breast cancer. N Engl J Med. 2017;377:122–31.
90. Masuda N, Lee S-J, Ohtani S, et al. Adjuvant capecitabine for breast cancer after preoperative chemotherapy. N Engl J Med. 2017;376:2147–59.
91. Early Breast Cancer Trialists' Cooperative Group. Adjuvant bisphosphonate treatment in early breast cancer: meta-analyses of individual patient data from randomised trials. Lancet. 2015;386:1353–61.

Chapter 7
Adjuvant Versus Neoadjuvant Systemic Therapy

Beth Overmoyer

Locally Advanced Breast Cancer: Embracing Neoadjuvant Systemic Therapy

Primary Local-Regional Therapy: Surgery and Radiation

Inoperable locally advanced breast cancer (LABC) classified as clinical T4 disease, bulky N2 or N3 disease, or inflammatory breast cancer (cT4d) was historically treated with radiation, either prior to or after surgery, i.e., radical mastectomy [1, 2]. The 5-year survival rate following the treatment of inoperable LABC ranged between 2% and 28% following a radical mastectomy and 10–30% after radiation therapy alone (Table 7.1). However, these older series were not well controlled for the clinical stage of patients treated with the two local-regional modalities, and often patients receiving primary radiation therapy had extensive disease not amenable to surgical resection [2].

Most patients with LABC treated in this fashion develop distant metastasis within 24 months of diagnosis; however local disease control is also poor, with local-regional recurrence (LRR) as high as 60% following surgery and 72% after radiation therapy alone [3, 4]. Among patients who experience LRR, more than 80% die of disease within 2 years [5]. Based upon these data and others, surgery alone or radiation therapy alone was not felt to be acceptable therapeutic modalities for the primary treatment of LABC. Combination radiation prior to or after surgical resection resulted in improved local-regional disease control; however this did not translate into an improvement in overall survival (OS) [2].

B. Overmoyer (✉)
Susan F. Smith Center for Women's Cancer, Dana Farber Cancer Institute, Boston, MA, USA

A. Soran, F. Nakhlis (eds.), *Management of the Breast and Axilla in the Neoadjuvant Setting*, https://doi.org/10.1007/978-3-030-88020-0_7

Table 7.1 Percent survival at 5 years for stage III breast cancer treated with local-regional therapy alone

Reference	Year	Number of patients	% survival
Surgery alone			
MacKay [6]	1970	587	32
Sicher [7]	1973	604	29
Haagensen [8]	1986	109	3
Radiation therapy alone			
Langlands [9]	1976	165	14
Zucali [10]	1976	321	21
Rubens [4]	1977	184	13
Surgery +/− radiation therapy			
Delarue [11]	1965	299	28
Fletcher [12]	1965	226	28
Zucali [10]	1976	133	45

Adapted from Hortobagyi [2]

Breast Cancer as a Systemic Disease

The concept of breast cancer as a systemic disease at its inception, consisting of both viable and dormant tumor cells, was promoted by Fisher and his colleagues in the 1960s [13]. This hypothesis was supported by results of the randomized trial NSABP B04, whose 25-year update continued to demonstrate no significant difference in disease-free or OS among women with lymph node-negative or node-positive disease, randomized to various local-regional therapies [14]. The hazard ratio (HR) for death among women with lymph node-negative disease was comparable between radical mastectomy vs. total mastectomy with radiation (1.08, 95%CI, 0.91–1.28) and radical mastectomy vs. total mastectomy without radiation (1.03, 95%CI, 0.87–1.23). The HR for death was also comparable when radical mastectomy was compared to total mastectomy with radiation for clinically lymph node-positive disease (1.06, 95%CI, 0.89–1.27). These results supported a biological basis for the systemic management of breast cancer which diverged from the anatomical principles proposed by Halstead [15].

Early clinical trials investigating the benefit of adjuvant chemotherapy administered after primary surgical treatment of operable breast cancer demonstrated significant improvements in disease-free survival (DFS) [16, 17]. The benefit of adjuvant chemotherapy varied based upon tumor burden, i.e., tumor size and axillary lymph node involvement, menopausal status, and estrogen receptor (ER) status [18]. These findings supported the theory of breast cancer tumor heterogeneity and divergent susceptibility of micrometastatic disease to chemotherapy [13]. Administering non-cross-resistant chemotherapy, both in combination and in sequence, functions to eradicate susceptible clones prior to their development of drug resistance and consequent metastasis. This approach does not consider the potential presence or detection of micrometastatic clones of breast cancer that possess a priori drug resistance, nor does it allow the identification of subsets of patients with highly sensitive disease that does not require aggressive systemic therapy.

The innate heterogeneity of breast cancer not only contributes to the therapeutic failure of systemic chemotherapy but also to directed targeted therapy and immunotherapy, given the interactions between the immune microenvironment of the host and the variation in tumor cells. The administration of adjuvant systemic therapy infers a belief that the treatment will be effective without immediate confirmation. Applying systemic therapy to an intact tumor (neoadjuvant), however, not only allows direct information about its susceptibility to treatment but also informs decisions on the need for subsequent management of the disease, including the modification of systemic therapy mid-treatment. This construct contributed to the broader application of neoadjuvant systemic therapy for patients not only with inoperable LABC but also earlier stage, operable disease.

Primary Systemic Therapy: Neoadjuvant Treatment

The concept of administering systemic chemotherapy preoperatively was developed almost simultaneously with the investigation of adjuvant chemotherapy for breast cancer. Initial studies applied neoadjuvant chemotherapy to patients with unresectable LABC with the therapeutic goal of converting the inoperable state of disease into one that was amenable to surgical resection. The additional benefit of neoadjuvant systemic therapy was the early dissemination of chemotherapy in the hope of eradicating micrometastatic disease in this high-risk population before cancer resistance develops [19].

Multiple studies evaluating the outcome of neoadjuvant chemotherapy demonstrated a substantial reduction in tumor volume in >50% of patients with LABC [20, 21]. This approach resulted in >70% of breast cancers being "downstaged," subsequently permitting standard local-regional treatment. A multimodality approach to stage III disease became acceptable in the early 1990s, with chemotherapy, surgery, and radiation considered to be the best therapeutic design.

Unlike the delayed acceptance of neoadjuvant therapy for non-inflammatory LABC, the use of neoadjuvant chemotherapy was promptly embraced for the treatment of inflammatory breast cancer (IBC). Historical series describe a 5-year overall survival (OS) of 1.5% when radical mastectomy alone was used to treat this disease [22]. The addition of radiation therapy with or without surgery improved local-regional disease control, but did not significantly impact OS, supporting the integration of neoadjuvant chemotherapy as primary treatment for IBC [10, 23]. Although the addition of neoadjuvant chemotherapy to radiation or surgery alone improved clinical outcomes, tri-modality therapy consisting of neoadjuvant systemic therapy, mastectomy, and radiation resulted in a significant improvement in overall survival, with 5- and 10-year rates equaling 55.4% and 37.3%, respectively [24–29] (Table 7.2). Current guidelines for IBC continue to support neoadjuvant

Table 7.2 Historical treatment of inflammatory breast cancer: supporting neoadjuvant systemic therapy

Study	No.	DFS	OS
Rouesse [26]		(4-yr)	(4-yr)
CT/RT/CT	170	32–54%	53–74%
RT	170	15%	42%
Fields [25]		(5-yr)	(5-yr)
CT/S/RT/CT	37	35%	44%
RT/CT	23	<10%	10%
Buzdar [24]		mDFS (mo)	mOS(mo)
CT/RT	32	22.8	30.1
RT (historical)	32	9	18
Rueth [29]		NA	(5-yr/10-yr)
CT/S/RT	6811		55.4%/37.3%
S	500		NA/16.5%
CT/S	2728		42.9%/28.5%
S/RT	158		40.7%/23.5%

No number, *DFS* disease-free survival, *OS* overall survival, *CT* chemotherapy, *S* surgery, *RT* radiation therapy, *yr* year, *mo* months, *mDFS* median disease-free survival, *mOS* median overall survival

therapy as the mainstay of treatment; however modified radical mastectomy followed by comprehensive radiation therapy continues to be the standard of care for local-regional disease control in this disease, regardless of the extent of clinical downstaging which may occur with optimal disease response to systemic therapy [30, 31].

Operable Breast Cancer: Benefits of Neoadjuvant Therapy

Neoadjuvant Therapy Facilitates Breast Conservation

The 20-year follow-up of NSABP B06 continued to support comparable survival among women with stage I or II breast cancer randomized to local therapy consisting of total mastectomy, lumpectomy, or lumpectomy with radiation [32]. NSABP B06 transformed the approach to the treatment of operable breast cancer and stimulated the development of future clinical trials using systemic therapy as a means of downstaging disease with the goal of achieving the ability to undergo breast-conserving surgery.

NSABP B18 was an early study which randomized 1523 women with operable breast cancer (T1-3, N1-0) to receive an identical chemotherapeutic regimen either prior to (neoadjuvant) or after surgery (adjuvant) with the objective of assessing the impact of neoadjuvant chemotherapy on clinical outcomes [33]. After 16 years of follow-up, there was no statistically significant difference in DFS or OS between the two chemotherapy schedules with HR of 0.99 (95%CI, 0.85–1.16; $P = .90$) and 0.93

(95%CI, 0.81–1.06; $P = .27$), respectively [34]. Multiple studies have confirmed these data, summarized by the Early Breast Cancer Trialists' Collaborative Group (EBCTCG) meta-analysis of individual patient data from 4756 women treated on clinical trials comparing clinical outcomes following neoadjuvant or adjuvant treatment of early-stage breast cancer from 1983 to 2002 [35]. No significant difference was found in 15-year distant disease recurrence rates (risk ratio (RR) = 1.02, 95%CI, 0.92–1.14; $P = .66$), breast cancer mortality (RR = 1.06, 95%CI, 0.95–1.18; $P = .31$), or death from any cause (RR = 1.04, 95%CI, 0.94–1.15; $P = .45$).

Given the comparable clinical outcomes when comparable chemotherapeutic regimens are administered prior to or after surgery, neoadjuvant therapy should be considered for early-stage breast cancer whenever the goal of treatment is to downstage the tumor and pursue de-escalation of surgery, i.e., breast conservation. Multiple studies have established the utility of neoadjuvant therapy in increasing the rate of breast conservation in operable breast cancer [36, 37]. NSABP B18 pioneered this approach by finding a greater number of women treated with lumpectomy and radiation therapy after neoadjuvant treatment compared with those who received adjuvant chemotherapy, 67.8% vs. 59.8%, respectively [33]. The EBCTCG confirmed an increased frequency of breast conservation when neoadjuvant therapy was given versus adjuvant treatment, 65% vs. 49%, respectively, with 33% of planned surgery converted from mastectomy to lumpectomy [35].

Neoadjuvant Therapy Downstages Axillary Lymph Node Disease

Complete axillary lymph node (ALND) dissection is associated with significant morbidity, including sensory deficits, lymphedema, limitation of arm movement, and a higher risk of infection [38]. Advances in surgical techniques have resulted in a de-escalation of axillary surgery so that sentinel lymph node (SLN) sampling has become the standard approach to the pathologic evaluation of the clinically node-negative axilla. Early studies supporting SLN sampling were associated with an accurate prediction of ALN status in 95.6–97.5% of cases where SLN sampling was followed by a completion ALN dissection [39–41]. Surgical morbidity was improved with the acceptance of SLN sampling, with less sensory loss, greater arm and shoulder function, reduced incidence of lymphedema, and an overall improvement in quality of life [42, 43]. More importantly, SLN sampling did not compromise clinical outcomes in lymph-node negative or positive breast cancer treated with primary surgery and radiation therapy [42, 44–46].

The receipt of neoadjuvant therapy not only results in reducing primary tumor size allowing the removal of less breast tissue and a higher frequency of negative surgical margins, but it also leads to effective clearing of nodal disease, converting positive to negative ALN [47, 48]. NSABP B18 showed a 16% increase in the number of patients with pathologic lymph node-negative disease after neoadjuvant therapy compared with the adjuvant therapy group [49]. This number increased by 6.9% with the administration of additional neoadjuvant chemotherapy in NSABP B27

[50]. The application of SLN sampling following neoadjuvant therapy was an anticipated next step in de-escalating surgery for early-stage breast cancer. Similar rates of identifying SLN are seen following neoadjuvant therapy compared with primary surgery among patients with clinically node-negative disease. A meta-analysis of 16 studies involving 1456 patients with clinically node-negative disease who received neoadjuvant therapy followed by SLN sampling confirmed the feasibility of this technique, with an identification rate of 96% and a false-negative rate of 6% [51].

Considering the data demonstrating significant downstaging of the axilla following neoadjuvant therapy, a natural extension of the acceptance of SLN sampling was in the exploration of performing this procedure for clinically node-positive disease after the completion of neoadjuvant therapy. Several clinical trials (ACOSOG Z1071, SENTINA, SN FNAC study, and GANEA2 study) confirmed downstaging to a pathologically node-negative status, but also established a satisfactory identification rate of SLN after neoadjuvant treatment: 92.7%, 80.1%, 87.6%, and 79.5%, respectively [52–55]. Improved techniques, such as dual tracer use and sampling a minimum of three SLN, have lowered the false-negative rate to <10%. Although a proportion of patients will have undetected micrometastatic nodal involvement, SLN post-neoadjuvant therapy is associated with an axillary recurrence rate of <2% [56, 57]. These studies stimulated a greater acceptance and use of neoadjuvant therapy with the goal of de-escalating surgery, i.e., greater ability to pursue breast conservation and SLN sampling.

Goal of Neoadjuvant Therapy: Complete Pathologic Response (pCR)

Improved Clinical Outcomes Associated with pCR

The use of neoadjuvant therapy eliminates the ability to utilize anatomic prognostic features of newly diagnosed breast cancer such as ALN involvement and tumor size. However, the tumor response from neoadjuvant therapy is a direct indication of therapeutic sensitivity, which can be used as a surrogate for disease prognosis [34]. The definition of complete pathologic response (pCR) has varied across clinical trials for neoadjuvant therapy making cross-trial comparisons of therapeutic efficacy challenging. The most rigorous criteria which discriminate favorable versus unfavorable clinical outcomes define pCR as the absence of invasive disease in the breast and ALN (ypT0/is, ypN0), and the presence of in situ disease in the breast (Tis) is allowed [58, 59].

Older studies not only differed in their definition of pCR, but clinical outcomes were not assessed based upon specific breast cancer subtypes, differentiated by hormone receptor (estrogen receptor (ER), progesterone receptor (PR)), and HER2 status. Recent data revealed a correlation between clinical outcomes and pCR rate most consistently seen in the HER2-positive and triple-negative (TN = ER negative,

PR negative, HER2 negative) subtypes [58–60]. A pooled analysis of 12 clinical trials involving neoadjuvant therapy administered to 11,955 patients with a wide range of clinical stages correlated longer event-free survival (EFS) and OS associated with a pCR [59]. Differences in pCR rates were seen among breast cancer subtypes, with the more proliferative subtypes, HER2 positive and TN, having higher rates compared with the hormone receptor-positive subtype. These subtypes also had a stronger association between pCR and OS with HR of 0.34 (95%CI, 0.24–0.47) and 0.16 (95%CI, 0.11–0.25), respectively, compared with the hormone receptor-positive subtype (HR = 0.49, 95%CI, 0.33–0.71). However, the prognostic strength of pCR was greater among the higher proliferative hormone receptor-positive subgroups, such as histologic grade 3 disease or ER and/or PR positive and HER2 positive (luminal B) [58, 59].

Optimizing Neoadjuvant Therapy: Use of Targets

Targeting HER2-Positive Disease

The NOAH trial was the first randomized trial evaluating the benefit of adding anti-HER2 blockade with trastuzumab to a standard neoadjuvant chemotherapy backbone for the treatment of LABC, IBC, and operable breast cancer [61]. The results demonstrated an increased ability to achieve a pCR (ypT0/is, ypN0) when targeted therapy, i.e., trastuzumab, was combined with chemotherapy versus chemotherapy alone, 87% vs. 55%, respectively. This translated into a statistically significant improvement in 5-year EFS with the addition of trastuzumab, 58% vs. 43% without trastuzumab (HR = 0.64, 95%CI 0.44–0.93; *P* = .016).

Since the NOAH trial was first published, several different classes of agents targeting HER2 have been developed, such as small molecule inhibitors (lapatinib, neratinib, tucatinib), drug antibody conjugates (trastuzumab emtansine (T-DM1), trastuzumab deruxtecan), and monoclonal antibodies against HER2 (trastuzumab, pertuzumab) [62]. This has led to the utilization of neoadjuvant studies as a mechanism to identify effective therapy against HER2-positive disease using pCR as a surrogate for prognosis and tumor response. The KRISTINE trial lends support to this method of exploring novel therapies, showing that regardless of which neoadjuvant treatment was administered to the 444 patients with stage II or III HER2-positive disease, a pCR (ypT0/is, ypN0) was associated with a decreased risk in invasive DFS (HR = 0.24, 95%CI, 0.09–0.60) [63].

Targeting Triple-Negative Disease

Unlike hormone receptor or HER2-positive disease, TN breast cancer has no known therapeutic target. In addition, TN disease is associated with a worse prognosis, not only due to limitations in treatment options available, i.e., chemotherapy alone, but also due to its underlying biology [64]. Given these two challenges, neoadjuvant therapy has been used to confirm disease response with pCR as a prognostic indicator. TN breast cancer is associated with a higher incidence of pCR following neoadjuvant chemotherapy resulting in comparable clinical outcomes to other subtypes if pCR is achieved [59, 65, 66].

Research in the underlying biology of this disease identified a *BRCA-ness* phenotype which is associated with deficiencies in DNA repair by homologous recombination [67, 68]. This led to an investigation of the clinical benefit of adding DNA-damaging agents, such as carboplatin, to standard neoadjuvant chemotherapy, and improving pCR rates, ranging from 6.7–60% to 3.3–46% with a non-platinum-containing regimen, respectively [69–71]. Although the addition of platinum-based neoadjuvant therapy results in higher rates of pCR, it is associated with greater toxicity and the effect on clinical outcomes remains mixed.

BRCA1 germline mutations are present in approximately 10% of TN breast cancers and convey an inherited deficiency in DNA repair by homologous recombination like that seen in the acquired *BRCA-ness* phenotype found in sporadic TN disease [72]. Neoadjuvant therapy provided the means to explore the potential benefit of non-chemotherapy regimens to treat BRCA-associated TN breast cancer. Talazoparib, a poly-adenosine diphosphate [ADP]-ribose polymerase (PARP) inhibitor, was administered as a single agent to a small number of patients ($n = 20$) with stage II or III BRCA-positive breast cancer, demonstrating a pCR rate of 53% overall and 57% in TN disease [73]. These results can be used to support larger clinical trials studying PARP inhibitors as a means of targeting early-stage TN breast cancer, without the need for chemotherapy.

Another potential therapeutic target that has been explored in TN breast cancer is the immune microenvironment. The presence of tumor-infiltrating lymphocytes (TILs) has been shown to be a favorable prognostic feature of TN breast cancer and supported subsequent investigation of immune checkpoint blockade to enhance chemotherapy efficacy [74, 75]. Several pivotal randomized clinical trials using anti-programmed death 1 (PD-1) inhibitors with chemotherapy in the neoadjuvant setting have resulted in 13.6–17% higher rates of pCR compared with standard chemotherapy [76, 77]. This has translated into improved EFS regardless of the presence of a marker for response, i.e., PD-L1 positivity. Although the challenge of identifying a subgroup of TN breast cancers best served by "targeted" therapies continues, neoadjuvant therapy in this high-risk patient population remains an important therapeutic strategy.

Targeting Hormone Receptor-Positive Disease

Hormone receptor-positive breast cancer is the most challenging subtype to treat with neoadjuvant therapy due to its lower frequency of downstaging in both the breast and ALN [50, 58, 59, 78]. There continues to be controversy concerning the optimal neoadjuvant therapy, i.e., chemotherapy versus endocrine therapy, which will result in the maximum pathological downstaging and pCR rate to warrant a change in the treatment paradigm for early-stage hormone receptor-positive disease which has traditionally favored adjuvant systemic therapy to neoadjuvant treatment.

In the adjuvant setting, genomic analysis can select patients with early-stage ER and/or PR-positive breast cancer who would benefit from chemotherapy in addition to endocrine therapy to reduce the risk of disease recurrence and increase overall survival [79–81]. Candidates for adjuvant chemotherapy as determined by genomic analysis may benefit from administering this treatment in the neoadjuvant setting, since this subgroup of hormone receptor-positive breast cancer falls into the more proliferative group (luminal B) where pCR has been shown to be predictive of clinical outcomes [58, 65]. Several studies have utilized genomic analysis performed on preoperative tumor biopsies to predict response to neoadjuvant chemotherapy and identify patients who would benefit from neoadjuvant chemotherapy followed by adjuvant endocrine therapy [82–85].

Conversely, genomic analysis performed on diagnostic biopsies may identify patients who could be treated with neoadjuvant endocrine therapy alone to downstage their disease, thus avoiding overtreatment with chemotherapy [86]. The TransNEOS study validated the use of the 21-gene test to predict response to neoadjuvant endocrine therapy among 295 postmenopausal patients with clinically node-negative disease [87]. Lower values of a 21-gene signature were associated with higher response rates with endocrine therapy resulting in 58% converting to breast conservation ($p = .009$). Refinements in the identification of subgroups within the 21-gene signature now include both node-negative and node-positive disease [80, 88, 89]. These results can be applied to the neoadjuvant setting not only to identify appropriate patients for neoadjuvant endocrine therapy but also to assist in the investigation of targeted therapies, such as CDK4/6 inhibitors and PIK3CA inhibitors combined with endocrine therapy in order to achieve greater disease response [90, 91].

Residual Disease Post-neoadjuvant Therapy Informs Adjuvant Treatment

Residual disease post-completion of neoadjuvant therapy is associated with an increased risk of disease relapse which varies among breast cancer subtypes [59]. For this reason, several investigators sought to improve clinical outcomes by modifying adjuvant treatment for those patients who did not achieve a pCR from neoadjuvant therapy. As in the neoadjuvant trials, these "post-neoadjuvant" studies are specific to each breast cancer subtype and identify a subset of patients who benefit from a modification of standard adjuvant therapies.

High-Risk Disease: Triple Negative and HER2 Positive

A meta-analysis of nine publications comparing neoadjuvant to adjuvant treatment among 36,480 patients with TN breast cancer found a significant benefit in OS when patients received neoadjuvant chemotherapy and achieved a pCR (HR = 0.53; 95%CI, 0.29–0.98; *P* = .04), whereas those with residual disease following neoadjuvant therapy fared poorly [92]. These results identified a patient population who would benefit from the addition of adjuvant therapy, since the standard of care was active observation regardless of pCR. The CREATE-X study involved the addition of six to eight cycles of capecitabine chemotherapy administered to patients with residual disease following neoadjuvant therapy [93]. In the subset of patients with the highest risk of disease relapse, i.e., those with triple-negative disease, the addition of adjuvant capecitabine resulted in a 13.7% improvement in 5-year DFS and an 8.5% improvement in OS compared with active observation. Similar treatment modifications were applied to HER2-positive disease in the KATHERINE trial which demonstrated an 11.3% improvement in 3-year invasive DFS and a 1.8% improvement in OS when T-DM1 was given as adjuvant maintenance anti-HER2 therapy compared with trastuzumab for patients who did not achieve a pCR from neoadjuvant therapy [94].

Hormone Receptor Positive

MonarchE focused on the approximately 30% of patients with high-risk hormone receptor-positive breast cancer who are at risk of disease recurrence and may benefit from targeted therapy with a CDK4/6 inhibitor added to standard endocrine therapy in the adjuvant setting [95]. Patients with high-risk disease, which included clinical stage prior to receiving neoadjuvant treatment, were randomized to standard adjuvant endocrine therapy with or without abemaciclib, a CDK4/6 inhibitor. The addition of abemaciclib for 2 years improved the 2-year invasive DFS by 3.5% which was statistically significant (HR = 0.75, 95%CI, 0.60–0.93, *P* = .01).

Who Should Receive Adjuvant Therapy Alone?

The use of neoadjuvant therapy is associated with the loss of initial prognostic indicators, such as pathologic stage, and thus there remains a risk of overtreating a segment of the breast cancer population if everyone was administered neoadjuvant therapy. Patients presenting with small tumors, T1a/T1b, have an excellent 5-year OS without adjuvant chemotherapy, with or without trastuzumab, exceeding 95% [96]. A prospective cohort study involving 4113 women from the NCCN Breast Cancer Outcomes Database, with node-negative, T1a/T1b disease demonstrated an

Table 7.3 Clinical outcomes in favorable breast cancer without neoadjuvant therapy

	T1a, N0		T1b, N0	
	No C or T	C w/wo T	No C	C w/wo T
Outcome	5-yr (%)	5-yr (%)	5-yr (%)	5 yr (%)
HR+/HER−	*N* = 972	*N* = 12	*N* = 2005	*N* = 241
OS	98	100	97	98
IDFS	93	96	91	95
HR+/HER2+	*N* = 102	*N* = 33	*N* = 89	*N* = 100
OS	95	100	95	99
IDFS	86	00	86	90
HR−/HER2+	*N* = 49	*N* = 32	*N* = 17	*N* = 88
OS	93	100	100	95
IDFS	84	89	68	94
TN	*N* = 74	*N* = 25	*N* = 94	*N* = 170
OS	94	100	91	96
IDFS	86	91	81	25

Adapted from Vaz-Luis [96]
C chemotherapy, *T* trastuzumab, *w/wo* with or without, *yr* year, *HR* hormone receptor, *OS* overall survival, *IDFS* invasive disease-free survival, *N* number, *TN* triple negative

excellent prognosis over a median follow-up of 5.5 years (Table 7.3). Among patients with TN breast cancer, the 5-year disease relapse-free survival (DRFS) was 93% and 90% for untreated T1a and T1b disease, respectively, and increased to 100% and 98% with treatment for the same respective tumor stage.

The Adjuvant Paclitaxel and Trastuzumab (APT) trial lent support for adjuvant therapy alone as systemic treatment for small, low-risk, HER2-positive breast cancer [97]. This phase II study involved 410 patients with HER2-positive disease measuring <3.0 cm, node negative, or microscopic node positive (N1mic), having completed primary surgical treatment. The receipt of 12 weeks of weekly paclitaxel with 1 year of trastuzumab resulted in a 93.3% (95%CI, 91.8–97.5) 7-year DFS and a 98.6% (95%CI, 97–100) 7-year breast cancer-specific survival (BCSS). These data support an adjuvant therapy approach to stage I and small stage II T1/T2 (N0/N1mic) HER2-positive breast cancer, resulting in excellent clinical outcomes and thus avoiding the potential for overtreatment if neoadjuvant therapy was offered.

Conclusion

The acceptance of neoadjuvant therapy for the treatment of breast cancer has evolved from historical criteria for inoperable disease to a more generalized approach involving several clinical objectives. Those patients with operable disease may benefit from downstaging their primary tumor to pursue breast-conserving surgery and/or clear ALN involvement allowing SLN sampling and limit potential surgical complications associated with complete ALN dissection. In addition to the surgical benefits of neoadjuvant therapy, this treatment modality can offer the ability to change systemic therapy midcourse if disease response is not seen and provide prognostic information based upon the amount of residual disease left at the time of surgery.

A more favorable cohort of patients who achieve a pCR following neoadjuvant treatment may not require aggressive adjuvant systemic therapy, whereas those with residual disease now have options for adjuvant treatment which will improve their clinical outcomes. Finally, neoadjuvant therapy affords the opportunity for clinical research of novel therapies in small numbers of patients, providing information about biologic activity, tumor response, and clinical efficacy.

For these reasons, neoadjuvant therapy is becoming the mainstay of treatment for early-stage breast cancer. However, there remains a subset of patients with small, highly favorable disease who can avoid overtreatment with neoadjuvant therapy by undergoing a standard surgical approach for their disease followed by minimal adjuvant therapy. Breast cancer treatment is rapidly evolving, and these guidelines may not be applicable in the future. If that is so, it will demonstrate advances in the treatment of this disease that provides even greater optimism.

References

1. Hortobagyi G, Connolly JL, D'Orsi C, Edge SB, Mittendorf EA, Rugo HS, et al. AJCC cancer staging manual. 8th ed. Chicago: The American College of Surgeons (ACS), Springer; 2017.
2. Hortobagyi G, Buzdar A. Locally advanced breast cancer: a review including the M.D. Anderson experience. In: Ragaz J, Ariel I, editors. High-risk breast cancer – therapy. Berlin: Springer; 1991. p. 382–415.
3. Davila E, Vogel CL. Management of locally advanced breast cancer (stage III): a review. Int Adv Surg Oncol. 1984;7:297–327.
4. Rubens RD, Armitage P, Winter PJ, Tong D, Hayward JL. Prognosis in inoperable stage III carcinoma of the breast. Eur J Cancer. 1977;13(8):805–11.
5. Wilson RE. Surgical management of locally advanced and recurrent breast cancer. Cancer. 1984;53(3 Suppl):752–7.
6. MacKay EN, Sellers AH. A prospective trial of the TNM classification of breast cancer by the regional cancer treatment centres in Ontario, 1960–1964. Int J Cancer. 1970;6(3):517–28.
7. Sicher K, Waterhouse JA. Evaluation of TNM classification of carcinoma of the breast. Br J Cancer. 1973;28(6):580–8.
8. Haagensen CD. Clinical classification of the stage of advancement of breast carcinoma. In: Haagensen CD, editor. Diseases of the breast. Philadelphia: Saunders; 1986. p. 851–63.
9. Langlands AO, Kerr GR, Shaw S. The management of locally advanced breast cancer by X-ray therapy. Clin Oncol. 1976;2(4):365–71.
10. Zucali R, Uslenghi C, Kenda R, Bonadonna G. Natural history and survival of inoperable breast cancer treated with radiotherapy and radiotherapy followed by radical mastectomy. Cancer. 1976;37(3):1422–31.
11. Delarue NC, Ash CL, Peters V, Fielden R. Preoperative irradiation in management of locally advanced breast cancer. Arch Surg. 1965;91(1):136–54.
12. Fletcher GH, Montague ED. Radical irradiation of advanced breast cancer. Am J Roentgenol Radium Therapy, Nucl Med. 1965;93:573–84.

13. Fisher B. Laboratory and clinical research in breast cancer--a personal adventure: the David A. Karnofsky memorial lecture. Cancer Res. 1980;40(11):3863–74.
14. Fisher B, Jeong JH, Anderson S, Bryant J, Fisher ER, Wolmark N. Twenty-five-year follow-up of a randomized trial comparing radical mastectomy, total mastectomy, and total mastectomy followed by irradiation. N Engl J Med. 2002;347(8):567–75.
15. Halsted W. The results of operations for the cure of cancer of the breast performed at the Johns Hopkins Hospital from June, 1889, to January, 1894. Ann Surg. 1894;20(5):497–555.
16. Bonadonna G, Brusamolino E, Valagussa P, Rossi A, Brugnatelli L, Brambilla C, et al. Combination chemotherapy as an adjuvant treatment in operable breast cancer. N Engl J Med. 1976;294(8):405–10.
17. Fisher B, Carbone P, Economou SG, Frelick R, Glass A, Lerner H, et al. 1-Phenylalanine mustard (L-PAM) in the management of primary breast cancer. A report of early findings. N Engl J Med. 1975;292(3):117–22.
18. Fisher B, Redmond C, Fisher ER. The contribution of recent NSABP clinical trials of primary breast cancer therapy to an understanding of tumor biology--an overview of findings. Cancer. 1980;46(4 Suppl):1009–25.
19. Goldie JH, Coldman AJ. A mathematic model for relating the drug sensitivity of tumors to their spontaneous mutation rate. Cancer Treat Rep. 1979;63(11–12):1727–33.
20. Hortobagyi GN. Multidisciplinary management of advanced primary and metastatic breast cancer. Cancer. 1994;74(1 Suppl):416–23.
21. Hortobagyi GN, Ames FC, Buzdar AU, Kau SW, McNeese MD, Paulus D, et al. Management of stage III primary breast cancer with primary chemotherapy, surgery, and radiation therapy. Cancer. 1988;62(12):2507–16.
22. Treves N. The inoperability of inflammatory carcinoma of the breast. Surg Gynecol Obstet. 1959;109(2):240–2.
23. Perez CA, Graham ML, Taylor ME, Levy JF, Mortimer JE, Philpott GW, et al. Management of locally advanced carcinoma of the breast. I Noninflammatory Cancer. 1994;74(1 Suppl):453–65.
24. Buzdar AU, Montague ED, Barker JL, Hortobagyi GN, Blumenschein GR. Management of inflammatory carcinoma of breast with combined modality approach – an update. Cancer. 1981;47(11):2537–42.
25. Fields JN, Perez CA, Kuske RR, Fineberg BB, Bartlett N. Inflammatory carcinoma of the breast: treatment results on 107 patients. Int J Radiat Oncol Biol Phys. 1989;17(2):249–55.
26. Rouesse J, Friedman S, Sarrazin D, Mouriesse H, Le Chevalier T, Arriagada R, et al. Primary chemotherapy in the treatment of inflammatory breast carcinoma: a study of 230 cases from the Institut Gustave-Roussy. J Clin Oncol. 1986;4(12):1765–71.
27. De Lena M, Zucali R, Viganotti G, Valagussa P, Bonadonna G. Combined chemotherapy-radiotherapy approach in locally advanced (T3b-T4) breast cancer. Cancer Chemother Pharmacol. 1978;1(1):53–9.
28. Jaiyesimi IA, Buzdar AU, Hortobagyi G. Inflammatory breast cancer: a review. J Clin Oncol. 1992;10(6):1014–24.
29. Rueth NM, Lin HY, Bedrosian I, Shaitelman SF, Ueno NT, Shen Y, et al. Underuse of trimodality treatment affects survival for patients with inflammatory breast cancer: an analysis of treatment and survival trends from the National Cancer Database. J Clin Oncol. 2014;32(19):2018–24.
30. Ueno NT, Espinosa Fernandez JR, Cristofanilli M, Overmoyer B, Rea D, Berdichevski F, et al. International consensus on the clinical management of inflammatory breast cancer from the Morgan Welch Inflammatory Breast Cancer Research Program 10th Anniversary Conference. J Cancer. 2018;9(8):1437–47.
31. NCCN clinical practice guidelines in oncology: breast cancer [Internet]. National Comprehensive Cancer Network (NCCN). [cited 12/06/20]. Available from: https://www.nccn.org/professionals/physician_gls/pdf/breast.pdf.

32. Fisher B, Anderson S, Bryant J, Margolese RG, Deutsch M, Fisher ER, et al. Twenty-year follow-up of a randomized trial comparing total mastectomy, lumpectomy, and lumpectomy plus irradiation for the treatment of invasive breast cancer. N Engl J Med. 2002;347(16):1233–41.
33. Fisher B, Bryant J, Wolmark N, Mamounas E, Brown A, Fisher ER, et al. Effect of preoperative chemotherapy on the outcome of women with operable breast cancer. J Clin Oncol. 1998;16(8):2672–85.
34. Rastogi P, Anderson SJ, Bear HD, Geyer CE, Kahlenberg MS, Robidoux A, et al. Preoperative chemotherapy: updates of National Surgical Adjuvant Breast and Bowel Project Protocols B-18 and B-27. J Clin Oncol. 2008;26(5):778–85.
35. Early Breast Cancer Trialists' Collaborative Group. Long-term outcomes for neoadjuvant versus adjuvant chemotherapy in early breast cancer: meta-analysis of individual patient data from ten randomised trials. Lancet Oncol. 2018;19(1):27–39.
36. van der Hage JA, van de Velde CJ, Julien JP, Tubiana-Hulin M, Vandervelden C, Duchateau L. Preoperative chemotherapy in primary operable breast cancer: results from the European Organization for Research and Treatment of Cancer trial 10902. J Clin Oncol. 2001;19(22):4224–37.
37. Golshan M, Loibl S, Wong SM, Houber JB, O'Shaughnessy J, Rugo HS, et al. Breast conservation after neoadjuvant chemotherapy for triple-negative breast cancer: surgical results from the BrighTNess randomized clinical trial. JAMA Surg. 2020;155(3):e195410.
38. Warmuth MA, Bowen G, Prosnitz LR, Chu L, Broadwater G, Peterson B, et al. Complications of axillary lymph node dissection for carcinoma of the breast: a report based on a patient survey. Cancer. 1998;83(7):1362–8.
39. Veronesi U, Paganelli G, Galimberti V, Viale G, Zurrida S, Bedoni M, et al. Sentinel-node biopsy to avoid axillary dissection in breast cancer with clinically negative lymph-nodes. Lancet. 1997;349(9069):1864–7.
40. Krag D, Weaver D, Ashikaga T, Moffat F, Klimberg VS, Shriver C, et al. The sentinel node in breast cancer--a multicenter validation study. N Engl J Med. 1998;339(14):941–6.
41. Giuliano AE, Kirgan DM, Guenther JM, Morton DL. Lymphatic mapping and sentinel lymphadenectomy for breast cancer. Ann Surg. 1994;220(3):391–8; discussion 8–401.
42. Mansel RE, Fallowfield L, Kissin M, Goyal A, Newcombe RG, Dixon JM, et al. Randomized multicenter trial of sentinel node biopsy versus standard axillary treatment in operable breast cancer: the ALMANAC Trial. J Natl Cancer Inst. 2006;98(9):599–609.
43. Veronesi U, Paganelli G, Viale G, Luini A, Zurrida S, Galimberti V, et al. A randomized comparison of sentinel-node biopsy with routine axillary dissection in breast cancer. N Engl J Med. 2003;349(6):546–53.
44. Langer I, Guller U, Viehl CT, Moch H, Wight E, Harder F, et al. Axillary lymph node dissection for sentinel lymph node micrometastases may be safely omitted in early-stage breast cancer patients: long-term outcomes of a prospective study. Ann Surg Oncol. 2009;16(12):3366–74.
45. Galimberti V, Cole BF, Zurrida S, Viale G, Luini A, Veronesi P, et al. Axillary dissection versus no axillary dissection in patients with sentinel-node micrometastases (IBCSG 23-01): a phase 3 randomised controlled trial. Lancet Oncol. 2013;14(4):297–305.
46. Giuliano AE, Hunt KK, Ballman KV, Beitsch PD, Whitworth PW, Blumencranz PW, et al. Axillary dissection vs no axillary dissection in women with invasive breast cancer and sentinel node metastasis: a randomized clinical trial. JAMA. 2011;305(6):569–75.
47. Woeste MR, Bhutiani N, Donaldson M, McMasters KM, Ajkay N. Evaluating the effect of neoadjuvant chemotherapy on surgical outcomes after breast conserving surgery. J Surg Oncol. 2021;123(2):439–45.
48. Weiss A, Wong S, Golshan M, Freedman RA, Metzger O, Bellon J, et al. Patterns of axillary management in stages 2 and 3 hormone receptor-positive breast cancer by initial treatment approach. Ann Surg Oncol. 2019;26(13):4326–36.
49. Fisher B, Brown A, Mamounas E, Wieand S, Robidoux A, Margolese RG, et al. Effect of preoperative chemotherapy on local-regional disease in women with operable breast cancer: findings from National Surgical Adjuvant Breast and Bowel Project B-18. J Clin Oncol. 1997;15(7):2483–93.

50. Bear HD, Anderson S, Brown A, Smith R, Mamounas EP, Fisher B, et al. The effect on tumor response of adding sequential preoperative docetaxel to preoperative doxorubicin and cyclophosphamide: preliminary results from National Surgical Adjuvant Breast and Bowel Project Protocol B-27. J Clin Oncol. 2003;21(22):4165–74.
51. Geng C, Chen X, Pan X, Li J. The feasibility and accuracy of sentinel lymph node biopsy in initially clinically node-negative breast cancer after neoadjuvant chemotherapy: a systematic review and meta-analysis. PLoS One. 2016;11(9):e0162605.
52. Classe JM, Loaec C, Gimbergues P, Alran S, de Lara CT, Dupre PF, et al. Sentinel lymph node biopsy without axillary lymphadenectomy after neoadjuvant chemotherapy is accurate and safe for selected patients: the GANEA 2 study. Breast Cancer Res Treat. 2019;173(2):343–52.
53. Boileau JF, Poirier B, Basik M, Holloway CM, Gaboury L, Sideris L, et al. Sentinel node biopsy after neoadjuvant chemotherapy in biopsy-proven node-positive breast cancer: the SN FNAC study. J Clin Oncol. 2015;33(3):258–64.
54. Kuehn T, Bauerfeind I, Fehm T, Fleige B, Hausschild M, Helms G, et al. Sentinel-lymph-node biopsy in patients with breast cancer before and after neoadjuvant chemotherapy (SENTINA): a prospective, multicentre cohort study. Lancet Oncol. 2013;14(7):609–18.
55. Boughey JC, Suman VJ, Mittendorf EA, Ahrendt GM, Wilke LG, Taback B, et al. Sentinel lymph node surgery after neoadjuvant chemotherapy in patients with node-positive breast cancer: the ACOSOG Z1071 (Alliance) clinical trial. JAMA. 2013;310(14):1455–61.
56. Piltin MA, Hoskin TL, Day CN, Davis J Jr, Boughey JC. Oncologic outcomes of sentinel lymph node surgery after neoadjuvant chemotherapy for node-positive breast cancer. Ann Surg Oncol. 2020;27(12):4795–801.
57. El Hage Chehade H, Headon H, El Tokhy O, Heeney J, Kasem A, Mokbel K. Is sentinel lymph node biopsy a viable alternative to complete axillary dissection following neoadjuvant chemotherapy in women with node-positive breast cancer at diagnosis? An updated meta-analysis involving 3,398 patients. Am J Surg. 2016;212(5):969–81.
58. von Minckwitz G, Untch M, Blohmer JU, Costa SD, Eidtmann H, Fasching PA, et al. Definition and impact of pathologic complete response on prognosis after neoadjuvant chemotherapy in various intrinsic breast cancer subtypes. J Clin Oncol. 2012;30(15):1796–804.
59. Cortazar P, Zhang L, Untch M, Mehta K, Costantino JP, Wolmark N, et al. Pathological complete response and long-term clinical benefit in breast cancer: the CTNeoBC pooled analysis. Lancet. 2014;384(9938):164–72.
60. Boughey JC, Ballman KV, McCall LM, Mittendorf EA, Symmans WF, Julian TB, et al. Tumor biology and response to chemotherapy impact breast cancer-specific survival in node-positive breast cancer patients treated with neoadjuvant chemotherapy: long-term follow-up from ACOSOG Z1071 (Alliance). Ann Surg. 2017;266(4):667–76.
61. Gianni L, Eiermann W, Semiglazov V, Lluch A, Tjulandin S, Zambetti M, et al. Neoadjuvant and adjuvant trastuzumab in patients with HER2-positive locally advanced breast cancer (NOAH): follow-up of a randomised controlled superiority trial with a parallel HER2-negative cohort. Lancet Oncol. 2014;15(6):640–7.
62. Patel A, Unni N, Peng Y. The changing paradigm for the treatment of HER2-positive breast cancer. Cancers (Basel). 2020;12(8):2081.
63. Hurvitz SA, Martin M, Jung KH, Huang CS, Harbeck N, Valero V, et al. Neoadjuvant trastuzumab emtansine and pertuzumab in human epidermal growth factor receptor 2-positive breast cancer: three-year outcomes from the phase III KRISTINE study. J Clin Oncol. 2019;37(25):2206–16.
64. Dent R, Trudeau M, Pritchard KI, Hanna WM, Kahn HK, Sawka CA, et al. Triple-negative breast cancer: clinical features and patterns of recurrence. Clin Cancer Res. 2007;13(15 Pt 1):4429–34.
65. Chaudhary LN, Wilkinson KH, Kong A. Triple-negative breast cancer: who should receive neoadjuvant chemotherapy? Surg Oncol Clin N Am. 2018;27(1):141–53.

66. Carey LA, Dees EC, Sawyer L, Gatti L, Moore DT, Collichio F, et al. The triple negative paradox: primary tumor chemosensitivity of breast cancer subtypes. Clin Cancer Res. 2007;13(8):2329–34.
67. Turner N, Tutt A, Ashworth A. Hallmarks of 'BRCAness' in sporadic cancers. Nat Rev Cancer. 2004;4(10):814–9.
68. Nanda R. "Targeting" triple-negative breast cancer: the lessons learned from BRCA1-associated breast cancers. Semin Oncol. 2011;38(2):254–62.
69. Sikov WM, Berry DA, Perou CM, Singh B, Cirrincione CT, Tolaney SM, et al. Impact of the addition of carboplatin and/or bevacizumab to neoadjuvant once-per-week paclitaxel followed by dose-dense doxorubicin and cyclophosphamide on pathologic complete response rates in stage II to III triple-negative breast cancer: CALGB 40603 (Alliance). J Clin Oncol. 2015;33(1):13–21.
70. Dieci MV, Del Mastro L, Cinquini M, Montemurro F, Biganzoli L, Cortesi L, et al. Inclusion of platinum agents in neoadjuvant chemotherapy regimens for triple-negative breast cancer patients: development of GRADE (Grades of Recommendation, Assessment, Development and Evaluation) Recommendation by the Italian Association of Medical Oncology (AIOM). Cancers (Basel). 2019;11(8):1137.
71. Pandy JGP, Balolong-Garcia JC, Cruz-Ordinario MVB, Que FVF. Triple negative breast cancer and platinum-based systemic treatment: a meta-analysis and systematic review. BMC Cancer. 2019;19(1):1065.
72. Couch FJ, Hart SN, Sharma P, Toland AE, Wang X, Miron P, et al. Inherited mutations in 17 breast cancer susceptibility genes among a large triple-negative breast cancer cohort unselected for family history of breast cancer. J Clin Oncol. 2015;33(4):304–11.
73. Litton JK, Scoggins ME, Hess KR, Adrada BE, Murthy RK, Damodaran S, et al. Neoadjuvant talazoparib for patients with operable breast cancer with a germline BRCA pathogenic variant. J Clin Oncol. 2020;38(5):388–94.
74. Denkert C, von Minckwitz G, Darb-Esfahani S, Lederer B, Heppner BI, Weber KE, et al. Tumour-infiltrating lymphocytes and prognosis in different subtypes of breast cancer: a pooled analysis of 3771 patients treated with neoadjuvant therapy. Lancet Oncol. 2018;19(1):40–50.
75. Hida AI, Watanabe T, Sagara Y, Kashiwaba M, Sagara Y, Aogi K, et al. Diffuse distribution of tumor-infiltrating lymphocytes is a marker for better prognosis and chemotherapeutic effect in triple-negative breast cancer. Breast Cancer Res Treat. 2019;178(2):283–94.
76. Schmid P, Cortes J, Pusztai L, McArthur H, Kummel S, Bergh J, et al. Pembrolizumab for early triple-negative breast cancer. N Engl J Med. 2020;382(9):810–21.
77. Mittendorf EA, Zhang H, Barrios CH, Saji S, Jung KH, Hegg R, et al. Neoadjuvant atezolizumab in combination with sequential nab-paclitaxel and anthracycline-based chemotherapy versus placebo and chemotherapy in patients with early-stage triple-negative breast cancer (IMpassion031): a randomised, double-blind, phase 3 trial. Lancet. 2020;396(10257):1090–100.
78. Livingston-Rosanoff D, Schumacher J, Vande Walle K, Stankowski-Drengler T, Greenberg CC, Neuman H, et al. Does tumor size predict response to neoadjuvant chemotherapy in the modern era of biologically driven treatment? A nationwide study of US breast cancer patients. Clin Breast Cancer. 2019;19(6):e741–e7.
79. Paik S, Tang G, Shak S, Kim C, Baker J, Kim W, et al. Gene expression and benefit of chemotherapy in women with node-negative, estrogen receptor-positive breast cancer. J Clin Oncol. 2006;24(23):3726–34.
80. Sparano JA, Gray RJ, Makower DF, Pritchard KI, Albain KS, Hayes DF, et al. Adjuvant chemotherapy guided by a 21-gene expression assay in breast cancer. N Engl J Med. 2018;379(2):111–21.
81. Cardoso F, van't Veer LJ, Bogaerts J, Slaets L, Viale G, Delaloge S, et al. 70-gene signature as an aid to treatment decisions in early-stage breast cancer. N Engl J Med. 2016;375(8):717–29.
82. Pease AM, Riba LA, Gruner RA, Tung NM, James TA. Oncotype DX((R)) recurrence score as a predictor of response to neoadjuvant chemotherapy. Ann Surg Oncol. 2019;26(2):366–71.

83. Bear HD, Wan W, Robidoux A, Rubin P, Limentani S, White RL Jr, et al. Using the 21-gene assay from core needle biopsies to choose neoadjuvant therapy for breast cancer: a multicenter trial. J Surg Oncol. 2017;115(8):917–23.
84. Prat A, Galvan P, Jimenez B, Buckingham W, Jeiranian HA, Schaper C, et al. Prediction of response to neoadjuvant chemotherapy using core needle biopsy samples with the prosigna assay. Clin Cancer Res. 2016;22(3):560–6.
85. Soliman H, Wagner S, Flake DD 2nd, Robson M, Schwartzberg L, Sharma P, et al. Evaluation of the 12-gene molecular score and the 21-gene recurrence score as predictors of response to neo-adjuvant chemotherapy in estrogen receptor-positive, HER2-negative breast cancer. Ann Surg Oncol. 2020;27(3):765–71.
86. Kantor O, Barrera E, Kopkash K, Pesce C, Barrera E, Winchester DJ, et al. Are we over-treating hormone receptor positive breast cancer with neoadjuvant chemotherapy? Role of OncotypeDx((R)) for hormone receptor positive patients undergoing neoadjuvant chemotherapy. Ann Surg Oncol. 2019;26(10):3232–9.
87. Iwata H, Masuda N, Yamamoto Y, Fujisawa T, Toyama T, Kashiwaba M, et al. Validation of the 21-gene test as a predictor of clinical response to neoadjuvant hormonal therapy for ER+, HER2-negative breast cancer: the TransNEOS study. Breast Cancer Res Treat. 2019;173(1):123–33.
88. Ramsey SD, Barlow WE, Gonzalez-Angulo AM, Tunis S, Baker L, Crowley J, et al. Integrating comparative effectiveness design elements and endpoints into a phase III, randomized clinical trial (SWOG S1007) evaluating oncotypeDX-guided management for women with breast cancer involving lymph nodes. Contemp Clin Trials. 2013;34(1):1–9.
89. Andre F, Ismaila N, Henry NL, Somerfield MR, Bast RC, Barlow W, et al. Use of biomarkers to guide decisions on adjuvant systemic therapy for women with early-stage invasive breast cancer: ASCO clinical practice guideline update-integration of results from TAILORx. J Clin Oncol. 2019;37(22):1956–64.
90. Cottu P, D'Hondt V, Dureau S, Lerebours F, Desmoulins I, Heudel PE, et al. Letrozole and palbociclib versus chemotherapy as neoadjuvant therapy of high-risk luminal breast cancer. Ann Oncol. 2018;29(12):2334–40.
91. Saura C, Hlauschek D, Oliveira M, Zardavas D, Jallitsch-Halper A, de la Pena L, et al. Neoadjuvant letrozole plus taselisib versus letrozole plus placebo in postmenopausal women with oestrogen receptor-positive, HER2-negative, early-stage breast cancer (LORELEI): a multicentre, randomised, double-blind, placebo-controlled, phase 2 trial. Lancet Oncol. 2019;20(9):1226–38.
92. Xia LY, Hu QL, Zhang J, Xu WY, Li XS. Survival outcomes of neoadjuvant versus adjuvant chemotherapy in triple-negative breast cancer: a meta-analysis of 36,480 cases. World J Surg Oncol. 2020;18(1):129.
93. Masuda N, Lee SJ, Ohtani S, Im YH, Lee ES, Yokota I, et al. Adjuvant capecitabine for breast cancer after preoperative chemotherapy. N Engl J Med. 2017;376(22):2147–59.
94. von Minckwitz G, Huang CS, Mano MS, Loibl S, Mamounas EP, Untch M, et al. Trastuzumab emtansine for residual invasive HER2-positive breast cancer. N Engl J Med. 2019;380(7):617–28.
95. Johnston SRD, Harbeck N, Hegg R, Toi M, Martin M, Shao ZM, et al. Abemaciclib combined with endocrine therapy for the adjuvant treatment of HR+, HER2-, node-positive, high-risk, early breast cancer (monarchE). J Clin Oncol. 2020;38(34):3987–98.
96. Vaz-Luis I, Ottesen RA, Hughes ME, Mamet R, Burstein HJ, Edge SB, et al. Outcomes by tumor subtype and treatment pattern in women with small, node-negative breast cancer: a multi-institutional study. J Clin Oncol. 2014;32(20):2142–50.
97. Tolaney SM, Guo H, Pernas S, Barry WT, Dillon DA, Ritterhouse L, et al. Seven-year follow-up analysis of adjuvant paclitaxel and trastuzumab trial for node-negative, human epidermal growth factor receptor 2-positive breast cancer. J Clin Oncol. 2019;37(22):1868–75.

Chapter 8
Molecular Testing and Personalized Neoadjuvant Treatment

Adrienne Waks

Introduction

Neoadjuvant administration of systemic therapy in early-stage breast cancer offers many advantages. For all three major breast cancer subtypes, neoadjuvant treatment can accomplish downstaging of the breast and/or axilla, optimizing surgical outcome and minimizing surgical morbidity. For patients with human epidermal growth factor receptor 2 (HER2)-positive (HER2+) and triple-negative breast cancers, the extent of residual disease at surgery following neoadjuvant systemic therapy correlates strongly with long-term breast cancer outcomes [1]. Accordingly, the presence or absence of residual disease at surgery (following neoadjuvant chemotherapy, plus anti-HER2 therapy for those with HER2+ tumors) is used to tailor adjuvant therapy recommendations, with adjuvant treatment escalation recommended for patients with residual disease. For patients with hormone receptor (HR)-positive/HER2-negative (HR+/HER2−) breast cancers, the presence or absence of pCR following neoadjuvant chemotherapy is a less strong predictor of long-term outcomes [1], and thus, at present, extent of residual disease at surgery is not a standard consideration in adjuvant treatment planning.

Beyond the three standard markers that drive nearly all systemic therapy recommendations in breast cancer (estrogen receptor, ER; progesterone receptor, PR; and, HER2), there is enormous potential utility in identifying additional molecular markers to individualize treatments offered to each patient. Neoadjuvant treatment offers a unique opportunity for observation of tumor response while the primary breast tumor remains in place. Therefore, the neoadjuvant setting is an ideal platform for development of such individualized molecular biomarkers. Here, we discuss the

A. Waks (✉)
Department of Medical Oncology, Breast Oncology Program, Dana-Farber Cancer Institute, Boston, MA, USA
e-mail: adrienne_waks@dfci.harvard.edu

A. Soran, F. Nakhlis (eds.), *Management of the Breast and Axilla in the Neoadjuvant Setting*, https://doi.org/10.1007/978-3-030-88020-0_8

development of biomarkers that can help to predict neoadjuvant treatment responses in patients with HR+/HER2− breast cancer (genomic risk scores and Ki67 staining), the neoadjuvant role of DNA-damaging therapies (platinum chemotherapy and inhibitors of poly-(adenosine diphosphate [ADP]-ribose) polymerase (PARP)) and associated biomarkers of DNA damage repair capacity, and the ongoing investigation of CDK4/6 inhibitors and immune checkpoint blockade in neoadjuvant regimens.

Genomic Risk Scores and Neoadjuvant Therapy for Hormone Receptor-Positive/HER2-Negative Breast Cancer

Genomic Risk Score and Response to Neoadjuvant Chemotherapy

A central question in the management of all early-stage HR+/HER2− breast tumors is whether chemotherapy will add benefit beyond endocrine therapy. Genomic risk scores are metrics derived from breast tumor gene expression profiling that serve as both prognostic biomarkers, corresponding with long-term outcomes, and in some cases predictive biomarkers of chemotherapy benefit for HR+/HER2− tumors. The 21-gene Onco*type* DX recurrence score (Genomic Health, Redwood City, CA) and 70-gene MammaPrint assay (Agendia, Irvine, CA) are predictive biomarkers in broad clinical use to guide decision-making about the benefit of adjuvant chemotherapy for many patients with early-stage HR+/HER2− breast cancer. The large, randomized, prospective clinical trials TAILORx, MINDACT, and RxPONDER demonstrated the clinical utility of genomic risk scores for determination of adjuvant chemotherapy benefit [2–4].

While the bulk of high-quality data supports the use of genomic risk scores in the adjuvant, as opposed to the neoadjuvant, setting, the correlation of gene expression profiling or genomic risk score with pathologic complete response (pCR) following neoadjuvant chemotherapy has been shown across multiple cohorts. The 21-gene recurrence score is derived from expression of four main gene sets: an estrogen receptor (ER)-related set, a proliferation set, a HER2 set, and an invasion set. In a landmark early analysis of 89 patients (both ER+ and ER−) from Istituto Nazionale dei Tumori in Milan published in 2005, the authors showed a significant positive association between 21-gene recurrence score and likelihood of pCR after neoadjuvant paclitaxel and doxorubicin (Fig. 8.1a). Unsupervised analysis of the same cohort showed a correlation between gene expression related to three main biological processes and pCR: proliferation- and immune-related genes were positively correlated with likelihood of pCR, while ER-related genes were negatively correlated [5]. The ADAPT study led by the West German Study Group was the first large prospective clinical trial to demonstrate a statistically significant association between high 21-gene recurrence score (defined as score >25) and likelihood of pCR following neoadjuvant chemotherapy [6].

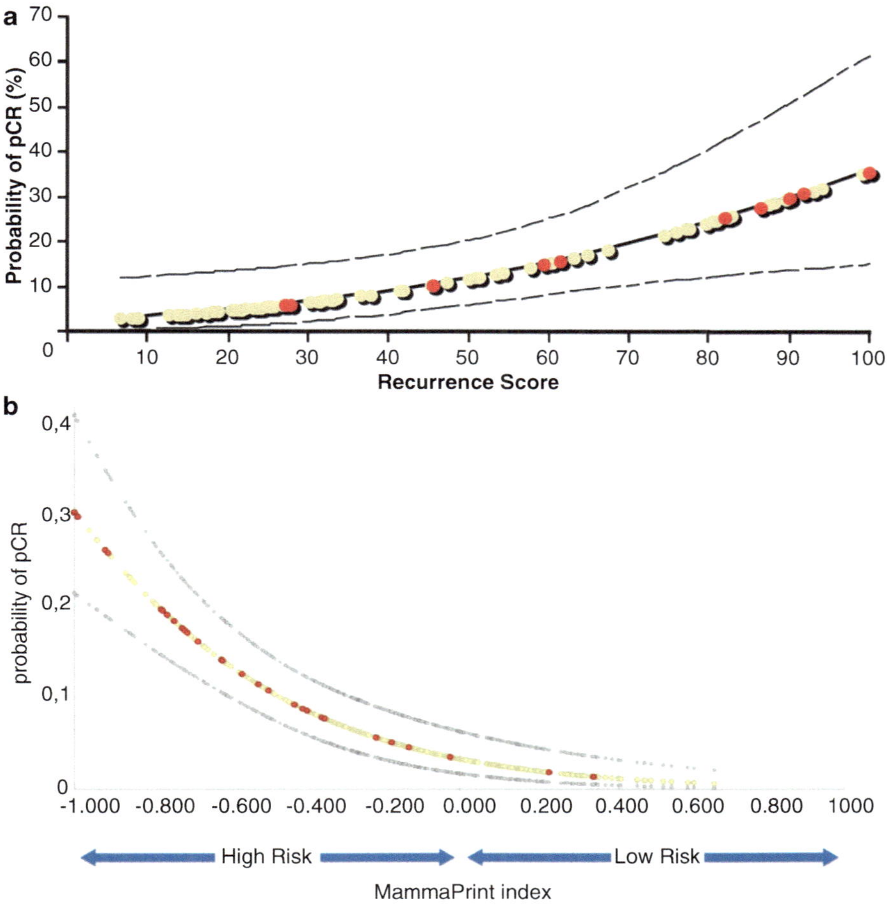

Fig. 8.1 (**a**) Probability of pathologic complete response (pCR; y-axis) and 21-gene recurrence score (x-axis) in the Insituto Nazionale dei Tumori-Milan cohort. Red circles represent patients who had pCR; yellow circles represent patients who did not have pCR. (Borrowed with permission from Gianni et al. [5]. https://pubmed.ncbi.nlm.nih.gov/16145055/ ©American Society of Clinical Oncology). (**b**) Probability of pathologic complete response (pCR; y-axis) and MammaPrint 70-gene recurrence score (x-axis) in the Neoadjuvant Breast Registry Symphony Trial cohort. Red circles represent patients who had pCR; yellow circles represent patients who did not have pCR. (Borrowed without modification from Whitworth et al. [8]. Link to the Creative Commons License: http://creativecommons.org/licenses/by/4.0/)

The role of the 21-gene recurrence score in predicting neoadjuvant chemotherapy response specifically within axillary lymph nodes has also been explored. A retrospective cohort study identified patients in the National Cancer Database with clinically lymph node-positive (cN1-N2) ER+/HER2− breast cancer who underwent 21-gene recurrence score testing and received neoadjuvant chemotherapy (N = 158). Patients were stratified into low (<18), intermediate (18–30), or high

(>31) recurrence score categories. The overall rate of axillary pCR was 14.6%. Axillary pCR rates among patients with low, intermediate, and high 21-gene recurrence scores were 10.7%, 9.7%, and 27.5%, respectively, which was a statistically significant correlation between higher 21-gene recurrence score and chance of achieving axillary pCR [7].

Like the 21-gene Onco*type* DX recurrence score, the 70-gene MammaPrint score has also been shown to correlate with likelihood of pCR to neoadjuvant chemotherapy. Among 405 patients with HR+/HER2− breast cancer who underwent 70-gene expression profiling and received neoadjuvant chemotherapy on the prospective Neoadjuvant Breast Registry Symphony Trial, a higher risk MammaPrint index was significantly associated with a higher chance of achieving pCR ($p < 0.001$; Fig. 8.1b). On this trial the overall pCR rate to neoadjuvant chemotherapy was 11%. Among patients with low-risk and high-print MammaPrint index, the pCR rates were 2% and 13%, respectively. Within the same cohort, intrinsic subtype determination (luminal type, HER2 type, or basal type; all tumors were HR+/HER2− by standard clinical testing) was performed using the 80-gene BluePrint gene profiling assay. pCR to neoadjuvant chemotherapy was significantly more likely among basal tumors (32% pCR rate) compared to luminal type (5% pCR rate) [8].

In summary, both retrospective and prospective data support higher genomic risk scores as a valid predictor of favorable response to neoadjuvant chemotherapy for HR+/HER2− breast cancers. However, the majority of data—including large, randomized, prospective trials incorporating over 15,000 patients—demonstrate the utility of genomic risk scores to guide chemotherapy decisions specifically in the adjuvant setting. Accordingly, the 2021 guidelines from the American Society of Clinical Oncology (ASCO) find that there is insufficient evidence to support using genomic risk scores when determining whether or not to use neoadjuvant chemotherapy [9]. In clinical practice, for patients with HR+/HER2− tumors who would benefit from downstaging prior to breast surgery, decisions must be made on a case-by-case basis in a multidisciplinary fashion.

Genomic Risk Score and Response to Neoadjuvant Endocrine Therapy

Separate from the question of how genomic risk scores may be used to predict response to neoadjuvant chemotherapy, which is aligned with these tests' main evidence-based role as predictors of long-term chemotherapy benefit, other analyses have sought to examine how genomic risk score may predict response to neoadjuvant endocrine therapy. The largest such effort is the TransNEOS study, a translational sub-cohort of the phase III New Primary Endocrine-Therapy Origination Study (NEOS) designed to investigate clinical response and surgical outcomes following 6 months of neoadjuvant letrozole on the basis of the 21-gene recurrence score. Of note, outside of a clinical trial, neoadjuvant endocrine therapy

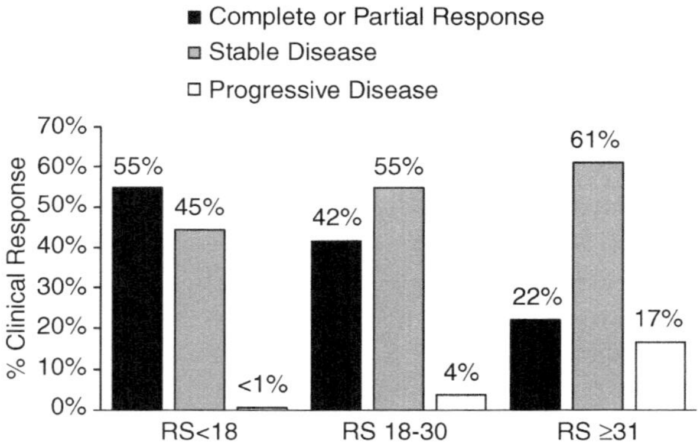

Fig. 8.2 Clinical responses to neoadjuvant letrozole according to 21-gene recurrence score in the TransNEOS study. (Borrowed without modification from Iwata et al. [10]. Link to the Creative Commons License: http://creativecommons.org/licenses/by/4.0/)

is standard only for postmenopausal women. TransNEOS evaluated 295 postmenopausal patients with ER+/HER2− clinically node-negative breast cancer. Recurrence score group (low, score <18; intermediate, score 18–30; high, score >31) was significantly associated with likelihood of clinical response to neoadjuvant letrozole. Patients with low, intermediate, and high recurrence scores experienced clinical response rates of 55%, 42%, and 22%, respectively (Fig. 8.2). There was also a significant difference in the risk of developing progressive disease on neoadjuvant hormonal therapy (<1% risk in patients with low recurrence score; 17% risk in patients with high recurrence score). Finally, patients with low recurrence score were significantly more likely than patients with high recurrence score to undergo breast-conserving surgery and more likely to experience a difference in posttreatment surgery received as opposed to pre-treatment surgery recommendation [10]. While these data are interesting and hypothesis-generating, it should be underscored that the important role of genomic risk scores is in predicting chemotherapy, not endocrine therapy, benefit.

Dynamic Testing of Ki67 to Guide Neoadjuvant Therapy for Hormone Receptor-Positive/HER2-Negative Breast Cancer

The proliferative protein Ki67 has been examined as a marker informing treatment decisions and long-term prognosis following neoadjuvant endocrine therapy. Dynamic measurement of Ki67 currently does not play a role in breast cancer treatment decisions outside of a clinical trial. However, it has been the focus of many completed and ongoing trials incorporating neoadjuvant endocrine therapy. One major advantage of Ki67 measurement as a prognostic tool is that it is more easily performed and much less expensive than genomic risk scores and therefore more widely available [11]. A low Ki67 value (<10%) measured in treatment-naïve HR+/HER2− correlates with better long-term breast cancer outcome [11]. When Ki67 is measured again following 2–4 weeks on neoadjuvant endocrine therapy, it serves as a metric of endocrine responsiveness (with greater suppression in Ki67 corresponding with greater endocrine sensitivity) and adds additional prognostic value to the baseline Ki67 measurement [11, 12]. Ki67 measurement is also incorporated into the Preoperative Endocrine Prognostic Index (PEPI), a validated prognostic marker calculated at surgery following (and while continuously on) neoadjuvant endocrine therapy, which is composed of pathologic stage, Ki67 level, and Allred score for ER expression. PEPI score of 0 (pT1/2, pN0, Ki67 <2.7%, and Allred ER score >2) correlates with a more favorable long-term breast cancer outcome compared to higher PEPI scores [12].

The prognostic value of dynamic Ki67 measurement during neoadjuvant endocrine therapy was well demonstrated in the POETIC trial (Peri-Operative Endocrine Therapy—Individualising Care) [11]. In this phase III trial, postmenopausal women with HR+ operable breast cancer were randomized to receive perioperative aromatase inhibitor for 2 weeks before and 2 weeks after surgery or no perioperative aromatase inhibitor. Ki67 was measured in breast tumor tissue at baseline and at surgery (i.e., 2 weeks following aromatase inhibitor initiation, if administered per randomization). At baseline, 33% of women with HR+/HER2− tumors ($N = 2235$) had low Ki67 (<10%) and 67% had high Ki67 (>10%). Women with low Ki67 at both baseline and following 2 weeks of aromatase inhibitor had the best long-term prognosis (4.3% 5-year breast cancer recurrence risk). Among women with high baseline Ki67, those with suppression of Ki67 following 2 weeks of aromatase inhibitor had significantly better long-term outcome than those with persistently high Ki67 following 2 weeks of aromatase inhibitor (8.4% vs. 21.5% 5-year recurrence rates, respectively). All patients in the POETIC trial were treated with standard adjuvant therapy according to United Kingdom Guidelines [11]. Overall, these data indicate that dynamic measurement of Ki67 can be used to assess endocrine therapy responsiveness following just 2 weeks of neoadjuvant exposure to aromatase inhibitor and carries prognostic significance.

Translating dynamic measurement of Ki67 into a biomarker guiding treatment decisions, specifically regarding which patients with HR+/HER2− breast tumors will benefit from chemotherapy, is a related area of active investigation. The ADAPT HR+/HER2− trial run by the West German Study Group enrolled pre- and post-menopausal women with cT1-T4 and cN0-N3 HR+/HER2− non-metastatic breast cancer who were candidates for chemotherapy by conventional criteria. The incorporation of premenopausal women in this trial population is notable as the large majority of evidence supporting both neoadjuvant endocrine therapy and the associated dynamic measurement of Ki67 is from postmenopausal women only. In the neoadjuvant endocrine therapy portion of the ADAPT trial, all tumors were assessed for 21-gene recurrence score and Ki67 at baseline, patients then received 2–4 weeks of neoadjuvant endocrine therapy, and Ki67 staining was repeated. The primary endpoint of the trial was to compare 5-year invasive disease-free survival (iDFS) between two groups ($N = 2290$): patients with cN0-N1 tumors and baseline 21-gene recurrence score of 01–1 who received neo/adjuvant endocrine therapy only per protocol and patients with cN0-N1 tumors, baseline recurrence score of 12–25, and

Ki67 <10% after 2–4 weeks on neoadjuvant endocrine therapy, who received neo/adjuvant endocrine therapy only per protocol. Patients with Ki67 >10% at the 2- to 4-week timepoint were switched to neoadjuvant chemotherapy. In other words, Ki67 suppression on neoadjuvant endocrine therapy was used as a marker for endocrine sensitivity to allow omission of chemotherapy for patients with recurrence scores of 21–25. Approximately 30% of enrolled patients were premenopausal. The trial met its primary endpoint, demonstrating non-inferior 5-year iDFS for those patients with recurrence score 21–25 and Ki67 suppression on endocrine therapy, compared to patients with recurrence score 0–11 (92.6% vs 93.9% 5-year iDFS, respectively) [13]. Overall, these results support the concept that dynamic Ki67 measurement in the neoadjuvant setting may be an adequate proxy for endocrine therapy sensitivity and, therefore, can aid in selection of patients who can be treated with endocrine therapy alone. However, this cannot be definitively concluded from the ADAPT trial data as the exposure to chemotherapy was not randomized.

Two prospective trials have evaluated chemosensitivity for those patients who do not experience Ki67 suppression on short-term neoadjuvant endocrine therapy, given concern that such patients do not have optimally endocrine-sensitive disease. In the small prospective American College of Surgeons Oncology Group (ACOSOG) Z1031B trial, postmenopausal women with ER+ stage II or III breast cancer and Ki67 >10% following 2–4 weeks of neoadjuvant aromatase inhibitor were switched to treatment with neoadjuvant chemotherapy. The pCR rate for patients switched to chemotherapy in this manner was quite low (5.7%; 2/35 patients) [12]. The larger follow-up ALTERNATE trial accrued postmenopausal patients with ER+/HER2− non-metastatic breast cancer. All were initially treated with neoadjuvant anastrozole, fulvestrant, or the combination. Patients with persistently high Ki67 (>10%) following 4 or 12 weeks on neoadjuvant endocrine therapy were switched to neoadjuvant chemotherapy (N = 168). Confirming the results of the ACOSOG Z1031B trial, the pCR rate was low (4.8%), as was the rate of minimal residual disease (Residual Cancer Burden score of I; an additional 9.8% of patients) [14]. The less favorable prognosis of patients who do not experience Ki67 suppression on neoadjuvant endocrine therapy, combined with the lack of significant chemosensitivity in this group, makes them an ideal target population for investigation of novel therapies.

DNA Damage Repair Status to Guide Neoadjuvant Therapy

Deficiency in homologous recombination, a type of DNA repair process, is a hallmark of cancers associated with germline mutations in *BRCA1* and *BRCA2*. Cancers associated with germline loss of *BRCA1/2* are sensitive to PARP inhibition, which interrupts other cellular DNA damage repair processes. PARP inhibitors demonstrate activity and are Food and Drug Administration (FDA) approved for use in multiple metastatic cancers associated with germline *BRCA1/2* mutation, including ovarian, prostate, pancreas, and breast cancers. Even in the absence of *BRCA1/2* mutation, it has been recognized that a significant proportion of triple-negative breast cancers share hallmarks of homologous recombination deficiency (HRD) at the molecular level, raising the question of whether DNA-damaging therapies (platinum chemotherapy and PARP inhibitors) may be effective treatments for tumors with this disease biology. A small pilot trial published in 2010 initially demonstrated the clinical activity of neoadjuvant cisplatin for triple-negative breast tumors [15]. Since then, multiple prospective trials have explored the activity of platinum chemotherapy or PARP inhibition in the neoadjuvant setting for tumors associated with *BRCA1/2* mutation and for triple-negative breast cancer more broadly.

Neoadjuvant PARP Inhibitor Therapy

A pilot trial showed promising activity of the PARP inhibitor talazoparib for neoadjuvant treatment of patients with operable HER2-negative breast cancers associated with germline *BRCA1/2* mutation. In this very small cohort of 20 patients (15 with triple-negative breast cancer; five with HR+/HER2− breast cancer), 53% experienced pCR following 6 months of neoadjuvant daily oral talazoparib [16]. These impressive preliminary findings are now being further explored in a larger phase II trial (NCT03499353). The phase III randomized BrighTNess trial randomized patients with triple-negative breast cancer (*BRCA1/2*-wildtype and *BRCA1/2*-mutant) to neoadjuvant paclitaxel, neoadjuvant paclitaxel/carboplatin, or neoadjuvant paclitaxel/carboplatin/veliparib (a PARP inhibitor). All patients also received neoadjuvant adriamycin/cyclophosphamide (AC). pCR rate was not significantly different between the paclitaxel/carboplatin and paclitaxel/carboplatin/veliparib arms (58% vs. 53%, respectively), indicating no activity of neoadjuvant veliparib in this patient population [17]. There are many possible explanations for the discordant results between these two neoadjuvant trials, including the majority of *BRCA1/2*-wild-type patients in the BrighTNess population, addition of veliparib to a chemotherapy backbone in BrighTNess, and differential pharmacodynamic effects of veliparib versus talazoparib on PARP enzymes [16]. Further investigation of neoadjuvant PARP inhibition in breast tumors associated with *BRCA1/2* mutation is warranted and ongoing. At present it does not appear that these agents will play a role in the overall triple-negative breast cancer population.

Neoadjuvant Platinum Chemotherapy and Biomarkers of DNA Repair Deficiency

It is clear that the addition of a platinum agent to multiagent neoadjuvant chemotherapy regimens for triple-negative breast cancer increases the likelihood of pathologic complete response. In the Cancer and Leukemia Group B (CALGB) 40,603 trial, patients ($N = 443$) with stage II–III triple-negative breast cancer were randomized to receive carboplatin or no carboplatin added to a neoadjuvant chemotherapy backbone of AC and paclitaxel (AC-T). The addition of carboplatin led to significant improvement in pCR rate (54% vs. 41% pCR rate with and without carboplatin, respectively; $p = 0.0029$) [18]. In the GeparSixto trial, a similar population of triple-negative breast cancer patients ($N = 315$) was randomized to receive carboplatin or no carboplatin with a backbone of neoadjuvant paclitaxel, non-pegylated liposomal doxorubicin, and bevacizumab. This cohort also demonstrated significant improvement in pCR with the addition of neoadjuvant carboplatin (53.2% vs. 42.7% pCR rate with and without carboplatin, respectively; $p = 0.015$) [19]. pCR in all cases referenced here indicates ypT0/isN0.

While the addition of a platinum agent to multiagent neoadjuvant chemotherapy for triple-negative breast cancer can facilitate a better response at the time of surgery, uncertainty remains regarding whether the addition of neoadjuvant platinum improves long-term breast cancer outcomes. In CALGB 40603, carboplatin did not improve 3-year event-free survival, whereas in GeparSixto, carboplatin significantly improved disease-free survival [20, 21]. The use of a nonstandard chemotherapy backbone in GeparSixto and the fact that CALGB 40603 was underpowered to assess event-free survival mean that uncertainty remains around a role for carboplatin in improving long-term outcomes in triple-negative breast cancers.

Following from the observation that the DNA-damaging platinum agents demonstrate activity in neoadjuvant therapy of triple-negative breast cancers, possibly due in part to these tumors' deficient DNA repair abilities, Translational Breast Cancer Research Consortium (TBCRC) 030 was a prospective phase II study evaluating whether homologous recombination deficiency (HRD) was a predictive biomarker for response to neoadjuvant chemotherapy (single-agent cisplatin or paclitaxel) in triple-negative tumors. HRD (Myriad Genetics, Inc.) is a sequencing-based assay that quantifies genomic instability, with preliminary retrospective data suggesting that HRD-high status correlated with favorable response to neoadjuvant platinum-containing chemotherapy regimens. Nearly all patients in the TBCRC 030 trial were germline *BRCA1/2* wild type, as the intent was to evaluate the HRD biomarker in the broader TNBC population. 71.1% of tumors were HRD-high. The pCR rate was 15.3% with 12 weeks of single-agent cisplatin and 11.9% with 12 weeks of single-agent paclitaxel. HRD-high status showed no significant correlation with pathologic response to either chemotherapy agent [22]. Evaluation of the same HRD biomarker in secondary analyses of the GeparSixto and BrighTNess trials also showed no interaction between HRD status and platinum benefit [21, 23]. Thus, the HRD biomarker should not play a role in selection of neoadjuvant platinum chemotherapy for triple-negative breast cancer patients.

A consistent role for neoadjuvant platinum chemotherapy specifically among patients with germline *BRCA1/2* mutations also has not been demonstrated. In the prospective phase II INFORM trial (TBCRC 031), patients with *BRCA1/2*-associated breast cancers were randomized to either neoadjuvant cisplatin or neoadjuvant AC, with a primary objective of comparing pCR rates between the two arms. The study population ($N = 117$) included both triple-negative and HR+/

HER2− breast cancers. Neoadjuvant cisplatin did not significantly improve pCR rates compared to AC in this cohort (18% pCR rate vs. 26% pCR rate for patients treated with neoadjuvant cisplatin or AC, respectively). The finding of numerically higher pCR rates with AC was consistent across the overall study population, participants with triple-negative tumors, and participants with HR+/HER2− tumors [24]. A secondary analysis of the GeparSixto trial evaluated whether germline *BRCA1/2* mutation affects the benefit of neoadjuvant carboplatin. In this substudy population ($N = 291$), 17.2% of patients harbored a germline *BRCA1/2* mutation. With the non-carboplatin-containing neoadjuvant chemotherapy regimen, patients with *BRCA1/2*-associated tumors were more likely to experience pCR compared to patients with *BRCA1/2* wild-type germline status. The addition of neoadjuvant carboplatin led to increased pCR rates among *BRCA1/2*-wild-type patients, but not among *BRCA1/2*-mutant patients [25]. These data argue against enhanced clinical activity of neoadjuvant platinum chemotherapy for patients with *BRCA1/2* mutations.

In summary, neoadjuvant platinum clearly improves pathologic responses in triple-negative breast cancer, but whether it impacts long-term outcome remains under investigation. Despite preliminary data suggesting that HRD or *BRCA1/2* mutational status could be predictive biomarkers of response to neoadjuvant platinum, this has not been borne out by the prospective data to date.

Evolving Neoadjuvant Treatment Strategies

Neoadjuvant CDK4/6 Inhibition in HR+/HER2− Breast Cancer

Given the need to identify more tools for downstaging HR+/HER2− breast tumors in the neoadjuvant setting, as well as the enormous benefit of inhibiting cyclin-dependent kinase 4 and 6 (CDK4/6) in the treatment of metastatic HR+/HER2− breast cancer, the activity of CDK4/6 inhibitors has been investigated in the neoadjuvant setting. Trials have consistently shown that the addition of a CDK4/6 inhibitor to neoadjuvant aromatase inhibitor significantly increases the suppression of Ki67 in on-treatment biopsies [26–28]. However, the addition of CDK4/6 inhibitor to neoadjuvant endocrine therapy has not been shown to increase clinical response rates or to facilitate increased rates of breast-conserving surgery. In the randomized phase II PALLET trial, 307 postmenopausal women with operable ER+/HER2− breast cancer were randomized to receive neoadjuvant treatment with letrozole alone or letrozole plus palbociclib for 14–16 weeks. Clinical response rates to the neoadjuvant regimen were 49.5% versus 54.4% for letrozole by itself or combined with palbociclib, respectively ($p = 0.20$ for comparison). The percentage of patients who converted from mastectomy to breast-conserving surgery candidates was the same across the two groups [26]. The reason that CDK4/6 inhibitors do not seem to improve clinical response when administered with endocrine therapy in the neoadjuvant setting, while consistently improving overall response rates in the metastatic setting, remains an unresolved question. At present there is no indication for neoadjuvant administration of a CDK4/6 inhibitor outside of a clinical trial.

Neoadjuvant Immune Checkpoint Inhibition in Triple-Negative Breast Cancer

Antibody drugs targeting the immune checkpoint proteins programmed cell death 1 (PD-1) and programmed cell death ligand 1 (PD-L1) have demonstrated efficacy in combination with chemotherapy in metastatic triple-negative breast cancer, leading to their FDA approval for use in the metastatic setting. Two large, randomized, phase III trials have also shown clinical activity of PD-1/PD-L1 inhibitors when added to chemotherapy in the neoadjuvant setting for triple-negative breast cancer, though follow-up remains immature to assess the agents' impact on event-free survival (EFS). The IMpassion031 trial randomized patients with stage II–III triple-negative breast cancer to neoadjuvant therapy with nab-paclitaxel followed by AC, with anti-PD-L1 antibody atezolizumab or placebo. Pathologic complete response (the primary endpoint of the trial) was observed in 58% versus 41% of patients in the atezolizumab and placebo arms, respectively, reaching the threshold for a statistically significant difference ($p = 0.0044$). Improvement in pCR rate with the addition of atezolizumab was seen in both PD-L1-positive and PD-L1-negative tumors (Fig. 8.3) [29], an interesting contrast to what is observed in the metastatic

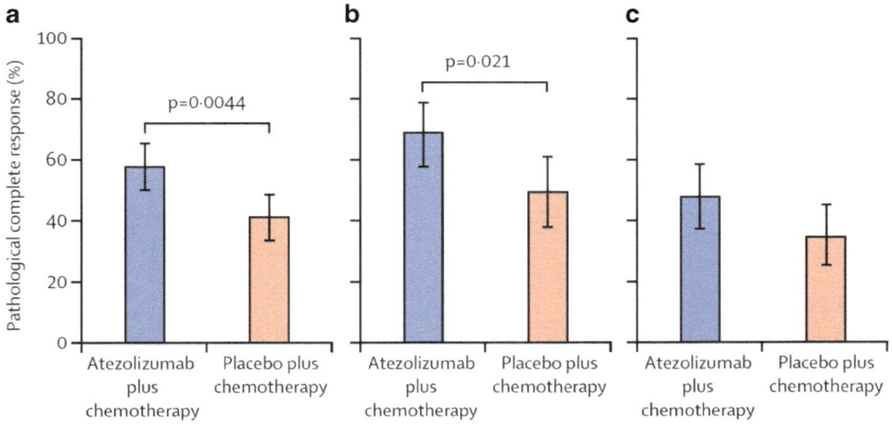

Fig. 8.3 Pathological complete response based on PD-L1 status in the IMpassion031 trial of atezolizumab or placebo in combination with standard neoadjuvant multiagent chemotherapy for triple-negative breast cancer. (**a**) All randomized population and PD-L1 population; (**b**) PD-L1-positive population; (**c**) PD-L1-negative population. Statistical comparison between the two groups was not performed in the PD-L1-negative population. (Reprinted from Mittendorf et al. [29]. Copyright 2020, with permission from Elsevier)

triple-negative breast cancer setting, where benefit of adding checkpoint inhibitor to chemotherapy is limited to patients with PD-L1-positive cancers [30, 31]. The KEYNOTE-522 trial randomized patients with stage II–III triple-negative breast cancer to neoadjuvant treatment with paclitaxel and carboplatin followed by AC with anti-PD-1 antibody pembrolizumab or placebo. As in IMpassion031, pCR rate was higher with the addition of pembrolizumab compared to placebo (64.8% vs. 51.2%, respectively, $p < 0.001$), and this was seen across PD-L1-positive and PD-L1-negative subgroups. EFS data from KEYNOTE-522 remain immature but suggest a possible EFS improvement with addition of pembrolizumab [32].

At present it remains unclear whether checkpoint inhibition will become part of the standard of care for neoadjuvant therapy of triple-negative breast cancer. While a favorable impact on response at surgery has been definitively demonstrated, the impact on long-term breast cancer outcome remains uncertain, and it does not appear that PD-L1 positivity is a biomarker of benefit. Identification of predictive biomarkers will be essential for delineating patient populations who may benefit, as it would be ideal for neoadjuvant checkpoint inhibition to be used selectively given the potential for rare but serious toxicities from these agents.

Conclusion

Neoadjuvant treatment offers an ideal platform for biomarker development. Preliminary activity profiles of novel agents and novel treatment approaches can be rapidly ascertained via quantification of responses in surgical pathology specimens. Biomarker evaluation can be similarly facilitated through correlation of surgical response and baseline or on-treatment tumor characteristics. Nonetheless, many of the neoadjuvant treatment approaches and associated biomarkers discussed here remain investigational, with their impact on long-term outcome unclear. With additional time and research, there is little doubt that biomarker-guided neoadjuvant therapy will play an increasingly large role in more individualized, and therefore more optimal, treatment of breast cancer across all subtypes.

References

1. Cortazar P, Zhang L, Untch M, Mehta K, Costantino JP, Wolmark N, et al. Pathological complete response and long-term clinical benefit in breast cancer: the CTNeoBC pooled analysis. Lancet. 2014;384(9938):164–72.
2. Sparano JA, Gray RJ, Makower DF, Pritchard KI, Albain KS, Hayes DF, et al. Adjuvant chemotherapy guided by a 21-gene expression assay in breast cancer. N Engl J Med. 2018;379(2):111–21.
3. Cardoso F, van't Veer LJ, Bogaerts J, Slaets L, Viale G, Delaloge S, et al. 70-gene signature as an aid to treatment decisions in early-stage breast cancer. N Engl J Med. 2016;375(8):717–29.
4. Kalinsky K, Barlow WE, Meric-Bernstam F, Gralow JR, Albain KS, Hayes D, et al. First results from a phase III randomized clinical trial of standard adjuvant endocrine therapy (ET)

+/− chemotherapy (CT) in patients (pts) with 1-3 positive nodes, hormone receptor-positive (HR+) and HER2-negative (HER2-) breast cancer (BC) with recurrence score (RS) < 25: SWOG S1007 (RxPonder). San Antonio Breast Cancer Symposium. 2020:GS3-00.
5. Gianni L, Zambetti M, Clark K, Baker J, Cronin M, Wu J, et al. Gene expression profiles in paraffin-embedded core biopsy tissue predict response to chemotherapy in women with locally advanced breast cancer. J Clin Oncol. 2005;23(29):7265–77.
6. Kuemmel S, Gluz O, Nitz U, Braun M, Ludtke-Heckenkamp K, von Schumann R, et al. Neoadjuvant nab-paclitaxel weekly versus dose-dense paclitaxel followed by dose-dense ED in high risk HR+/HER2- early BC: results from the neoadjuvant part of the ADAPT HR+/HER2- trial. San Antonio Breast Cancer Symposium. 2020:GS4-03.
7. Pardo JA, Fan B, Mele A, Serres S, Valero MG, Emhoff I, et al. The role of oncotype DX(®) recurrence score in predicting axillary response after neoadjuvant chemotherapy in breast cancer. Ann Surg Oncol. 2021;28(3):1320–5.
8. Whitworth P, Beitsch P, Mislowsky A, Pellicane JV, Nash C, Murray M, et al. Chemosensitivity and endocrine sensitivity in clinical luminal breast cancer patients in the prospective Neoadjuvant Breast Registry Symphony Trial (NBRST) predicted by molecular subtyping. Ann Surg Oncol. 2017;24(3):669–75.
9. Korde LA, Somerfield MR, Carey LA, Crews JR, Denduluri N, Hwang ES, et al. Neoadjuvant chemotherapy, endocrine therapy, and targeted therapy for breast cancer: ASCO guideline. J Clin Oncol. 2021:Jco2003399.
10. Iwata H, Masuda N, Yamamoto Y, Fujisawa T, Toyama T, Kashiwaba M, et al. Validation of the 21-gene test as a predictor of clinical response to neoadjuvant hormonal therapy for ER+, HER2-negative breast cancer: the TransNEOS study. Breast Cancer Res Treat. 2019;173(1):123–33.
11. Smith I, Robertson J, Kilburn L, Wilcox M, Evans A, Holcombe C, et al. Long-term outcome and prognostic value of Ki67 after perioperative endocrine therapy in postmenopausal women with hormone-sensitive early breast cancer (POETIC): an open-label, multicentre, parallel-group, randomised, phase 3 trial. Lancet Oncol. 2020;21(11):1443–54.
12. Ellis MJ, Suman VJ, Hoog J, Goncalves R, Sanati S, Creighton CJ, et al. Ki67 proliferation index as a tool for chemotherapy decisions during and after neoadjuvant aromatase inhibitor treatment of breast cancer: results from the American College of Surgeons Oncology Group Z1031 Trial (Alliance). J Clin Oncol. 2017;35(10):1061–9.
13. Harbeck N, Gluz O, Kuemmel S, Christgen M, Braun M, Aktas B, et al. Endocrine therapy alone in patients with intermediate or high-risk luminal early breast cancer (0-3 lymph nodes), recurrence score <26 and Ki67 response after preoperative endocrine therapy: primary outcome analysis from the ADAPT HR+/HER2- trial. San Antonio Breast Cancer Symposium. 2020:GS4-04.
14. Ma CX, Suman VJ, Leitch M, Sanati S, Vij K, Unzeitig G, et al. Neoadjuvant chemotherapy (NCT) response in postmenopausal women with clinical stage II or III estrogen receptor-positive (ER+) and HER2 negative (HER2-) breast cancer (BC) resistance to endocrine therapy (ET) in the ALTERNATE trial (Alliance A011106). San Antonio Breast Cancer Symposium. 2020:GS4-05.
15. Silver DP, Richardson AL, Eklund AC, Wang ZC, Szallasi Z, Li Q, et al. Efficacy of neoadjuvant Cisplatin in triple-negative breast cancer. J Clin Oncol. 2010;28(7):1145–53.
16. Litton JK, Scoggins ME, Hess KR, Adrada BE, Murthy RK, Damodaran S, et al. Neoadjuvant talazoparib for patients with operable breast cancer with a germline BRCA pathogenic variant. J Clin Oncol. 2020;38(5):388–94.
17. Loibl S, O'Shaughnessy J, Untch M, Sikov WM, Rugo HS, McKee MD, et al. Addition of the PARP inhibitor veliparib plus carboplatin or carboplatin alone to standard neoadjuvant chemotherapy in triple-negative breast cancer (BrighTNess): a randomised, phase 3 trial. Lancet Oncol. 2018;19(4):497–509.
18. Sikov WM, Berry DA, Perou CM, Singh B, Cirrincione CT, Tolaney SM, et al. Impact of the addition of carboplatin and/or bevacizumab to neoadjuvant once-per-week paclitaxel followed by dose-dense doxorubicin and cyclophosphamide on pathologic complete response

rates in stage II to III triple-negative breast cancer: CALGB 40603 (Alliance). J Clin Oncol. 2015;33(1):13–21.
19. von Minckwitz G, Schneeweiss A, Loibl S, Salat C, Denkert C, Rezai M, et al. Neoadjuvant carboplatin in patients with triple-negative and HER2-positive early breast cancer (GeparSixto; GBG 66): a randomised phase 2 trial. Lancet Oncol. 2014;15(7):747–56.
20. Sikov WM, Berry DA, Perou CM, Singh B, Cirrincione CT, Tolaney SM, et al. Event-free and overall survival following neoadjuvant weekly paclitaxel and dose-dense AC +/− carboplatin and/or bevacizumab in triple-negative breast cancer: outcomes from CALGB 40603 (Alliance). San Antonio Breast Cancer Symposium. 2015:abstr S2-05.
21. Loibl S, Weber KE, Timms KM, Elkin EP, Hahnen E, Fasching PA, et al. Survival analysis of carboplatin added to an anthracycline/taxane-based neoadjuvant chemotherapy and HRD score as predictor of response-final results from GeparSixto. Ann Oncol. 2018;29(12):2341–7.
22. Mayer EL, Abramson V, Jankowitz R, Falkson C, Marcom PK, Traina T, et al. TBCRC 030: a phase II study of preoperative cisplatin versus paclitaxel in triple-negative breast cancer: evaluating the homologous recombination deficiency (HRD) biomarker. Ann Oncol. 2020;31(11):1518–25.
23. Telli ML, Metzger O, Timms K, Evans B, Vogel D, Wei H, et al. Evaluation of homologous recombination deficiency (HRD) status with pathological response to carboplatin −/− veliparib in BrighTNess, a randomized phase 3 study in early stage TNBC. J Clin Oncol. 2018;36(15_suppl):519.
24. Tung N, Arun B, Hacker MR, Hofstatter E, Toppmeyer DL, Isakoff SJ, et al. TBCRC 031: randomized phase II study of neoadjuvant cisplatin versus doxorubicin-cyclophosphamide in germline BRCA carriers with HER2-negative breast cancer (the INFORM trial). J Clin Oncol. 2020;38(14):1539–48.
25. Hahnen E, Lederer B, Hauke J, Loibl S, Kröber S, Schneeweiss A, et al. Germline mutation status, pathological complete response, and disease-free survival in triple-negative breast cancer: secondary analysis of the GeparSixto randomized clinical trial. JAMA Oncol. 2017;3(10):1378–85.
26. Johnston S, Puhalla S, Wheatley D, Ring A, Barry P, Holcombe C, et al. Randomized phase II study evaluating palbociclib in addition to letrozole as neoadjuvant therapy in estrogen receptor-positive early breast cancer: PALLET trial. J Clin Oncol. 2019;37(3):178–89.
27. Hurvitz SA, Martin M, Press MF, Chan D, Fernandez-Abad M, Petru E, et al. Potent cell-cycle inhibition and upregulation of immune response with abemaciclib and anastrozole in neoMONARCH, phase II neoadjuvant study in HR(+)/HER2(−) breast cancer. Clin Cancer Res. 2020;26(3):566–80.
28. Ma CX, Gao F, Luo J, Northfelt DW, Goetz M, Forero A, et al. NeoPalAna: neoadjuvant palbociclib, a cyclin-dependent kinase 4/6 inhibitor, and anastrozole for clinical stage 2 or 3 estrogen receptor-positive breast cancer. Clin Cancer Res. 2017;23(15):4055–65.
29. Mittendorf EA, Zhang H, Barrios CH, Saji S, Jung KH, Hegg R, et al. Neoadjuvant atezolizumab in combination with sequential nab-paclitaxel and anthracycline-based chemotherapy versus placebo and chemotherapy in patients with early-stage triple-negative breast cancer (IMpassion031): a randomised, double-blind, phase 3 trial. Lancet (London, England). 2020;396(10257):1090–100.
30. Schmid P, Adams S, Rugo HS, Schneeweiss A, Barrios CH, Iwata H, et al. Atezolizumab and nab-paclitaxel in advanced triple-negative breast cancer. N Engl J Med. 2018;379(22):2108–21.
31. Cortes J, Cescon DW, Rugo HS, Nowecki Z, Im SA, Yusof MM, et al. Pembrolizumab plus chemotherapy versus placebo plus chemotherapy for previously untreated locally recurrent inoperable or metastatic triple-negative breast cancer (KEYNOTE-355): a randomised, placebo-controlled, double-blind, phase 3 clinical trial. Lancet (London, England). 2020;396(10265):1817–28.
32. Schmid P, Cortes J, Pusztai L, McArthur H, Kümmel S, Bergh J, et al. Pembrolizumab for early triple-negative breast cancer. N Engl J Med. 2020;382(9):810–21.

Part IV
Surgical Considerations in a Patient Receiving Neoadjuvant Systemic Therapy

Chapter 9
Breast Cancer Imaging Pre- and Post-Neoadjuvant Systemic Therapy

Stephanie Chung and Sughra Raza

Background

As a result of breast cancer screening and improved therapies, breast cancer mortality has decreased from an annual death rate of 33.2 out of 100,000 in 1989 to 19.9 out of 100,000 in 2017 for women of all ages and races [1, 2]. For non-metastatic breast cancer, goals of therapy are to eliminate disease from the breast and axillary lymph nodes and to prevent disease spread. Local-regional treatment for non-metastatic breast cancer includes surgery, radiation, and systemic therapies with goals to completely resect tumor and minimize recurrence risk. Systemic therapies can be given either in the adjuvant or neoadjuvant setting based on cancer subtype, stage, and patient-specific factors. In general, treatment for patients with hormone receptor (HR) expressing tumors includes endocrine therapies and possible cytotoxic chemotherapy. For other molecular sub-types of breast cancer with different bio-marker profiles, including over-expression of tumoral ERBB2 (HER2) biomarkers, or absence of hormonal and ERBB2(HER2) (triple negative), cytotoxic chemotherapy and targeted antibody therapy maybe added or used exclusively [3]. Imaging plays an important role in all steps of loco-regional management of breast cancer, including identifying the index lesion, delineating the extent of disease in the breast and axilla, and monitoring the effect of treatment given prior to surgery.

While neoadjuvant therapy was traditionally used in locally advanced disease (stage III, T3 or T4 tumors of all subtypes) or inflammatory breast cancer, in recent years, there has been a dramatic increase in treatment administered in the neoadjuvant setting. It is now frequently offered to patients with breast cancers judged to be operable even at initial diagnosis to improve tumor-to-breast ratios or to assess

S. Chung (✉) · S. Raza
Division of Breast Imaging, Department of Radiology, Brigham and Women's Hospital, Boston, MA, USA
e-mail: chung-stephanie@cooperhealth.edu; sughra.raza1@umassmed.edu

A. Soran, F. Nakhlis (eds.), *Management of the Breast and Axilla in the Neoadjuvant Setting*, https://doi.org/10.1007/978-3-030-88020-0_9

response to specific systemic therapies. An additional important practical benefit of neoadjuvant therapy is that it allows direct assessment of an administered systemic therapy's effect on the existing tumor through clinical assessment and imaging, not afforded in the adjuvant setting when treatment is given after tumor resection. Observing this response may allow more precise and individually tailored selection of postoperative treatment options. Another clinically significant benefit of neoadjuvant treatment is that patients with positive lymph nodes may be spared postsurgical radiation to the axilla if nodal disease is cleared. Patients who may not be considered appropriate surgical candidates at the time of diagnosis may be offered neoadjuvant therapy to make surgery possible if there is significant reduction in tumor size as well as nodal burden. Finally, neoadjuvant treatment can allow time for more thorough patient evaluation, including genetic testing and counseling. If genetic mapping places the patient at high risk for future breast cancer, consideration of prophylactic contralateral mastectomy may be added to surgical management.

As knowledge regarding the behavior of specific molecular subtypes of breast cancer continues to grow, identifying receptor subtypes helps determine the optimal neoadjuvant therapy for each specific cancer. Importantly, neoadjuvant therapy has been shown to have implications for prognosis as a useful surrogate for tumor responsiveness, characterized by pathologic responsiveness. For example, triple negative cancers and those with HER2-postive receptor expression respond more robustly to chemotherapy. These cancers are more likely to resolve completely with treatment, and pathologic complete response (pCR) after neoadjuvant therapy has been found a suitable surrogate end point for patients with luminal B/HER-2 negative, HER-2 positive, and triple negative disease [4]. Additionally, in the Collaborative Trials in Neoadjuvant Breast Cancer (CTNeoBC) pooled analysis of 11 international clinical trials of neoadjuvant treatment of breast cancer, pathological complete response defined as eradication of all tumor from the breast and lymph nodes had improved survival [5]. Therefore, the role of neoadjuvant therapy is continuing to expand, with concurrent increased role of imaging for frequent monitoring of tumor response.

Monitoring Response

Determination of tumor burden is based on clinical assessment and imaging. When neoadjuvant treatment is administered, assessing change in tumor burden requires objective measurement of tumor size as well as potential disease progression. In order to standardize widely accepted methods of such assessment, a World Health Organization-sponsored effort led to the development of Response Evaluation Criteria in Solid Tumors or RECIST in 2000, subsequently revised in 2009 [5]. However, this was found to be useful primarily in non-breast solid tumors and more in a research setting. The more commonly used clinical method of assessing treatment response in breast oncology is to determine Residual Cancer Burden (RCB), which has been shown to be a reliable prognostic indicator [7–9]. RCB is based on multiple factors, including primary tumor size, proportion of invasive versus in situ components of the primary tumor, and lymph node involvement. A web-based calculator hosted by MD Anderson Cancer Center is used to calculate the individual patient's residual disease, classifying the pathologic response as RCB-I (minimal), RCB-II (moderate), or RCB-III (extensive) [7]. The gold standard for tumor response of course is based on histopathology, with the ideal pCR defined as no residual viable tumor.

Clinical Assessment

Clinical breast examination remains important in assessing tumor size at diagnosis and after neoadjuvant treatment. Tumor measurements may be made by palpation or with calipers for precision and better reproducibility. However, in comparison with imaging, physical examination has been shown to be less accurate. In a retrospective study of 61 patients, Croshow et al. reported 54% accuracy for physical assessment when determining pCR after neoadjuvant therapy in patients with locally advanced breast cancer compared to 74% for mammography and 79% for ultrasound [10]. In determining relative accuracy of mammography, sonography, and MRI in predicting residual tumor after NAT compared with physical examination and pathology, Yeh et al. demonstrated agreement with pathology was 19% for physical examination, 26% for mammography, 35% for ultrasound, and 71% for magnetic resonance imaging (MRI) [11]. Other studies have corroborated the higher accuracy of breast MRI in assessment of neoadjuvant response [12–16]. Clinical evaluation of tumor size may be more difficult in patients with inherently dense breast tissue, or those in whom the treatment causes fibrosis around the tumor, which can make measurements difficult and even result in an apparent erroneous enlargement of the mass.

Imaging

Imaging guidelines for patients who will receive neoadjuvant treatment for newly diagnosed breast cancer are not well established. All imaging modalities may both under- and overestimate residual disease. The American College of Radiology (ACR) publishes criteria regarding monitoring response to neoadjuvant systemic therapy for breast cancer, which are evidenced-based, annually reviewed guidelines (Table 9.1) [17]. Conventional breast imaging prior to beginning neoadjuvant therapy is performed with mammography and ultrasound. At the time of diagnosis, a bilateral mammogram is performed to determine the extent of disease and to stage the affected breast, as well as screen the contralateral breast for unsuspected occult disease. Ultrasound is used for more detailed characterization of masses and, if clinically indicated, to assess the ipsilateral axillary lymph nodes for possible regional involvement [18]. MRI is the most sensitive imaging modality for breast cancer detection and for establishing extent of disease, including loco-regional involvement of axillary and internal mammary lymph nodes, as well as extra-mammary extension such as skin, chest wall, and occasionally, hepatic or pulmonary involvement. It is also the most sensitive for contralateral breast screening with studies showing a diagnostic yield of 3–5% in finding unsuspected, mammographically and sonographically occult contralateral cancers [19, 20]. However, breast MRI use varies widely based on access and clinical preference. Per the most recent NCCN breast cancer treatment guidelines, breast MRI may be of benefit before and after systemic therapy to determine disease extent, treatment response, and surgical candidacy. Additionally, they advise imaging during neoadjuvant therapy should be not be

Table 9.1 ACR appropriateness criteria: monitoring response to neoadjuvant systemic therapy for breast cancer

Scenario	Imaging	Appropriateness[a]	Relative radiation level[b]	Comments
Initial determination of tumor size and extent within the breast prior to neoadjuvant chemotherapy	Diagnostic mammogram/DBT[c]	9	0.1–1	Often combined with ultrasound and MRI
	Ultrasound	9	0	Often combined with mammogram, of benefit if cancer is mammographically occult
	MRI with and without IV contrast	9	0	If post-treatment MRI will be obtained
	BSGI (Tc-99m)[d]	2	1–10	
	^{18}FDG-PET/CT whole body	1	10–30	To evaluate for extra-mammary disease
	^{18}FDG-PEM	1	10–30	
Initial imaging examination of the breast after initiation or completion of neoadjuvant chemotherapy	MRI with and without IV contrast	9	0	Requires pre-treatment MRI
	Ultrasound	8	0	Most helpful when pre-treatment exam is performed
	Diagnostic mammogram/DBT	7	0.1–1	
	BSGI (Tc-99m)	2	1–10	
	MRI breast without IV contrast	1	0	
	^{18}FDG-PET/CT whole body	1	10–30	
	^{18}FDG-PEM[e]	1	10–30	

Table 9.1 (continued)

Scenario	Imaging	Appropriateness[a]	Relative radiation level[b]	Comments
Initial imaging examination in breast cancer with clinical suspicion of metastatic disease. Staging or assessment of response to neoadjuvant chemotherapy	Whole body bone scan (Tc-99m)	9	1–10	
	^{18}FDG-PET/CT whole body	9	10–30	
	CT chest abdomen pelvis with IV contrast	8	10–30	Concern for distant metastasis
	CT chest abdomen pelvis with and without IV contrast	7	10–30	With and without contrast generally not needed for staging
	CT chest abdomen pelvis without IV contrast	1	10–30	
	MRI chest abdomen pelvis with and without IV contrast	1	0	
	MRI chest abdomen pelvis without IV contrast	1	0	

[a]1,2,3 = usually not appropriate; 4,5,6 = may be appropriate; 7,8,9 = usually appropriate
[b]Adult effective dose range (mSv)
[c]Digital breast tomosynthesis
[d]Breast-specific gamma imaging (Technetium 99m)
[e]Positron emission mammography

performed routinely, only when progression is suspected. Preoperative imaging should be determined based on a multidisciplinary team. They note accurate assessment to pre-operative systemic therapy is difficult, and imaging studies performed for assessment should include those modalities abnormal at the time of initial staging, in addition to physical examination [21]. It should be noted that there are multiple ongoing drug trials for NAT in breast cancer, which include prescribed pretreatment, interval, and presurgical imaging with various imaging modalities, including conventional 2D mammography, digital breast tomosynthesis (3D mammography), ultrasound, and contrast-enhanced MRI (CE-MRI). A special scenario to mention here is invasive lobular carcinoma (ILC) which, due to its growth pattern, frequently presents with subtle imaging findings on all modalities. It follows then that it remains difficult to image when looking for changes based on treatment. Since most ILC subtypes are hormone receptor positive, upfront treatment prior to surgery is only offered to those patients in whom it would be a surgical advantage to decrease the axillary nodal burden. In such cases, even if the primary tumor is not well imaged on any modality, US evaluation of the axilla can be helpful.

Mammography

Complete diagnostic evaluation of both breasts with mammography should be performed in a patient with a new breast cancer diagnosis prior to commencing any treatment, including neoadjuvant therapy. This should include extent of disease assessment of the affected breast, with full-field mediolateral oblique (MLO) (Fig. 9.1) and craniocaudal (CC) views, possible full-field lateral view and spot compression or spot magnification views for optimal assessment of malignant masses and/or calcifications. If the disease manifestation includes calcifications, high-quality spot compression magnification views are important, and should cover the entire quadrant or expected ductal distribution area so as to include any potential skip lesions or extensive intraductal component (EIC). Complete screening evaluation of the contralateral breast with full-field MLO and CC views should be obtained at diagnosis, if not performed within the past 6 months. Digital breast tomosynthesis, if available, can improve accuracy of lesion detection and characterization, as well as mammographic tumor measurement over 2D mammographic technique [22].

Limitations of mammography include dense tissue which can obscure masses, difficulty outlining tumor margins when mass margins are highly spiculated, incomplete axillary assessment, and inability to determine if calcifications represent active

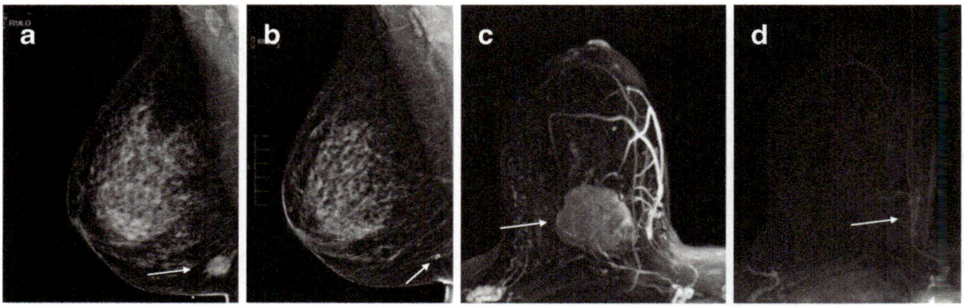

Fig. 9.1 42-year-old woman with right lower inner breast palpable lump. Right mediolateral oblique (MLO) mammogram (**a**) with a high-density oval mass at the site of palpable concern (arrow). Biopsy yielded invasive ductal carcinoma (IDC), poorly differentiated, ER/PR positive and HER-2/NEU negative. Right MLO mammogram after NAT with Lupron (**b**) reveals complete resolution of the mass and only the post-biopsy clip (arrow) at the site. At this point the patient was lost to follow-up, returning to care 12 months later. Maximum intensity projection (MIP) image from CE-MRI performed at this time (**c**) demonstrates a 4.0 cm mass (arrow). She was again treated with Lupron and follow-up MRI after 5 months of treatment (**d**) shows resolution of the mass with only subtle residual nonmass enhancement (NME) measuring up to 2.7 cm at the tumor bed (arrow). Lumpectomy confirmed complete pathologic response (pCR) with no residual invasive or in situ carcinoma identified in the tumor bed

disease versus treatment-related cell death. Microcalcifications do not normally resolve after treatment, regardless of pathologic response. Therefore, even with pCR, microcalcifications will remain visible and may even increase in areas of previously uncalcified tumor cells due to treatment-related necrosis (Figs. 9.2, 9.3, and 9.4) [23]. Residual mammographic calcifications do not correlate with the pathologic extent of disease, and have been shown to overestimate disease in 22–40% of patients [23, 24].

At the time of diagnostic core needle biopsy and/or prior to commencement of neoadjuvant therapy, it is standard of care to place a radio-opaque tissue marker clip

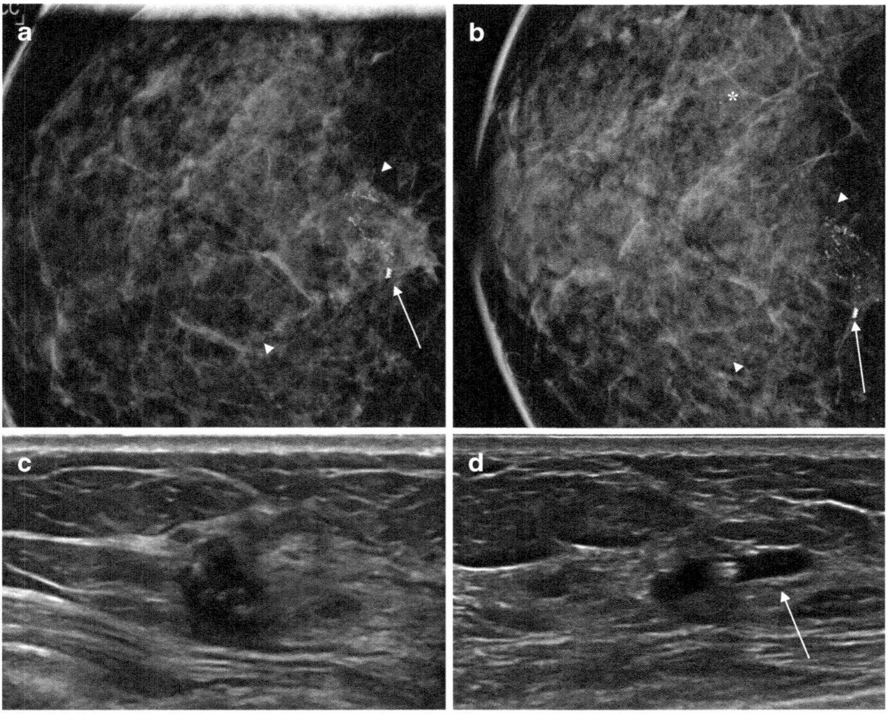

Fig. 9.2 60-year-old woman with right upper breast palpable lump. Magnification craniocaudal (MCC) mammogram (**a**) shows a spiculated mass at the site of palpable lump in the mid upper breast at posterior depth (arrow) with associated pleomorphic microcalcifications (arrowheads). US showed a corresponding irregular 1.2 cm hypoechoic mass (**b**, arrows) and US-guided core needle biopsy yielded IDC, poorly differentiated, ER weakly positive, PR and HER-2/NEU negative, treated as triple negative. A Hydromark clip was placed within the mass at the time of biopsy (arrow). Additional suspicious calcifications extend anteriorly from the mass (arrowheads). Mammographic magnification view after NAT (AC-T) (**c**) reveals resolution of the mass with clip remaining in place (arrow), and unchanged calcifications (arrowheads) as well as new calcifications laterally possibly representing previously uncalcified malignancy (asterisk). US (**d**) of the tumor site after NAT demonstrates only the clip without residual mass. (arrow). Mastectomy revealed multifocal residual IDC and DCIS within a 4.8 cm tumor bed

at the site of biopsy (Fig. 9.1), or multiple clips placed to mark the extent of disease. This allows correlation with imaging findings across modalities, evaluation of potential radiology–pathology discordance, ability to accurately assess the malignant site on post-treatment imaging, a target to perform post-treatment image guided localization to direct surgical resection of the tumor or residual tumor bed, and indication of the precise site for pathologic assessment of the surgical specimen.

Accuracy of post-treatment mammography in predicting preoperative extent of disease depends on the tumor's original mammographic visibility and multiple

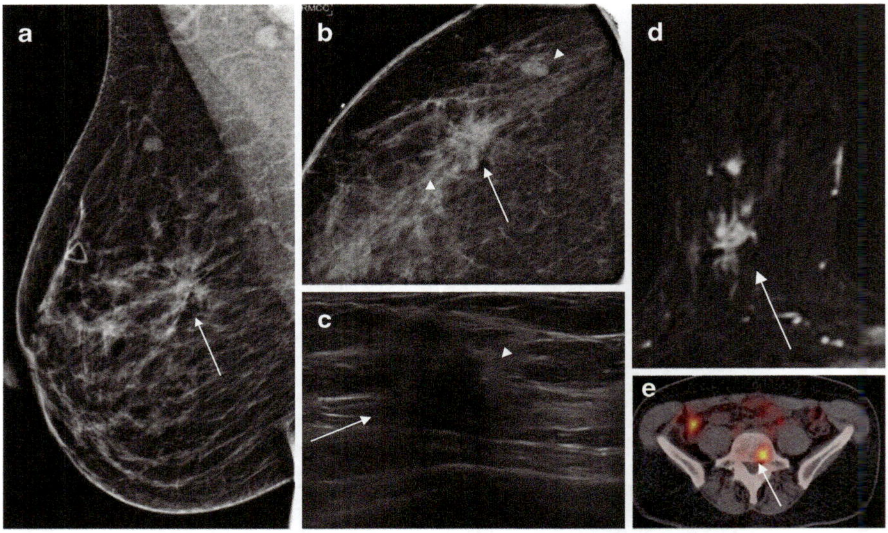

Fig. 9.3 45-year-old woman with oligometastatic right breast cancer initially presenting as a palpable lump. Right MLO (**a**) with triangular palpable marker and right magnification CC (**b**) views demonstrate a spiculated mass (arrows) with associated pleomorphic calcifications spanning up to 7.1 cm AP (arrowheads). US demonstrates a corresponding 1.9 cm irregular hypoechoic mass (**c**, arrow) with indistinct margins and hyperechoic halo (arrowheads). Biopsy showed poorly differentiated, ER/PR/HER2 positive IDC. An intramammary and axillary node were positive (not shown). Axial T1-weighted (T1-W) subtraction image of the right breast (**d**) demonstrates a corresponding irregular dominant enhancing mass (arrow). Additional enhancing masses and non-mass enhancement extend anteriorly from the index lesion, with overall extent of 6.6 cm antero-posteriorly. Axial fused 18FDG-PET/CT image (**e**) with avid lesion in the left L5 vertebral body (arrow), subsequently biopsy proven solitary metastasis. Given no other sites of metastatic disease, the option of local therapy including surgery to reach a no-evidence of disease state was offered. Treatment was initiated with paclitaxel, pertuzumab and trastuzumab, and tumor response monitored with imaging. Right MLO (**f**) and magnification CC (**g**) images demonstrate decrease of the mass marked by the open coil clip (arrow), and new subareolar calcifications (arrowheads). Sampled metastatic node is also marked with clip (asterisk). Axial T1-W subtraction MIP (**h**) shows no residual enhancement suggesting pCR. Given this imaging response to therapy, the patient has decided to forego mastectomy

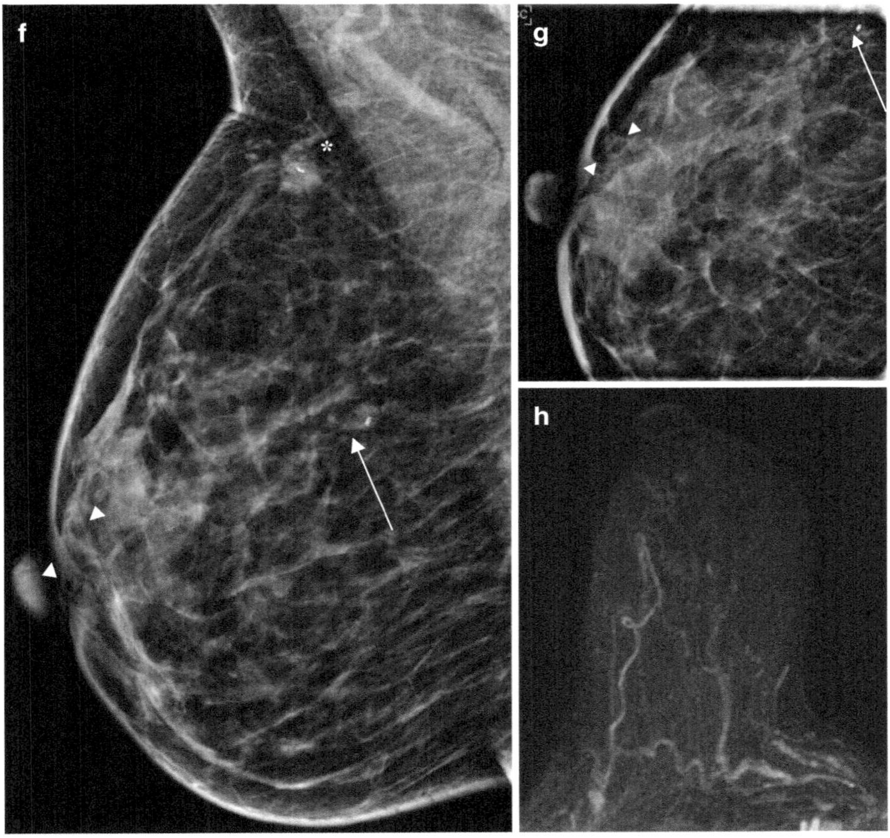

Fig. 9.3 (continued)

potential treatment responses, including fibrosis, necrosis, and tumor fragmentation (Fig. 9.1). In women with dense breast tissue, masking of malignant masses can limit initial detection as well as accurate assessment of tumor response (Fig. 9.5). Huber et al. showed a high correlation between mammographic tumor size and pathology if >50% of the margin was defined ($r = 0.77$) [25]. Helvie et al. found mammography to have 79% sensitivity and 77% specificity in predicting residual tumor in 56 women undergoing neoadjuvant chemotherapy; compared with clinical examination, mammography had higher sensitivity (79% vs. 49%), but lower specificity (77% vs. 92%); for patients with inflammatory carcinoma, mammographic sensitivity was 78% and specificity 83% (vs. 39% and 83% for physical examination, respectively) [26].

Ultrasound

Ultrasound has been shown to be a better predictor of pathologic tumor size compared to mammography [10, 27, 28], with accuracy of predicting residual tumor size ranging from 59.6–80% vs. 31.7–70% with mammography [10, 29]. When measuring a mass on ultrasound, the longest measurement should be obtained in relation to the longest axis of the mass visualized (Fig. 9.6). Additionally, calipers should extend to include a hyperechoic halo (Fig. 9.3), if present, as this has been shown to be more accurate than just measuring the hypoechoic portion (Fig. 9.6). As with clinical assessment and mammography, ultrasound can be challenging to interpret in the post-treatment setting as residual hypoechoic findings may represent treatment effect, residual viable tumor, or both (Fig. 9.5). Additionally, if the tumor resolves dramatically, it may be impossible to even identify the residual mass or the

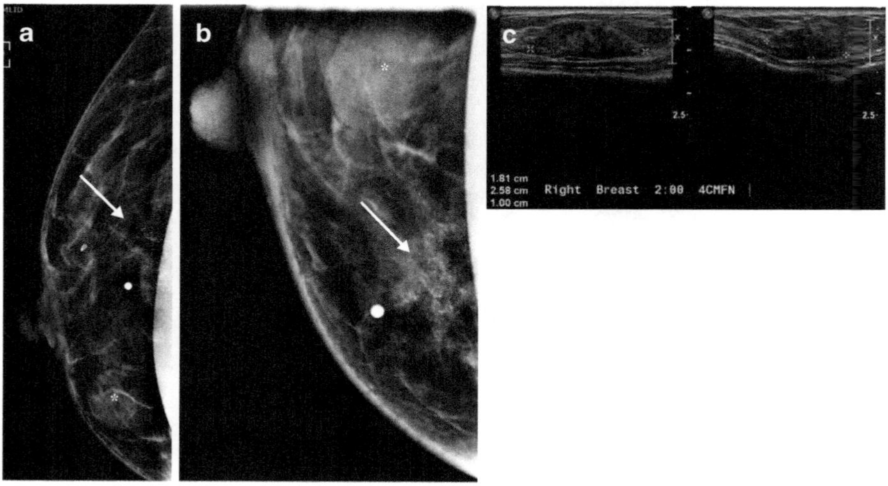

Fig. 9.4 34-year-old woman with history of cosmetic implant augmentation and newly diagnosed right ILC and DCIS, presenting as a palpable lump with positive ipsilateral axillary node. Right implant-displaced ML (**a**) and implant-displaced spot CC (**b**) mammograms show vague density and innumerable pleomorphic calcifications (arrow) at the site of palpable concern marked by a BB. The partially seen circumscribed mass (**a**, **b** asterisk) in the lower mid breast, was subsequently biopsied yielding fibroadenoma. US showed an irregular heterogeneous mass with indistinct margins (**c**, calipers) correlating with mammogram. Biopsy yielded moderately differentiated ILC, ER/PR/HER2 positive and intermediate nuclear grade DCIS, cribriform type. Axial T1-W subtraction MR image (**d**) shows an irregular enhancing mass at 2:00 measuring 4.2 cm (arrow), corresponding to mammographic and US findings. After treatment with anti-HER2 therapy (THP × 12 weeks and lupron), imaging showed 2.8 cm residual NME on MRI (**e**, arrows), consistent with partial imaging response. Spot ML (**f**) and CC (**g**) images show decreased density but interval increase in extent of calcifications (arrows). US shows no residual mass (**h**), and none was palpable on clinical exam. Patient underwent nipple sparing mastectomy and sentinel node biopsy, with pathology showing 1.5 cm residual IDLC and 1 of 3 sentinel lymph nodes positive. Subsequent full ALND was negative

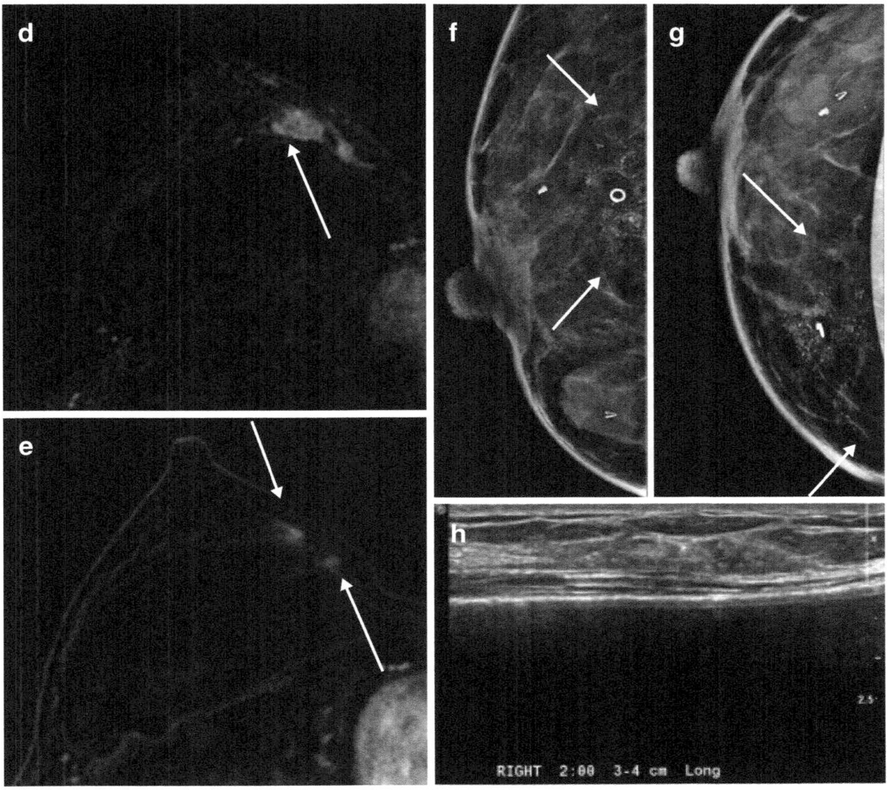

Fig. 9.4 (continued)

post biopsy tissue marker clip sonographically as placed to identify the tumor. Whole breast ultrasound may infrequently be used to assess extent of disease in the affected breast, or for screening of the contralateral breast, especially when the patient is unable to undergo breast MRI.

Ultrasound is the best modality for imaging the axilla. Criteria for morphologically abnormal lymph nodes are well established [30–35] and sonography allows visualization of multiple axillary nodes which can be assessed for morphologic abnormality. Specifically, focal thickening of the nodal cortex greater than the normal 3 mm is an early sign of metastatic deposition as the afferent lymphatics deliver tumor cells directly into the cortex. Thus, even focal bulging or prominence of an otherwise normal cortex, reliably imaged using ultrasound, can represent tumor deposits [32, 35, 36]. It is important to scan the axilla thoroughly and to document the number of abnormal lymph nodes as this will help guide surgical planning. Abnormal lymph nodes usually undergo sampling with either fine needle aspiration or core needle biopsy of the most abnormal or the most accessible node, with

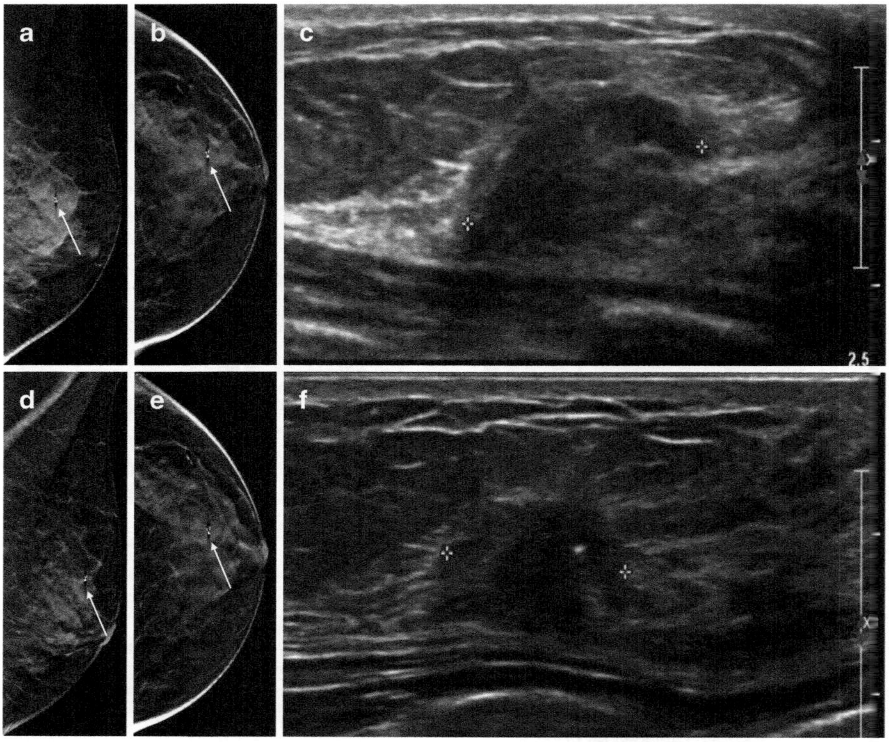

Fig. 9.5 62-year-old woman with left breast triple negative IDC presenting as a palpable area. Left tomosynthesis MLO (**a**) and CC (**b**) projections demonstrate a post-biopsy clip (arrow) within a mammographically occult biopsied mass in the upper breast. On US this was a 2.2 cm mass (**c**, calipers). Left MLO and CC views after NAT (AC-T) (**d**, **e**) reveal the clip (arrow) and US shows a residual 1.4 cm irregular mass (**f**, calipers). Lumpectomy revealed no residual carcinoma and changes consistent with treated tumor bed (0.9 cm × 0.6 cm), including stromal fibrosis, chronic inflammation, pigment-laden macrophages and biopsy site change, consistent with pCR

immediate post-procedure placement of a high visibility tissue marker or localization device within the abnormal cortex. If the node normalizes dramatically after treatment, the clip or localizing device will allow identification and serve as the target for preoperative localization for resection.

Magnetic Resonance Imaging

Contrast-enhanced breast MRI has been described as the most accurate imaging modality for assessment of neoadjuvant treatment response, and is reported to be more accurate than mammography, ultrasound, or clinical breast examination.

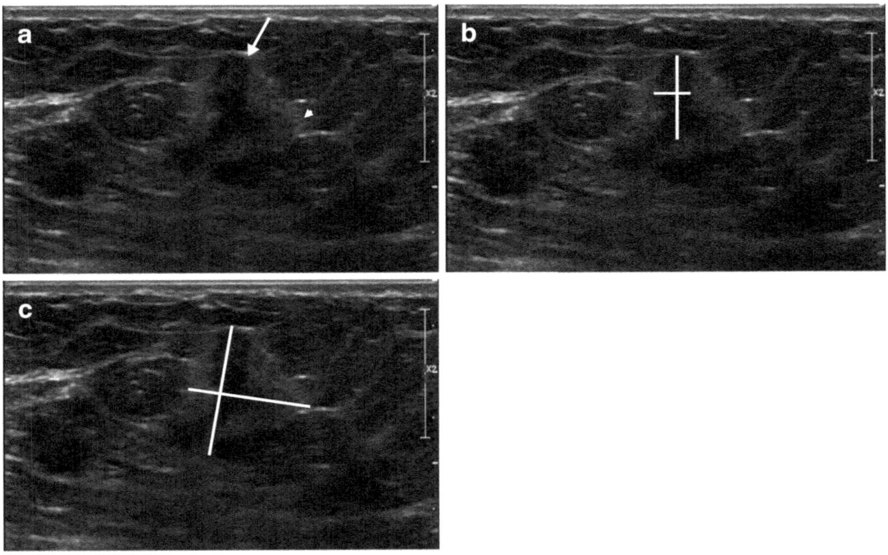

Fig. 9.6 83-year-old woman with history of left breast cancer status-post breast conserving therapy, and new left breast palpable abnormality. (**a**) Static greyscale transverse image demonstrates a left 2:00, 8–9 cm from the nipple, irregular hypoechoic mass (arrow) with hyperechoic halo (arrowhead) correlating with the palpable concern and suspicious mammographic mass (not shown). (**b**) The same static greyscale transverse image with incorrect measurement technique, with long axis measurement parallel to the frame of the image and the hypoechoic component only measured (lines). (**c**) The same static greyscale transverse image with the correct technique to measure this mass, with the axis measurements parallel to the axis of the mass, and the hyperechoic halo included (lines). Subsequent biopsy confirmed invasive ductal carcinoma

Multiple studies have demonstrated sensitivity for extent of disease assessment up to approximately 90%, specificity ranging from 60–100%, and accuracy of up to 91% [11–13, 15, 17, 37–40]. MRI has been noted to be particularly sensitive in women under age 50, who more commonly have mammographically dense tissues (Fig. 9.4). MRI detects otherwise occult multifocal and multicentric ipsilateral disease in up to 16% of patients [41], and in a study by Lehman et al., contralateral malignancy was present in 3.1% of 969 patients with MRI sensitivity of 91% and specificity of 88% [42]. MRI is the only breast imaging modality which can assess internal mammary lymph nodes for possible involvement, and also demonstrates the relationship of posteriorly located malignant lesions to the pectoralis muscle and chest wall showing abnormal enhancement in either when there is tumor involvement.

After NAT, breast cancer response is not necessarily uniform or identical among patients. Even if the original cancer was a uniformly solid mass, it may shrink concentrically in largest dimension or fragment into multiple components. MRI has been shown to visualize tumor response to NAT differently based on subtypes. In a study, triple-negative tumors were shown more likely to shrink concentrically, and HER-2 positive lesions were mutifocal and also demonstrated a large change in tumor diameter. In this study, residual tumors on pathology in ER-positive/HER-2 negative lesions did not correlate with the change in post-NAT largest enhancement diameter [43]. The type of shrinkage may then affect imaging appearance and imaging correlation with pathology, with DCE change in largest diameter of late enhancement significantly associated with residual tumor in the TN and HER-2 positive groups [43, 44]. In a 2018 retrospective study evaluating tumor shrinkage pattern (concentric vs. non-concentric) in patients with low-grade luminal (HR-positive, HER-2 negative, nuclear grades 1 or 2) cancers undergoing neoadjuvant chemotherapy, concentric shrinkage was associated with significantly longer disease-free survival (DFS), and this pattern was the only significant independent association with DFS [45]. Neoadjuvant treatment is not routinely added to the management of luminal breast cancers as pCR is rarely demonstrated on post-treatment imaging; however, this study correlated the pattern of shrinkage with long-term outcomes and therefore, describing the treatment response as a pattern may identify women who might benefit from NAT, and allow for modification of treatment based on pattern of response [46].

A pretreatment MRI should be obtained for patients in whom MRI is to be used subsequently to assess NAT response, such as for patients enrolled in investigational treatment protocols with prescribed specific MRI requirements for initial pretreatment, inflammatory breast cancer (Fig. 9.7) interval, and post-treatment presurgical MRI.

In a combined analysis, Crowshaw et al. reported MRI accuracy of positively predicting residual disease (PPV) of 93%, but a negative predictive value (correctly predicting absence of disease, NPV) of 65%. In the 2008 European Society of Breast Cancer Specialists (EUSOMA) guidelines with meta-analysis of 40 studies, (1513 patients), prediction of pathological response with MRI was evaluated. MRI was obtained pre-NAT, 2 weeks after last NAT, and within 2 weeks before surgery, and 36 of the 40 studies concluded that MRI was helpful and correlated better with pathology than clinical exam, mammography, and ultrasound. However, both over- and underestimation of treatment response was observed, especially for malignancies initially presenting as non-mass enhancement (NME) or tumors fragmenting into multiple foci (EUSOMA) [47].

The American College of Radiology Imaging Network (ACRIN) 6657 trial prospectively evaluated MRI in predicting treatment response and risk of recurrence in patients with stage 2 or 3 breast cancer undergoing neoadjuvant chemotherapy. Results comparing preoperative measurements showed the longest diameter of abnormal enhancement on MRI was the most accurate measure of pCR compared with the MRI volume or the longest diameter on mammography or clinical examination. This was true for all malignant lesions investigated, including single and multiple masses, nonmass enhancements and lesions with or without associated DCIS. The areas under the Receiver Operator Curve (AUC) used to assess CR in all lesion types, was 0.76 for all MR findings, and 0.84 for nonmass enhancements (NME). In patients with pathologic residual disease, longest MRI diameter had the highest correlation with pathology size [48]. Results from the I-SPY 1 trial showed that functional tumor volume, the semiautomated analysis of contrast-enhancement on MR using enhancement thresholds, predicted pCR and recurrence-free survival [49, 50].

Despite its advantages, MR is not uniformly considered a standard modality to include in routine evaluation of a patient with newly diagnosed breast cancer. As such, use varies widely by geographic location, institutional setting, clinical culture, and insurance coverage issues. A persistent issue has remained the question of lower specificity and higher false positive rates on breast MRI. The latter can lead to objectionable delay in treatment as additional biopsies in the same or the contralateral breast may need to be performed before definitive treatment can commence. Some studies have found mixed results in MRI serving as a surrogate marker for pCR. A recent single-institution retrospective study of 102 patients showed an accuracy of 78.6%, with 27.3% of patients with imaging complete response found to have residual cancer on surgical pathology [51]. Finally, some patients are not able to undergo MRI due to claustrophobia, presence of implanted devices considered unsafe in the specific magnetic field strength, or conditions which make the risk of contrast-related concerns more significant. Therefore, additional functional MRI techniques are being investigated to better monitor response to neoadjuvant therapy

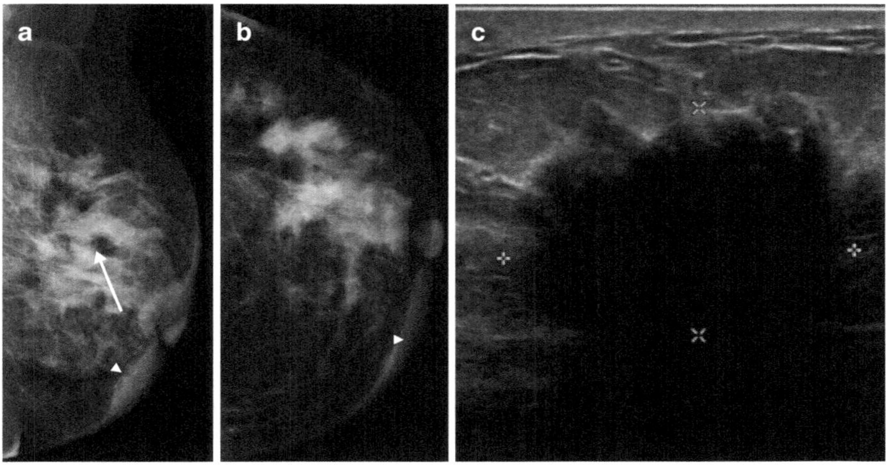

Fig. 9.7 59-year-old woman presenting with diffuse left breast skin thickening and extensive erythema, treated with antibiotics for presumed mastitis with persistent symptoms. Left MLO (**a**) and CC (**b**) views demonstrate marked peri-areolar skin thickening (arrowheads). A focal asymmetry was seen at 12:00 (arrow). US showed a hypoechoic mass with spiculated margins and dense shadowing, measuring 4.0 cm (**c**, calipers). Skin punch biopsy showed dermal lymphovascular invasion from poorly differentiated IDC. US guided biopsy of the mass confirmed micropapillary, ER+/PR−/HER2+ IDC. Axial T1-W subtraction MIP (**d**, **e**) shows a large confluent mass involving the anterior and outer left breast (arrow), and overlying skin., with pectoral muscle involvement (arrow) and axillary and pre-pectoral adenopathy (arrowheads) on sagittal T1-W fat-suppressed CE sequence (**e**). Post-treatment axial T1-W MIP (**f**) and sagittal T1-W image (**g**) shows small residual tumor (arrow) and no additional abnormal enhancement in the breast, with resolution of adenopathy and abnormal pectoralis enhancement. Mastectomy pathology demonstrated no residual carcinoma present including in the nipple and skin

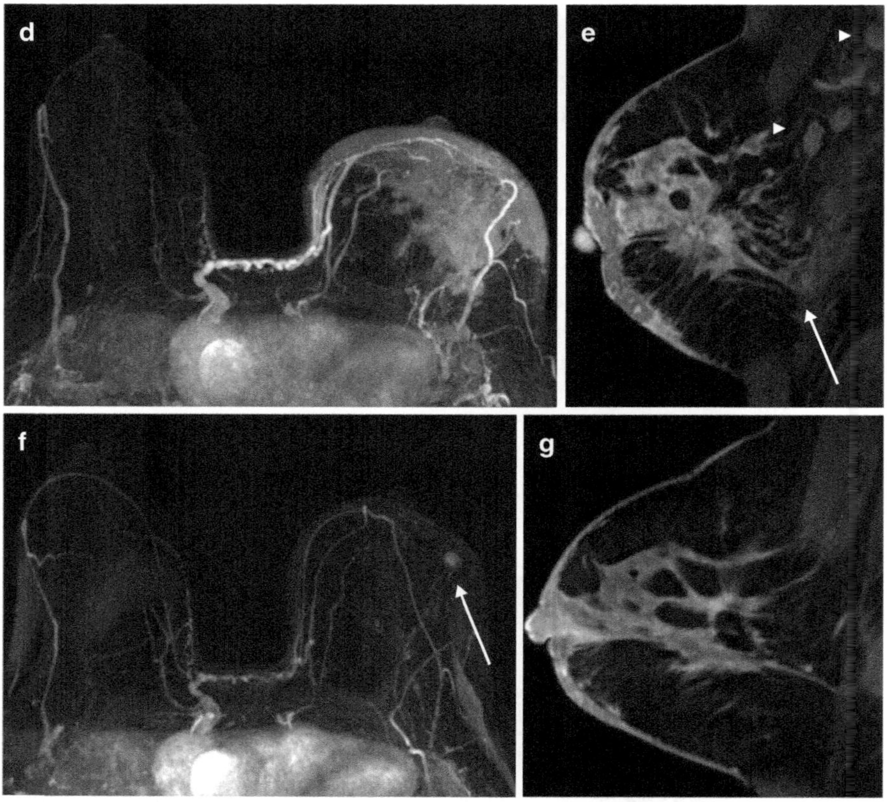

Fig. 9.7 (continued)

in breast cancer. Diffusion-weighted imaging (DWI) is an MRI sequence that generates signal based on differences in Brownian motion of water molecules and exploits aberrant cellularity and tumoral edema. This relative motion of water molecules in a tumor is measured as Apparent Diffusion Coefficient, or ADC. As no contrast is necessary, DWI may be of use in patients who cannot receive gadolinium contrast agents due to renal insufficiency or other reasons. In a 2012 meta-analysis by Wu et al. in prediction of pathological response to NAT, diffusion weighted-MRI (DW-MRI) was found to be highly sensitive and CE-MRI was highly specific [14]. The two combined can improve prediction of pathologic response to NAT. A 2010 study by Woodhams et al. found a higher accuracy for residual cancer burden with DW-MRI vs. CE-MRI (96% vs. 89%, respectively) [52]. Despite small studies providing promising results, including prediction of complete pathologic response to therapy, DW-MRI has not yet been validated and remains in analysis in the ACRIN 6698 trial, which aims to evaluate the utility of DWI and ADC as biomarkers of tumor characterization and NAT response [53].

Functional Imaging Methods and Future Directions

The most frequently used imaging modalities in monitoring response to neoadjuvant therapy, mammography, ultrasound, and MRI primarily utilize changes in lesion size as a surrogate for tumor response, which may be a delayed effect as therapies must first reach a level to induce changes, cause cell death, and tumor shrinkage. Functional imaging techniques, which allow assessment of physiologic changes in tissue, may allow an earlier identification of tumor responsiveness to guide patients to surgery or to modify current treatment regimens [18]. Currently, functional imaging techniques include standard CE-MRI, but additional specialized MR studies with multi-parametric imaging sequences have been under investigation and are being optimized for routine use. In addition, contrast-enhanced spectral mammography (CESM) and radionuclide-based imaging, such as breast-specific gamma imaging (BSGI), are also under investigation and being used clinically in parts of the world where access to MRI is limited. In the future, these modalities may play an increased role in the routine assessment of the physiologic response to systemic therapy.

Contrast-Enhanced Spectral Mammography

This technique is based on the hypothesis that, by combining intravenous iodinated contrast enhancement with digital mammography, occult cancers can be made visible. The currently optimized technique utilizes dual energy subtraction mammographic imaging after contrast administration. CESM has been shown to have cancer detection sensitivity equal to or better than breast MRI, and equal to MRI for estimating tumor size [54]. It stands to reason then that it is also highly accurate at demonstrating extent of disease as well as monitoring response to neoadjuvant treatment. For places where MRI availability or cost is limiting, this modality should be considered an alternative for diagnostic evaluation, extent of disease assessment, and monitoring response to NAT, in patients without contraindication to intravenous iodinated contrast administration.

Molecular Breast Imaging

Breast-specific gamma imaging (BSGI) using technetium 99m (99mTc)-sestamibi and dedicated breast-specific gamma cameras, with uptake of tracer related to blood flow and cellular metabolism [55] has been shown to have a high diagnostic performance as an adjunct to conventional breast imaging, with sensitivity of 95%, and specificity of 80–84% [56, 57]. BSGI is not widely used for two main reasons, one being the radiation dose associated with this modality, which remains a concern even it continues to decrease with technological advances. The second is that any radionuclide imaging requires expensive facilities and manpower to maintain all required radiation safety regulations and quality control. Still, there may be circumstances where BSGI is more easily put in place than MRI, and can then be used for detection, staging, and monitoring treatment response. In a 2016 meta-analysis including 14 studies and 503 breast cancer patients, Guo et al. showed a pooled sensitivity of 86%, specificity of 69% and AUC of 0.86, with most studies using whole body SPECT imaging and only three using breast specific systems [58]. These results have been corroborated by a subsequent 2018 meta-analysis which analyzed the ability of this modality to predict non-responsiveness to NAT [59].

While structural imaging modalities such as mammogram, ultrasound, and MRI depict anatomic changes to tissues, molecular imaging uses injectable materials to reflect and quantify biologic processes and cellular activity in vivo. Fluorodeoxyglucose positron emission tomography (FDG-PET) is the most well-known and clinically utilized imaging method, using a radioisotope of glucose as a marker of cellular metabolism. This is often fused with a CT scan of anatomically diagnostic quality to precisely localize the metabolic information. PET/CT is most often used for breast cancer staging (Fig. 9.3). However, numerous radioisotopes and molecules are being explored to target specific receptors and intracellular molecules specific to certain breast cancer sub-types. For example, fluoro-estradiol (FES), an estrogen analogue with a PET-emitting fluoride-18 tag, has been shown to identify and characterize tumors with variable levels of estrogen receptor (ER) expression [60, 61]. This can allow prediction of endocrine therapy response with FES positivity. Measurements of the metabolic avidity measured by PET can quantify ER expression concentration. In the setting of multifocal, multicentric, bilateral, or heterogeneous disease, the ER expression can be compared between or among lesions. Studies have shown early changes in FES-PET when monitoring response to neoadjuvant treatment [62]. Similarly, specific targeted functional imaging is being investigated for the progesterone receptors, HER2 receptors, cell proliferation (Ki-67), and many other cellular level functions [63].

Optical Imaging

Diffuse optical spectroscopic imaging (DOSI) uses near infrared (NIR) light with 650–1000 nm wavelength to characterize tumor metabolism, blood supply and oxygen consumption in vivo and in real time. It depicts molar concentrations of oxyhemoglobin, deoxyhemoglobin, water, and fat. Importantly, this technology is portable and non-invasive. The American College of Radiology Imaging Network (ACRIN) 6691 study, a national 7-center clinical study evaluated DOSI as a non-invasive monitor of preoperative chemotherapy. They used tissue optical index (TOI = deoxyhemoglobin x water/fat) assessed at baseline and mid-therapy and found the percent change of the TOl ratio of tumor-to-normal tissue (%TOI_{TN}) was useful to predict final pCR in 34 women undergoing NAT for breast cancer. Although a small study, they found the %TOI_{TN} AUC was 0.60, and in the smaller cohort of patients with baseline tumor oxygen saturation (%StO2) greater than the 77% median, %TOI_{TN} AUC improved to 0.83. The data suggest baseline and dynamic optical characteristics taken together may have utility in response prediction. However, this technology remains investigational, while larger studies are pursued, and the technology becomes more widely accessible.

Additional Considerations

Despite long-standing standardization of breast imaging reporting with the American College of Radiology Breast Imaging Reporting and Data (BI-RADS) lexicon, there are currently no published standards for reporting post-treatment tumor response. Indeed, the current BI-RADS manual does not include reporting guidelines for follow-up imaging in NAT. Suggestions of imaging descriptors in the literature, aside from size measurements, include changes in mammographic density, sonographic echotexture, and concentric versus fragmented tumor shrinkage [18].

The Response Evaluation Criteria in Solid Tumors (RECIST) or Residual Cancer Burden (RCB) are frequently used for standardization of tumor response in prospective clinical trials and allow categorization of complete and partial response, stable disease, or disease progression. However, this system does not include mammography and advises against ultrasound [64].

Imaging is important to delineate the extent of disease in breast cancer, with mammography, ultrasound, and contrast-enhanced MRI as the three primary imaging modalities at present. These modalities have importance in the neoadjuvant setting and help to optimize patient management and refine treatment decisions when incorporated into the comprehensive care management with regular collaboration and communication with breast oncologists and surgeons. Current clinical imaging trials in the neoadjuvant setting, and emerging imaging technologies will help continue to refine personalized treatment strategies for patients with varied pathologic subtypes and diverse clinical needs.

References

1. Howlader N, Noone A, Krapcho M, et al. SEER cancer statistics review, 1975–2017 SEER cancer statistics. Bethesda: National Cancer Institute; 2017.
2. Berry DA, Cronin KA, Plevritis SK, et al. Effect of screening and adjuvant therapy on mortality from breast cancer. N Engl J Med. 2005;353(17):1784–92.
3. Waks AG, Winer EP. Breast cancer treatment: a Review. JAMA. 2019;321(3):288–300.
4. Von Minckwitz G, Untch M, Blohmer JU, et al. Definition and impact of pathologic complete response on prognosis after neoadjuvant chemotherapy in various intrinsic breast cancer subtypes. J Clin Oncol. 2012;30(15):1796–804.

5. Cortazar P, Zhang L, Untch M, et al. Pathological complete response and long-term clinical benefit in breast cancer: the CTNeoBC pooled analysis. Lancet. 2014;384(9938):164–72.
6. Schwartz LH, Litière S, De Vries E, et al. RECIST 1.1 – update and clarification: from the RECIST committee. Eur J Cancer. 2016;62:132–7.
7. Symmans WF, Wei C, Gould R, et al. Long-term prognostic risk after neoadjuvant chemotherapy associated with residual cancer burden and breast cancer subtype. J Clin Oncol. 2017;35(10):1049–60.
8. Hamy AS, Darrigues L, Laas E, et al. Prognostic value of the residual cancer burden index according to breast cancer subtype: validation on a cohort of bc patients treated by neoadjuvant chemotherapy. PLoS One. 2020;15(6):e0234191.
9. Yau C, van der Noordaa M, Wei J, et al. Abstract GS5-01: Residual cancer burden after neoadjuvant therapy and long-term survival outcomes in breast cancer: A multi-center pooled analysis. Am Assoc Cancer Res. 2020:GS5-01.
10. Croshaw R, Shapiro-Wright H, Svensson E, Erb K, Julian T. Accuracy of clinical examination, digital mammogram, ultrasound, and MRI in determining postneoadjuvant pathologic tumor response in operable breast cancer patients. Ann Surg Oncol. 2011;18(11):3160–3.
11. Yeh E, Slanetz P, Kopans DB, et al. Prospective comparison of mammography, sonography, and MRI in patients undergoing neoadjuvant chemotherapy for palpable breast cancer. Am J Roentgenol. 2005;184(3):868–77.
12. Lobbes MBI, Prevos R, Smidt M, et al. The role of magnetic resonance imaging in assessing residual disease and pathologic complete response in breast cancer patients receiving neoadjuvant chemotherapy: a systematic review. Insights Imaging. 2013;4:163–75.
13. Yuan Y, Chen XS, Liu SY, Shen KW. Accuracy of MRI in prediction of pathologic complete remission in breast cancer after preoperative therapy: a meta-analysis. Am J Roentgenol. 2010;195(1):260–8.
14. Wu LM, Hu JN, Gu HY, Hua J, Chen J, Xu JR. Can diffusion-weighted MR imaging and contrast-enhanced MR imaging precisely evaluate and predict pathological response to neoadjuvant chemotherapy in patients with breast cancer? Breast Cancer Res Treat. 2012;135:17–28.
15. Marinovich ML, Houssami N, MacAskill P, et al. Meta-analysis of magnetic resonance imaging in detecting residual breast cancer after neoadjuvant therapy. J Natl Cancer Inst. 2013;105(5):321–33.
16. Sheikhbahaei S, Trahan TJ, Xiao J, et al. FDG-PET/CT and MRI for evaluation of pathologic response to neoadjuvant chemotherapy in patients with breast cancer: a meta-analysis of diagnostic accuracy studies. Oncologist. 2016;21(8):931–9.
17. Slanetz PJ, Moy L, Baron P, et al. ACR appropriateness criteria® monitoring response to neoadjuvant systemic therapy for breast cancer. J Am Coll Radiol. 2017;14(11):S462–75.
18. Fowler AM, Mankoff DA, Joe BN. Imaging neoadjuvant therapy response in breast cancer. Radiology. 2017;285(2):358–75.
19. Debruhl ND, Lee S-J, Mahoney MC, et al. MRI evaluation of the contralateral breast in women with recently diagnosed breast cancer: 2-year follow-up. J Breast Imaging. 2020;2(1):50–5.
20. Liberman L, Morris EA, Kim CM, et al. MR imaging findings in the contralateral breast of women with recently diagnosed breast cancer. Am J Roentgenol. 2003;180(2):333–41.
21. National Comprehensive Cancer Network. Breast Cancer (Version 1.2022). https://www.nccn.org/professionals/physician_gls/pdf/breast.pdf Accessed Nov 29, 2021. Pages 25, 26, 40, 137.
22. Förnvik D, Zackrisson S, Ljungberg O, et al. Breast tomosynthesis: accuracy of tumor measurement compared with digital mammography and ultrasonography. Acta Radiol. 2010;51(3):240–7.
23. Weiss A, Lee KC, Romero Y, et al. Calcifications on mammogram do not correlate with tumor size after neoadjuvant chemotherapy. Ann Surg Oncol. 2014;21(10):3310–6.
24. Adrada BE, Huo L, Lane DL, Arribas EM, Resetkova E, Yang W. Histopathologic correlation of residual mammographic microcalcifications after neoadjuvant chemotherapy for locally advanced breast cancer. Ann Surg Oncol. 2015;22(4):1111–7.

25. Huber S, Wagner M, Zuna I, Medl M, Czembirek H, Delorme S. Locally advanced breast carcinoma: evaluation of mammography in the prediction of residual disease after induction chemotherapy. Anticancer Res. 2000;20(1 B):553–9.
26. Helvie MA, Joynt LK, Cody RL, Pierce LJ, Adler DD, Merajver SD. Locally advanced breast carcinoma: accuracy of mammography versus clinical examination in the prediction of residual disease after chemotherapy. Radiology. 1996;198(2):327–32.
27. Keune JD, Jeffe DB, Schootman M, Hoffman A, Gillanders WE, Aft RL. Accuracy of ultrasonography and mammography in predicting pathologic response after neoadjuvant chemotherapy for breast cancer. Am J Surg. 2010;199(4):47.
28. Chagpar AB, Middleton LP, Sahin AA, et al. Accuracy of physical examination, ultrasonography, and mammography in predicting residual pathologic tumor size in patients treated with neoadjuvant chemotherapy. Ann Surg. 2006;243(2):257–64.
29. Aarsvold JN, Alazraki NP. Update on detection of sentinel lymph nodes in patients with breast cancer. Semin Nucl Med. 2005;35(2):116–28.
30. Deurloo EE, Tanis PJ, Gilhuijs KGA, et al. Reduction in the number of sentinel lymph node procedures by preoperative ultrasonography of the axilla in breast cancer. Eur J Cancer. 2003;39(8):1068–73.
31. Choi YJ, Ko EY, Han BK, Shin JH, Kang SS, Hahn SY. High-resolution ultrasonographic features of axillary lymph node metastasis in patients with breast cancer. Breast. 2009;18(2):119–22.
32. Bedi DG, Krishnamurthy R, Krishnamurthy S, et al. Cortical morphologic features of axillary lymph nodes as a predictor of metastasis in breast cancer: in vitro sonographic study. Am J Roentgenol. 2008;191(3):646–52.
33. Mainiero MB, Cinelli CM, Koelliker SL, Graves TA, Chung MA. Axillary ultrasound and fine-needle aspiration in the preoperative evaluation of the breast cancer patient: an algorithm based on tumor size and lymph node appearance. Am J Roentgenol. 2010;195(5):1261–7.
34. Dialani V, James DF, Slanetz PJ. A practical approach to imaging the axilla. Insights Imaging. 2015;6:217–29.
35. Abe H, Schmidt RA, Kulkarni K, Sennett CA, Mueller JS, Newstead GM. Axillary lymph nodes suspicious for breast cancer metastasis: sampling with US-guided 14-gauge core-needle biopsy – clinical experience in 100 patients. Radiology. 2009;250(1):41–9.
36. Ecanow JS, Abe H, Newstead GM, Ecanow DB, Jeske JM. Axillary staging of breast cancer: what the radiologist should know. Radiographics. 2013;33(6):1589–612.
37. Hylton N. Dynamic contrast-enhanced magnetic resonance imaging as an imaging biomarker. J Clin Oncol. 2006;24(20):3293–8.
38. Belli P, Costantini M, Malaspina C, Magistrelli A, LaTorre G, Bonomo L. MRI accuracy in residual disease evaluation in breast cancer patients treated with neoadjuvant chemotherapy. Clin Radiol. 2006;61(11):946–53.
39. Hollingsworth AB, Stough RG, O'Dell CA, Brekke CE. Breast magnetic resonance imaging for preoperative locoregional staging. Am J Surg. 2008;196(3):389–97.
40. Semiglazov V. RECIST for response (clinical and imaging) in neoadjuvant clinical trials in operable breast cancer. J Natl Cancer Inst – Monogr. 2015;2015(51):21–3.
41. Houssami N, Turner RM, Morrow M. Meta-analysis of pre-operative magnetic resonance imaging (MRI) and surgical treatment for breast cancer. Breast Cancer Res Treat. 2017;165:273–83.
42. Lehman CD, Gatsonis C, Kuhl CK, et al. MRI evaluation of the contralateral breast in women with recently diagnosed breast cancer. N Engl J Med. 2007;356(13):1295–303.
43. Loo CE, Straver ME, Rodenhuis S, et al. Magnetic resonance imaging response monitoring of breast cancer during neoadjuvant chemotherapy: relevance of breast cancer subtype. J Clin Oncol. 2011;29(6):660–6.
44. Aglietta M, Regge D. Imaging tumor response to therapy. Milano: Springer; 2012.
45. Fukada I, Araki K, Kobayashi K, et al. Pattern of tumor shrinkage during neoadjuvant chemotherapy is associated with prognosis in low-grade luminal early breast cancer. Radiology. 2018;286(1):49–57.

46. Moy L. Do tumor shrinkage patterns at breast MR imaging predict survival? Radiology. 2018;286(1):58–9.
47. Sardanelli F, Boetes C, Borisch B, et al. Magnetic resonance imaging of the breast: recommendations from the EUSOMA working group. Eur J Cancer. 2010;46(8):1296–316.
48. Scheel JR, Kim E, Partridge SC, et al. MRI, clinical examination, and mammography for preoperative assessment of residual disease and pathologic complete response after neoadjuvant chemotherapy for breast cancer: ACRIN 6657 trial. Am J Roentgenol. 2018;210(6):1376–85.
49. Hylton NM, Blume JD, Bernreuter WK, et al. Locally advanced breast cancer: MR imaging for prediction of response to neoadjuvant chemotherapy - Results from ACRIN 6657/I-SPY TRIAL. Radiology. 2012;263(3):663–72.
50. Hylton NM, Gatsonis CA, Rosen MA, et al. Neoadjuvant chemotherapy for breast cancer: functional tumor volume by MR imaging predicts recurrencefree survival-results from the ACRIN 6657/CALGB 150007 I-SPY 1 TRIAL. Radiology. 2016;279(1):44–55.
51. Sener SF, Sargent RE, Lee C, et al. MRI does not predict pathologic complete response after neoadjuvant chemotherapy for breast cancer. J Surg Oncol. 2019;120(6):903–10.
52. Woodhams R, Kakita S, Hata H, et al. Identification of residual breast carcinoma following neoadjuvant chemotherapy: diffusion-weighted imaging - comparison with contrast-enhanced MR imaging and pathologic findings. Radiology. 2010;254(2):357–66.
53. Partridge SC, Zhang Z, Newitt DC, et al. Diffusion-weighted MRI findings predict pathologic response in neoadjuvant treatment of breast cancer: the ACRIN 6698 multicenter trial. Radiology. 2018;289(3):618–27.
54. Fallenberg EM, Dromain C, Diekmann F, et al. Contrast-enhanced spectral mammography versus MRI: initial results in the detection of breast cancer and assessment of tumour size. Eur Radiol. 2014;24(1):256–64.
55. Muzahir S. Molecular breast cancer imaging in the era of precision medicine. AJR Am J Roentgenol. 2020;215(6):1512–9.
56. Narayanan D, Berg WA. Dedicated breast gamma camera imaging and breast PET: current status and future directions. PET Clin. 2018;13(3):363–81.
57. Sun Y, Wei W, Yang HW, Liu JL. Clinical usefulness of breast-specific gamma imaging as an adjunct modality to mammography for diagnosis of breast cancer: a systemic review and meta-analysis. Eur J Nucl Med Mol Imaging. 2013;40(3):450–63.
58. Guo C, Zhang C, Liu J, Tong L, Huang G. Is Tc-99m sestamibi scintimammography useful in the prediction of neoadjuvant chemotherapy responses in breast cancer? A systematic review and meta-analysis. Nucl Med Commun. 2016;37(7):675–88.
59. Collarino A, de Koster EJ, Valdés Olmos RA, de Geus-Oei LF, Pereira Arias-Bouda LM. Is technetium-99m sestamibi imaging able to predict pathologic nonresponse to neoadjuvant chemotherapy in breast cancer? A meta-analysis evaluating current use and shortcomings. Clin Breast Cancer. 2018;18(1):9–18.
60. Kurland BF, Peterson LM, Lee JH, et al. Estrogen receptor binding (18F-FES PET) and glycolytic activity (18F-FDG PET) predict progression-free survival on endocrine therapy in patients with ER+ breast cancer. Clin Cancer Res. 2017;23(2):407–15.
61. Miladinova D. Molecular imaging in breast cancer. Nucl Med Mol Imaging (2010). 2019;53(3):313–9.
62. Linden HM, Dehdashti F. Novel methods and tracers for breast cancer imaging. Semin Nucl Med. 2013;43(4):324–9.
63. Gebhart G, Gámez C, Holmes E, et al. 18F-FDG PET/CT for early prediction of response to neoadjuvant lapatinib, trastuzumab, and their combination in HER2-positive breast cancer: results from neo-ALTTO. J Nucl Med. 2013;54(11):1862–8.
64. Eisenhauer EA, Therasse P, Bogaerts J, et al. New response evaluation criteria in solid tumours: revised RECIST guideline (version 1.1). Eur J Cancer. 2009;45:228–47.

Chapter 10
Surgical Management of the Axilla in Node-Negative and Node-Positive Disease at Diagnosis

Joanna S. Lee, Priscilla F. McAuliffe, and Ronald R. Johnson

Introduction

Accurate nodal staging is important in breast cancer treatment because nodal involvement is a major prognostic predictor for breast cancer outcome. Nodal disease status widely determines the extent of systemic therapy, surgical treatment, radiation therapy, and reconstructive surgery. Historically, axillary lymph node dissection (ALND) was used to stage the axilla in all patients with breast cancer. However, axillary management has now evolved to utilize sentinel lymph node biopsy (SLNB), a less extensive surgery that still allows accurate staging of the axilla. The safety of SLNB alone in clinically node negative (cN0) patients with presumed low axillary disease burden is well established in the upfront surgery setting. The success of less extensive surgical intervention in the axilla is likely a factor of improved systemic and radiation therapy options, which also contribute to local disease control and improved overall oncologic outcomes.

In patients presenting with cN0 axilla, who are then found to have limited pathologic sentinel lymph node involvement, three clinical trials demonstrate that ALND is not necessary for all patients undergoing upfront surgery. The American College of Surgeons Oncology Group (ACOSOG) Z0011 trial was a practice-changing study that demonstrated no significant differences in locoregional recurrence (LRR), disease-free survival (DFS), and overall survival (OS) in patients with cN0 breast cancer with confirmed metastases in 1 or 2 sentinel lymph nodes (SLN), who were treated with breast conservation therapy (BCT) and whole breast radiation (WBRT), without ALND [1]. The International Breast Cancer Study Group (IBCSG) 23-01 trial demonstrated that ALND may be safely omitted in cN0 patients with limited

J. S. Lee · P. F. McAuliffe · R. R. Johnson (✉)
Breast Surgical Oncology, University of Pittsburgh, Pittsburgh, PA, USA
e-mail: leejs7@upmc.edu; mcauliffepf@upmc.edu; johnrr@upmc.edu

A. Soran, F. Nakhlis (eds.), *Management of the Breast and Axilla in the Neoadjuvant Setting*, https://doi.org/10.1007/978-3-030-88020-0_10

SLN involvement, showing no difference in 5-year DFS, but more surgery related toxicities, like lymphedema and neuropathy, in the ALND group [2]. The European Organization for Research and Treatment of Cancer (EORTC) 10981-22023 AMAROS trial also showed that, in patients with cT1-T2 N0 primary breast cancers treated with upfront surgery, radiation therapy is non-inferior to ALND. It is compelling that the patients in the axillary radiation group without ALND had significantly less lymphedema [3].

Axillary management following neoadjuvant chemotherapy (NAC) is also evolving. Use of NAC in early-stage breast cancer has increased over time with the goal to downstage the extent of surgery in both the breast and axilla. Depending on tumor biology, achieving pathologic complete response (pCR) following NAC is an important prognostic factor, especially for triple negative breast cancer (TNBC) and HER2 positive (HER2+) breast cancer. Although there is no overall survival difference between administration of chemotherapy in the neoadjuvant versus the adjuvant setting, a survival benefit has been demonstrated in the subset of patients with residual invasive disease following NAC who receive additional adjuvant chemotherapy.

Axillary management following neoadjuvant endocrine therapy (NET) is not well-known and there is paucity of information on this topic. Per the American Society of Breast Surgeons practice guidelines for the use of NST, NET produces the best response rates in postmenopausal women with clinical stage 2–3 breast cancer with strongly hormone receptor positive (HR+) breast cancer. Significant tumor downstaging using NET usually requires 4–6 months of continuous therapy, but pCR is rarely observed. Because pCR is rarely observed following NET, the clinical utility in axillary management is unknown. There is no established role for NET in premenopausal women currently. This chapter will review available literature regarding the optimal surgical management of axilla following NAC and will also briefly discuss surgical axillary management following NET. A different chapter in this book will go into more depth regarding the role of NET.

Benefit of NAC

Depending on tumor phenotype, NAC can effectively downstage the extent of surgery both in the breast and in the axilla. Even for patients with relatively smaller cN0 cancers at diagnosis, NAC may foster breast conservation by improving the tumor to breast size ratio. NAC also allows for in vivo assessment of tumor response. Furthermore, earlier data have shown that NAC receipt can result in downstaging of nodal involvement in patients presenting with cN+ disease which may consequently lead to less extensive axillary surgery. The National Surgical Adjuvant Breast and Bowel Project (NSABP) B-18 trial compared preoperative and postoperative doxorubicin and cyclophosphamide for operable breast cancer. This study showed that, regardless of the presenting clinical nodal status or tumor size, NAC resulted in significant reduction in nodal positivity, 59% with NAC vs. 43% with adjuvant therapy, $p < 0.001$ [4]. Following this study, NSABP B-27 reported an even greater reduction in nodal involvement following NAC with the addition of preoperative docetaxel to the regimen described in B-18—50.8% for NAC versus 58.2% for adjuvant therapy, $p < 0.001$ [5]. Long-term updates of NSABP B-18 and B-27 also confirmed that the addition of docetaxel to NAC with doxorubicin and cyclophosphamide significantly increased the rate of pCR and that those patients who achieved pCR had superior DFS and OS [6]. A study from the University of Texas MD Anderson Cancer Center (MDACC) also showed significant reduction in nodal disease after NAC compared with up-front surgery group, particularly in patients with T2–T3 primary tumor (T1: 12.7% vs. 19%, $p = 0.2$; T2: 20.5% vs. 36.5%, $p < 0.0001$; and T3: 30.4% vs. 51.4%, $p = 0.04$) [7].

An additional benefit of NAC is the assessment of end-chemotherapy response, which could open the door for additional adjuvant systemic therapy options for the appropriate patients. Several recent studies showed a survival benefit with additional adjuvant chemotherapy for those patients who do not achieve pCR following NAC. The CREATE-X UNIM Clinical Trial showed that the addition of adjuvant capecitabine prolonged DFS and OS among patients with HER2-negative (HER2−) breast cancer who had residual invasive disease following standard NAC regimens containing anthracycline, taxane, or both [8]. The study demonstrated improved DFS and OS in the capecitabine group (DFS: 74.1% vs. 67.6%, $p = 0.01$; OS: 89.2% vs. 83.6%, $p = 0.01$). The KATHERINE trial showed a 50% reduction in risk of recurrence of invasive breast cancer or death with adjuvant trastuzumab emtansine (T-DM1) compared to with adjuvant trastuzumab alone (HR 0.50, $p < 0.001$) in patients with HER2+ breast cancer who had residual disease following standard NAC containing taxane, with or without anthracycline and trastuzumab [9].

Benefit of NET

Endocrine therapy in adjuvant setting is a widely accepted, important component of breast cancer treatment for the luminal subtype, hormone receptor positive (HR+), HER2− breast cancer as per NCCN guidelines. Similar to NAC, the use of endocrine therapy in neoadjuvant setting can potentially downstage the extent of disease and provide in vivo information about the cancer's responsiveness to endocrine therapy. ACOSOG Z1031 is a randomized phase II NET trial comparing response rates between letrozole, anastrozole, and exemestane that reported overall clinical response rate of 69% with no differences between the three different aromatase inhibitors. This study showed that NET increases BCT rate as 51.5% of the patients who were not BCT candidates at initial surgical consultation were able to successfully undergo BCT following NET [10].

In regard to the axilla, there is scarce data in literature looking at the role of NET on the downstaging of axillary surgical management. A study from Memorial

Sloan Kettering Cancer Center (MSKCC) reports the nodal pCR rate was 11% following NET. The nodal downstaging rates with NET and NAC were not significantly different (11% with NET vs. 18% with NAC, $p = 0.37$). Patients who achieved nodal pCR with NET were older, $p = 0.004$ and had greater progesterone expression, $p = 0.031$ [11]. A recent NCDB analysis looking at 4580 patients undergoing NET showed that the overall axillary pCR was 14.5%. The patients who achieved a pCR were more likely to have smaller axillary disease burden ($p = 0.008$), have a higher grade ($p = 0.003$), and have a ductal histology ($p = 0.04$) [12]. Another NCDB analysis looking at 4495 patients who received NET, raises an interesting question of the oncologic significance of residual nodal disease after NET, whether this has the same prognostic implications as residual disease following NAC. This analysis reports very low rates of pCR overall, 1.4% pCR in the breast and 1.2% pCR in both breast and axilla. Regardless of the low rates of pCR, there was no significant different in OS between patients who achieved axillary pCR and those who had residual small volume axillary disease, isolated tumor cells (ITCs), or micrometastases. Additionally, survival outcomes for the patients following NET were more similar to patients undergoing upfront surgery than those who received NAC [13].

Feasibility of SLNB After NAC

Because nodal status is a key prognostic predictive factor for breast cancer, accurate assessment of the extent of axillary disease following NAC is very important. For those patients who have excellent response to NAC, less invasive axillary surgery can minimize surgical morbidity.

Historically, there were concerns that SLNB may inaccurately represent the axilla following NAC, due to altered lymphatic drainage, secondary to treatment-related tissue changes, including fibrosis [14, 15]. Due to these concerns, some investigators performed SLNB prior to initiation of NAC [16]. The potential benefit of performing SLNB before NAC is that the knowledge of pathologic nodal status before NAC could help streamline the need for adjuvant radiotherapy and facilitate the planning for reconstructive surgery in appropriate patients. However, a potential drawback of performing SLNB before NAC is the loss of the ability to downstage microscopic axillary disease. Combined data from the NSABP B-18 and B-27 trials demonstrate that the pathologic response post-NAC is more important than pre-NAC stage in terms of predicting oncologic outcomes. Specifically, the lack of nodal pCR is the strongest predictor of 10-year LRR, HR 4.5, $p < 0.001$. These findings suggest that the decision to proceed with SLNB pre-NAC should only be considered for unique situations with multidisciplinary consensus [17].

Clinically Node-Negative Patients

Despite initial concerns about the accuracy of SLNB following NAC, recent studies demonstrate similar SLN identification rates and also similar false negative rates (FNR) as those seen in the upfront surgery setting for cN0 patients after NAC. Results from NSABP B-27 concluded that SLNB is applicable following NAC with an 84.8% identification rate and an FNR of 10.7%. The study reports a non-significant trend toward improved identification rate among surgeons who performed a higher number of sentinel node procedures [15]. The GANEA 1 study was designed to look at the detection rate, the FNR, and the accuracy of SLNB following NAC. In the cN0 group, the SLN identification rate was 95% with an FNR of 9%, confirming the feasibility of SLNB after NAC. However, for the cN+ group, a significantly lower identification rate of 82% was reported ($p = 0.08$) [18]. The GANEA 2 study goes on to elaborate that among the patients in the cN0 group treated with SLNB alone, only one axillary relapse occurred during the follow-up period from 2010 to 2014, confirming that negative SLNB after NAC allows for safe omission of ALND in patients with no initial nodal involvement prior to NAC [19]. A study from MDACC reported similar SLN identification rates for up-front surgery compared to NAC: 98.7% and 97.4%, respectively. The FNR was 4.1% for up-front surgery and 5.8% for NAC; $p = 0.4$ [7]. The Netherlands Cancer Registry study also showed comparable SLN identification rates: 98% for up-front surgery versus 95% for NAC [20].

Although studies show comparable SLN identification rates and FNR, another concern that is raised is the long-term consequences of possibly leaving lymph nodes with potentially chemotherapy-resistant disease. Unfortunately, literature on this particular topic is scarce. A MDACC study showed a low regional recurrence of 1.2% in patients with a negative SLNB after NAC who underwent SLNB alone without ALND, with a median follow up of 47 months [7]. Similarly, the University of California at Los Angeles also reported low axillary recurrence of 0.7%, at a median follow up of 52 months [21].

Clinically Node-Positive Patients

Patients who are cN+ can achieve nodal pCR after NAC in up to 20–70%, based on their tumor biology. The highest rate of nodal pCR is seen in TNBC and HER2– breast cancer patients [22]. Three large, multicenter, prospective trials demonstrated the feasibility of SLNB in patients with cN+ disease at diagnosis following NAC (Table 10.1).

The ACOSOG Z1071 evaluated the FNR of SLNB after NAC in cN+ patients with overall reported FNR of 12.6%. Further subset analysis showed that the use of

Table 10.1 Trials demonstrating feasibility of SLNB in cN+ patients following NAC

Studies	Total patients	Pre-NAC biopsy	SLN identification rate (%)	Overall FNR (%)
ACOSOG Z1071 [23]	637	Yes	92.7	12.6
SENTINA [26]	592	No	87.8	14.2
SN FNAC [27]	153	Yes	87.6	13.4

dual-tracer technique reduced the FNR to 10.8% ($p = 0.05$). Additionally, removal of three or more SLN further improved FNR to 9.1% ($p = 0.007$) [23]. Lastly, the use of immunohistochemistry (IHC) further reduced the FNR to 8.7% [24]. It is interesting to note that a follow-up study on Z1071 showed that post-NAC ultrasound (US) alone was not predictive of pathologic nodal response after NAC. When the US demonstrates normal lymph node morphology, 56.3% of these patients still had residual disease on final surgical pathology. On the other hand, 28.2% of patients with persistently suspicious nodal morphology on US demonstrated nodal pCR on final surgical pathology [25].

The SENTinel NeoAdjuvant (SENTINA) trial was a 4-arm, multicenter trial from Europe. Unlike in ACOSOG Z1071, pathologic confirmation of metastases in clinically suspicious nodes with percutaneous biopsy pre-NAC was not mandatory in this study. One of the arms looked at patients who converted from cN+ to cN− status following NAC. Overall FNR was 14.2%. Dual-tracer technique reduced the FNR to 8.6%, $p = 0.15$ and removal of three or more SLN further improved FNR to 7.3%, $p = 0.008$. The use of IHC was not discussed in this study [26].

Sentinel Node Biopsy Following Neoadjuvant Chemotherapy (SN-FNAC) trial was the last of the three prospective trials looking at SLNB for cN+ patients following NAC. This Canadian trial was closed early with the publications of the SENTINA and ACOSOG Z1071 trials. The overall FNR was 13.4%. As shown in ACOSOG Z1071, the use of IHC improved the FNR to 8.4%. This trial also demonstrated dual-tracer technique and the removal of two or more SLN were important [27]. The surgical techniques that are shown to improve FNR are organized and reviewed again later (Table 10.2).

Evaluation of Clipped Node

In the subset analysis of the ACOSOG Z1071 trial, FNR was reduced to 6.8% when the biopsy-proven metastatic lymph node was clipped and removed at the time of surgery [28]. With this finding, MDACC proposed the procedure called targeted axillary dissection (TAD), where the clipped lymph node is localized with ^{125}I radioactive seed to ensure removal at the time-planned SLNB. In this study, the FNR for

Table 10.2 Modifications on the technique to improve FNR

Studies	IHC (%)	Single tracer (%)	Dual tracer (%)	1 SLN (%)	2 SLN (%)	≥3 SLN (%)
ACOSOG Z1071 [23, 24]	8.7	20.3	10.8	Not reported	21.1	9.1
SENTINA [26]	Not reported	16	8.6	24.3	18.5	7.3
SN FNAC [27]	8.4	16	5.2	18.2	≥2 SLN removed 4.9	Not reported

SLNB alone was 10.1% and the FNR for the clipped lymph node alone was 4.2%. When TAD is utilized, the FNR was reduced to 2% [29, 30]. A similar study from the University of Pittsburgh also demonstrated that SLNB combined with directed removal of the clipped axillary lymph node with a ^{125}I radioactive seed, termed directed-SLNB, accurately reflected the axillary nodal status following NAC, as those patients who had residual nodal disease all had disease seen in the clipped node [31]. These studies demonstrated that the clipped lymph node was not an SLN in 9–27% of the cases indicating that SLNB alone may potentially miss the previously known biopsy-proven positive lymph node [28–31]. The National Comprehensive Cancer Network (NCCN) guidelines endorse the use of SLNB for patients with cN+ disease who convert to cN0 following NAC. The NCCN guidelines also state that the FNR with SLNB following NAC can be improved by marking biopsied lymph nodes to document their removal, using dual tracer, and removing >2 SLN [32].

With these trials showing feasibility and low FNR of SLNB following NAC, the trend in clinical practice is clearly changing. A recent survey of the American Society of Breast Surgeons showed that 85% of the practitioners now offer SLNB to their patients following NAC, compared to 45% before these trials. The majority of the practitioners consider the following components of the surgical technique to be important: dual-tracer technique (86%), clipping the lymph node to ensure removal (82%), and removal of >2 SLN (70%) [33]. A National Cancer Database (NCDB) review done by Dana Farber Cancer Center also shows that the recent trend reveals a significant increase in the use of SLNB for cN+ patients following NAC, increased from 31.8% in 2012 to 49% in 2015 ($p < 0.001$). In this study, factors associated with SLNB following NAC were age < 45 at diagnosis, treatment facility, clinical N1 vs. N2 status, HER2+ and TNBC subtype, and choice of breast conservation therapy versus mastectomy. In this study, ALND was omitted in 36.9% of patients with isolated tumor cells (ITCs), 23.6% with micrometastatic disease, and 13% with macrometastatic disease [34]. The GANEA 3 study is a prospective multicenter diagnostic study currently ongoing to further assess the benefit of targeting the initially involved, clipped node.

Role of Radiation Therapy

Nodal basin radiation after SLNB is an accepted, non-inferior alternative to ALND among patients with limited nodal disease burden (1 or 2 positive nodes) undergoing up-front surgery [1, 3]. However, the indications for radiation therapy following NAC is not as standardized as in up-front surgery setting. The traditional approach is that the decision for radiation therapy would be made based on the pre-NAC stage. A large NCDB review looked at the role of post-mastectomy radiation therapy (PMRT) in patients with cN+ disease with nodal pCR following NAC. There was no statistical OS with PMRT. However on the subset analyses, PMRT was associated with a significant improvement in OS for patients with clinical stage IIIB/IIIC disease, or residual invasive disease in the breast following NAC ($p < 0.05$) [35]. A multicenter study from South Korea also showed that there was no statistical difference in OS with PMRT for patients who achieved nodal pCR following NAC [36].

Future Directions

Although overall clinical practice is heading toward downstaging axillary surgery following NAC to minimize surgical morbidity, there are still no published prospective data evaluating the long-term oncologic safety of omitting ALND. There are several clinical trials ongoing to further investigate this further (Table 10.3).

Table 10.3 Ongoing clinical trials

Studies	Country	Primary outcome	Accrual period (start date – primary completion date – completion date)	Estimated enrollment	Accrual
Alliance A011202 [37]	USA (NCT01901094)	Invasive breast cancer-recurrence free interval (IBC-RFI)	2/2014–1/2024 – -not reported	1660	Recruiting
ATNEC [38]	United Kingdom (NCT04109079)	DFS Patient reported lymphedema	12/2020–2/2030–2/2030	1900	Recruiting
TAXIS [39]	Switzerland (NCT03513614)	DFS	8/2018–3/2029–12/2043	1500	Recruiting
NSABP B-51 / RTOG 1304 [40]	USA (NCT01872975)	IBC-RFI	8/2013–7/2023–8/2028	1636	Recruiting
NEONOD 2 [41]	Italy (NCT04019678)	DFS	6/2019–6/2022–6/2027	850	Recruiting

The Alliance A011202 trial (NCT01901094) is looking at cN+ patients whose sentinel nodes remain persistently positive following NAC. The participants are then randomized to ALND or no further axillary surgery. All patients receive regional nodal irradiation. The primary end point of this study is ipsilateral locoregional invasive cancer recurrence with secondary endpoints looking at OS, lymphedema rate, adequacy of radiation fields, and residual cancer burden [37]. There are two similar European trials ongoing. First is the British ATNEC trial (NCT04109079), a prospective multicenter randomized trial looking at patients with 1–2 positive nodes following NAC with randomization to ALND vs. radiation therapy [38]. Second is the Swiss TAXIS trial (NCT03513614), a prospective multicenter randomized trial looking at ALND vs. excision of clinically suspicious clipped nodes and radiation therapy to the axilla [39]. The primary endpoint is DFS at 5 years for both of these European trials.

NSABP B-51/Radiation Therapy Oncology Group (RTOG) 1304 trial (NCT01872975) is a study looking at the benefit of regional nodal irradiation in cN+ patients who achieve nodal pCR following NAC. Patients with clinical T1-T3, biopsy-proven N1 disease undergo the scheduled axillary staging, SLNB vs. SLNB with ALND vs. ALND, following NAC. Patients who achieve nodal pCR will then be randomized to no regional nodal irradiation vs. regional nodal irradiation. The only field that is affected by this trial is the regional nodal basin. For patients undergoing breast conservation, everyone will receive the planned whole breast radiation and boost. For patients undergoing mastectomy, no chest wall radiation will be administered in patients who are randomized to no regional nodal irradiation. The primary endpoint is to assess recurrence-free interval, with secondary endpoints looking at OS, cosmetic outcome, toxicity, molecular predictors of recurrence, etc. [40].

The Italian NEONOD 2 trial (NCT04019678) is a multicenter non-inferiority trial designed to assess whether or not completion ALND could be omitted safely for patients micrometastatic disease in the SLN following NAC. The primary endpoint is DFS [41].

The results of these ongoing trials will likely further develop optimal axillary management strategies following NAC, and perhaps be able to individualize each patient's axillary treatment, based on response to NAC. When making these important treatment decisions, it is important to keep the tumor biology information in mind, as there is clear data showing the failure to achieve pCR in patients with triple negative breast cancer is associated with worse prognosis, while it is not the case for hormone receptor-positive breast cancer [42].

Conclusion

Accurate axillary staging following NST is important for adjuvant treatment planning and decision making. In terms of surgical axillary management following NAC, literature has demonstrated that SLNB is able to accurately stage the axilla following NAC for both cN0 and cN+ patients. For cN+ patients, there are modified techniques to minimize the FNR with SLNB as described before (using dual tracer, removal of >2 lymph nodes, and localizing the clipped lymph node if possible). Therefore, it is also important for the surgeons treating breast cancer to clearly understand and learn the important technical aspects of axillary staging following NAC for optimal oncologic outcome and to minimize surgical morbidity. At this time, while awaiting the results of the ongoing clinical trials, ALND remains the standard for patients with any residual axillary disease after NAC, regardless of the quantity of residual disease. In determining the optimal treatment plan for those patients who achieve nodal pCR with SLNB alone following NAC, there needs to be careful multidisciplinary evaluation of each patient's pre-NAC stage, tumor biology, response in the breast, age, and presence of other aggressive features like lymphovascular invasion, as the rate of regional recurrence in this subset of patients is unknown. The key question remains whether the pre-NAC stage vs. post-NAC stage determines the risk of LRR and the patient's overall oncologic outcome in the long run. Ongoing clinical trials as discussed before will address these difficult questions in the near future.

NET can be a safe and effective option for postmenopausal patients with strongly HR+, HER2− breast cancer. As mentioned before, NET allows for the opportunity to assess the endocrine responsiveness which may be important for overall oncologic prognosis. Given the low toxicity profile associated with NET, the use of endocrine therapy should be considered as a valuable treatment option in neoadjuvant setting for the correct patient population. It is well accepted that NET increases BCT rate with clinically significant partial response with tumor downstaging in the breast. However, the role of NET in surgical axillary management is limited as it rarely results in axillary pCR, hence not able to downstage axillary management. Further investigation is needed and dedicated randomized clinical trials are indicated to better utilize NET for axillary management in the future.

References

1. Giuliano AE, et al. Axillary dissection vs no axillary dissection in women with invasive breast cancer and sentinel node metastasis: a randomized clinical trial. JAMA. 2011;305(6):569–75.
2. Galimberti V, et al. Axillary dissection versus no axillary dissection in patients with sentinel-node micrometastases (IBCSG 23-01): a phase 3 randomised controlled trial. Lancet Oncol. 2013;14(4):297–305.
3. Donker M, et al. Radiotherapy or surgery of the axilla after a positive sentinel node in breast cancer (EORTC 10981-22023 AMAROS): a randomised, multicentre, open-label, phase 3 non-inferiority trial. Lancet Oncol. 2014;15(12):1303–10.
4. Fisher B, et al. Effect of preoperative chemotherapy on local-regional disease in women with operable breast cancer: findings from National Surgical Adjuvant Breast and Bowel Project B-18. J Clin Oncol. 1997;15(7):2483–93.
5. Bear HD, et al. The effect on tumor response of adding sequential preoperative docetaxel to preoperative doxorubicin and cyclophosphamide: preliminary results from National Surgical Adjuvant Breast and Bowel Project Protocol B-27. J Clin Oncol. 2003;21(22):4165–74.

6. Rastogi P, et al. Preoperative chemotherapy: updates of National Surgical Adjuvant Breast and Bowel Project Protocols B-18 and B-27. J Clin Oncol. 2008;26(5):778–85.
7. Hunt KK, et al. Sentinel lymph node surgery after neoadjuvant chemotherapy is accurate and reduces the need for axillary dissection in breast cancer patients. Ann Surg. 2009;250(4):558–66.
8. Masuda N, et al. Adjuvant capecitabine for breast cancer after preoperative chemotherapy. N Engl J Med. 2017;376(22):2147–59.
9. von Minckwitz G, et al. Trastuzumab emtansine for residual invasive HER2-positive breast cancer. N Engl J Med. 2019;380(7):617–28.
10. Ellis MJ, et al. Randomized phase II neoadjuvant comparison between letrozole, anastrozole, and exemestane for postmenopausal women with estrogen receptor-rich stage 2 to 3 breast cancer: clinical and biomarker outcomes and predictive value of the baseline PAM50-based intrinsic subtype–ACOSOG Z1031. J Clin Oncol. 2011;29(17):2342–9.
11. Montagna G, et al. How effective is neoadjuvant endocrine therapy (NET) in downstaging the axilla and achieving breast-conserving surgery? Ann Surg Oncol. 2020;27(12):4702–10.
12. Stafford A, et al. Axillary response in patients undergoing neoadjuvant endocrine treatment for node-positive breast cancer: systematic literature review and NCDB analysis. Ann Surg Oncol. 2020;27(12):4669–77.
13. Kantor O, et al. Prognostic significance of residual nodal disease after neoadjuvant endocrine therapy for hormone receptor-positive breast cancer. NPJ Breast Cancer. 2020;6:35.
14. King TA, Morrow M. Surgical issues in patients with breast cancer receiving neoadjuvant chemotherapy. Nat Rev Clin Oncol. 2015;12(6):335–43.
15. Mamounas EP, et al. Sentinel node biopsy after neoadjuvant chemotherapy in breast cancer: results from National Surgical Adjuvant Breast and Bowel Project Protocol B-27. J Clin Oncol. 2005;23(12):2694–702.
16. Pilewskie M, Morrow M. Axillary nodal management following neoadjuvant chemotherapy: a review. JAMA Oncol. 2017;3(4):549–55.
17. Mamounas EP, et al. Predictors of locoregional recurrence after neoadjuvant chemotherapy: results from combined analysis of National Surgical Adjuvant Breast and Bowel Project B-18 and B-27. J Clin Oncol. 2012;30(32):3960–6.
18. Classe JM, et al. Sentinel lymph node biopsy after neoadjuvant chemotherapy for advanced breast cancer: results of Ganglion Sentinelle et Chimiotherapie Neoadjuvante, a French prospective multicentric study. J Clin Oncol. 2009;27(5):726–32.
19. Classe JM, et al. Sentinel lymph node biopsy without axillary lymphadenectomy after neoadjuvant chemotherapy is accurate and safe for selected patients: the GANEA 2 study. Breast Cancer Res Treat. 2019;173(2):343–52.
20. de Munck L, Sonke GS, van Dalen T, van Diest PJ, van den Bongard HJ, Peeters PH, Rutgers EJ. Population based study on sentinel node biopsy before or after neoadjuvant chemotherapy in clinically node negative breast cancer patients: identification rate and influence on axillary treatment. Eur J Cancer. 2015;51(8):915–21.
21. Dauphine C, et al. Axillary recurrence after sentinel lymph node biopsy for breast cancer. Am Surg. 2010;76(10):1127–9.
22. Boughey JC, et al. Tumor biology correlates with rates of breast-conserving surgery and pathologic complete response after neoadjuvant chemotherapy for breast cancer: findings from the ACOSOG Z1071 (Alliance) Prospective Multicenter Clinical Trial. Ann Surg. 2014;260(4):608–14. discussion 614-6
23. Boughey JC, et al. Sentinel lymph node surgery after neoadjuvant chemotherapy in patients with node-positive breast cancer: the ACOSOG Z1071 (Alliance) clinical trial. JAMA. 2013;310(14):1455–61.
24. Boughey JC, et al. Abstract P2-01-02: methods impacting the false negative rate of sentinel lymph node surgery in patients presenting with node positive breast cancer (T0-T4,N1-2) who receive neoadjuvant chemotherapy – results from a prospective trial – ACOSOG Z1071 (Alliance). Cancer Res. 2015;75(9 Supplement):P2. -01-02-P2-01-02

25. Boughey JC, et al. Axillary ultrasound after neoadjuvant chemotherapy and its impact on sentinel lymph node surgery: results from the American College of Surgeons Oncology Group Z1071 Trial (Alliance). J Clin Oncol. 2015;33(30):3386–93.
26. Kuehn T, et al. Sentinel-lymph-node biopsy in patients with breast cancer before and after neoadjuvant chemotherapy (SENTINA): a prospective, multicentre cohort study. Lancet Oncol. 2013;14(7):609–18.
27. Boileau JF, et al. Sentinel node biopsy after neoadjuvant chemotherapy in biopsy-proven node-positive breast cancer: the SN FNAC study. J Clin Oncol. 2015;33(3):258–64.
28. Boughey JC, et al. Identification and resection of clipped node decreases the false-negative rate of sentinel lymph node surgery in patients presenting with node-positive breast cancer (T0-T4, N1-N2) who receive neoadjuvant chemotherapy: results from ACOSOG Z1071 (Alliance). Ann Surg. 2016;263(4):802–7.
29. Caudle AS, et al. Improved axillary evaluation following neoadjuvant therapy for patients with node-positive breast cancer using selective evaluation of clipped nodes: implementation of targeted axillary dissection. J Clin Oncol. 2016;34(10):1072–8.
30. Caudle AS, et al. Selective surgical localization of axillary lymph nodes containing metastases in patients with breast cancer: a prospective feasibility trial. JAMA Surg. 2015;150(2):137–43.
31. Diego EJ, et al. Axillary staging after neoadjuvant chemotherapy for breast cancer: a pilot study combining sentinel lymph node biopsy with radioactive seed localization of pre-treatment positive axillary lymph nodes. Ann Surg Oncol. 2016;23(5):1549–53.
32. National Comprehensive Cancer Network (NCCN). Breast cancer (Version 6.2020). Accessed 27 Nov 2020. Available from: https://www.nccn.org/professionals/physician_gls/pdf/breast.pdf
33. Caudle AS, et al. Use of sentinel lymph node dissection after neoadjuvant chemotherapy in patients with node-positive breast cancer at diagnosis: practice patterns of American Society of Breast Surgeons Members. Ann Surg Oncol. 2017;24(10):2925–34.
34. Wong SM, et al. Surgical management of the axilla in clinically node-positive patients receiving neoadjuvant chemotherapy: a national cancer database analysis. Ann Surg Oncol. 2019;26(11):3517–25.
35. Liu J, et al. The role of postmastectomy radiotherapy in clinically node-positive, stage II-III breast cancer patients with pathological negative nodes after neoadjuvant chemotherapy: an analysis from the NCDB. Oncotarget. 2016;7(17):24848–59.
36. Cho WK, et al. The benefit of post-mastectomy radiotherapy in ypN0 patients after neoadjuvant chemotherapy according to molecular subtypes. J Breast Cancer. 2019;22(2):285–96.
37. A011202 trial. Accessed 23 Jan 2021. Available from: https://clinicaltrials.gov/ct2/show/NCT01901094
38. ATNEC trial. Accessed 23 Jan 2021. Available from: https://clinicaltrials.gov/ct2/show/NCT04109079
39. TAXIS trial. Accessed 23 Jan 2021. Available from: https://clinicaltrials.gov/ct2/show/NCT04109079
40. NSABP B-51/RTOG 1304 trial. Accessed 23 Jan 2021. Available from: https://clinicaltrials.gov/ct2/show/NCT01872975
41. NEONOD2 trial. Accessed 23 Jan 2021. Available from: https://clinicaltrials.gov/ct2/show/NCT04019678
42. Cortazar P, et al. Pathological complete response and long-term clinical benefit in breast cancer: the CTNeoBC pooled analysis. Lancet. 2014;384(9938):164–72.

Chapter 11
Surgical Considerations and Expectations in Patients Receiving Neoadjuvant Chemotherapy and Neoadjuvant Endocrine Therapy

Olga Kantor and Anna Weiss

Surgical Considerations After Neoadjuvant Chemotherapy

Neoadjuvant chemotherapy (NAC) is an appealing approach to optimize surgical outcomes. Preoperative therapy has the potential to decrease tumor burden in both the breast and axilla, allowing for downstaging of the planned surgical intervention to include increased use of breast conserving therapy (BCT) in the breast, and sentinel lymph node biopsy (SLNB) in the axilla. In early randomized trials of NAC, there was a definite increase in the rates of BCT compared to adjuvant chemotherapy. The NSABP B-18 trial randomized 1523 patients to NAC or adjuvant chemotherapy from 1988 to 1993 and demonstrated an 8% increased rate of BCT in the NAC arm, with close to a threefold increase in BCT amongst those patients with tumors >5 cm [1]. The EORTC 10902 study randomized 698 patients to NAC or adjuvant chemotherapy from 1991 to1999 and found 23% of patients initially planned for mastectomy in the NAC arm were successfully downstaged to BCT [2]. The Early Breast Cancer Trialists' Collaborative Group (EBCTCG) performed a patient-level data meta-analysis of 4756 patients in 10 randomized trials comparing NAC to adjuvant chemotherapy from 1983 to 2002. Overall, BCT occurred in 65% of patients assigned to NAC compared to 49% of patients assigned to adjuvant chemotherapy (rate ratio 1.28 in favor of NAC, 95% confidence interval [CI] 1.22–1.34, $p < 0.05$). Of 684 patients with initially planned mastectomy who underwent NAC, 33% were downstaged to BCT [3].

O. Kantor · A. Weiss (✉)
Division of Breast Surgery, Department of Surgery, Brigham and Women's Hospital, Boston, MA, USA

Breast Oncology Program, Dana-Farber/Brigham and Women's Cancer Center, Boston, MA, USA
e-mail: okantor@bwh.harvard.edu; aweiss5@bwh.harvard.edu

A. Soran, F. Nakhlis (eds.), *Management of the Breast and Axilla in the Neoadjuvant Setting*, https://doi.org/10.1007/978-3-030-88020-0_11

Overwhelmingly, the literature supports the safety of BCT after NAC. A meta-analysis of 22 comparative studies of surgical outcomes after NAC compared to patients without NAC suggest similar rates of positive margins and lower excision volumes in tumors >2 cm at presentation treated with NAC [4]. A review of the Dutch National Breast Cancer Audit from 2011 to 2016 found similar margin positivity rates for patients with clinical T2 tumors (14% vs. 14%, $p = 0.05$) and lower margin positivity rates for patients with clinical T3 tumors (28% vs. 31%, $p < 0.01$) who underwent BCT after NAC compared to adjuvant chemotherapy [5]. However, some data suggest rates of local recurrence (LR) are higher after NAC and this may be related to increased rates of BCT. The basis for this concern is that not all tumors shrink concentrically, but rather some may have a more patchy or scattered response across the entirety of the tumor bed [6, 7] which could result in leaving behind microscopic disease when treated with BCT. The EBCTCG patient-level meta-analysis of randomized trials of NAC compared to adjuvant chemotherapy found a 5.5% absolute increase in LR after NAC at 15 years (risk ratio [RR] 1.37, 95% CI 1.17–1.61, $p < 0.01$), although this did not translate to a difference in distant or disease-free survival (RR 1.02, 95% CI 0.92–1.14, $p = 0.66$ for distant recurrence; 1.06, 95% CI 0.95–1.18, $p = 0.31$ for breast cancer mortality) [3]. In contrast, analysis of LR in 3088 patients in the NAC arms of the randomized NSABP B-18 and B-27 trials found a 10-year LR incidence of 9% for mastectomy patients and 8% for BCT patients. A reduction in locoregional recurrence (LRR) was seen with the addition of neoadjuvant docetaxel in the B-27 trial (from 12% to 9%, $p = 0.02$) [8]. Long-term follow up of the EORTC 1092 randomized trial found no difference in LRR rates after BCT following NAC between patients that were BCT candidates initially or those that were downstaged to BCT by NAC (hazard ratio 1.10, 95% CI 0.50–2.39, $p = 0.97$) [9]. A patient-level meta-analysis of 4125 patients in nine studies that had BCT following NAC found a 10-year LRR rate of 6.5%. Factors associated with increased LRR were hormone receptor (HR)-negative subtype (hazard ratio 1.89, $p < 0.01$), clinically node-positive disease (hazard ratio 1.37, $p = 0.01$), and lack of axillary pCR (hazard ratio 1.53, $p < 0.01$) [10].

A few studies have also examined whether negative lumpectomy margins after NAC should be defined differently than the up-front surgery consensus guidelines of "no tumor on ink" for invasive disease [11]. An Austrian study of 406 patients that had BCT after NAC found no difference in LR between patients with margins of 1 mm compared to >1 mm (5-year local recurrence-free survival [LRFS] 94% for ≤1 mm vs. 91% >1 mm, $p = 0.94$) [12]. A study of 382 BCT patients who had NAC at the Dana-Farber Cancer Institute examined multiple margin widths, including no tumor on ink, 1 mm, and 2 mm margins with findings suggesting no differences in LR at any margin width (5-year LRFS 96% for margins ≤2 mm, 94% for margins >2 mm, 100% for pCR, $p = 0.37$) [13]. Taken together, these findings suggest that downsizing the breast tumor with NAC to optimize surgical outcomes, specifically to achieve breast conservation, is a safe option.

Tumor downstaging after NAC is most effective in the tumor subtypes that have the highest rates of pathologic complete response (pCR). A meta-analysis of 11,695 patients in 30 studies of NAC found a pooled pCR rate of 19%, with the highest pCR rate of 39% in patients with hormone receptor-negative (HR-negative), HER2-positive subtype and the lowest pCR rate of 8% in patients with HR-positive HER2-negative subtype. The analysis included patients from 1995 to 2008, most of whom were treated before the routine use of targeted anti-HER2 therapies, with increasing rates of pCR noted over time (pCR increased with increasing midpoint year of study time frame, $p = 0.02$) [14]. In more modern series, including the use of targeted anti-HER2 therapy, the rates of pCR are higher across subtypes. Subtype-specific data from 694 patients with clinically node-positive breast cancer treated with NAC from the American College of Surgeons Oncology Group (ACOSOG)/Alliance Z1071 trial demonstrated breast pCR rates of 16% for HR-positive HER2-negative, 48% for triple-negative breast cancer (TNBC), and 50% for HER2-positive tumors. Although clinical response rates of the breast tumors were similar across subtypes, BCT was significantly correlated with breast pCR; rates of BCT were 35% for HR-positive HER2-negative, 43% for TNBC, and 47% for HER2-positive tumors ($p = 0.02$) [15]. A large prospective series of patients who had NAC at Memorial Sloan Kettering Cancer Center found that among 600 patients who were not initially BCT candidates, 69% of BCT-ineligible and 87% of BCT-borderline patients became candidates for BCT after NAC. Of those in whom BCT was attempted, it was successful in over 90%. Both breast pCR (odds ratio 2.62, $p < 0.01$) and TNBC or HER2-positive subtype (OR 2.26, $p < 0.01$ for TNBC; 1.63, $p < 0.05$ for HER2-positive) were associated with successful downstaging to BCT [16]. Table 11.1 summarizes rates of breast pCR and BCT after NAC in selected studies.

Table 11.1 Breast response and breast conserving therapy rates after NAC and NET in selected clinical trials

Neoadjuvant chemotherapy			
Trial	***Years of enrollment***	***Breast response after NAC***	***BCT after NAC***
B-18 [1]	1988–1993	80% clinical tumor response 13% pCR	67% overall 22% in cT3 tumors
EORTC 10902 [2]	1991–1998	4% pCR	37% overall 23% of planned mastectomy had BCT
B-27 [89]	1995–2000	13% pCR with AC 6% in ER+, 14% in ER− 26% pCR with ACT 14% in ER+, 23% in ER−	48% with AC 51% with ACT
Z1071 [15]	2009–2011	16% pCR in ER+HER2− 48% pCR in ER−HER2− 50% pCR in HER2+	35% of ER+HER2− 47% of ER-HER2− 43% of HER2+
Criscitiello et al. meta-analysis [24]	17 trials 1996–2014	24% overall (range 7–66%)	57% overall (range 13–76%)

(continued)

Table 11.1 (continued)

Neoadjuvant endocrine therapy			
Trial	***Years of enrollment***	***Breast response after NET***	***BCT after NET***
P024 [51]	1998–1999	55% clinical response by palpation after letrozole 36% after tamoxifen 1% pCR after letrozole 2% pCR after tamoxifen	45% after letrozole 35% after tamoxifen
IMPACT [52]	1997–2002	37% clinical objective response by caliper measurement after anastrozole 36% tamoxifen 39% combination	44% of mastectomy-only patients underwent BCT after anastrozole 31% tamoxifen 24% combination 46% were eligible for BCT after anastrozole 22% tamoxifen 26% combination
PROACT [53]	2000–2002	39% objective response by ultrasound after anastrozole 35% tamoxifen	41% of mastectomy-only or inoperable patients at baseline, surgery was feasible after anastrozole 36% tamoxifen
ACOSOG Z1031 [54, 90]	2006–2009	63% clinical response by caliper measurement after exemestane 75% letrozole 69% anastrozole 5.7% pCR after NAC (ACOSOG Z1031 Cohort B)	51% of mastectomy-only patients 83% of marginal BCT candidates
Semiglazov et al. [55]	Not specified	70% clinical objective response after NET 60% after NAC 3% pCR NET 6% pCR NAC	43% NET 24% NAC
GEICAM 2006–03 [56]	2007–2008	48% clinical response rate after NET 66% NAC 0% pCR NET 2% pCR NAC	56% NET 47% NAC

pCR pathologic complete response, *AC* Adriamycin, cyclophosphamide, *ACT* Adriamycin, cyclophosphamide, taxol, *BCT* breast conserving therapy

Neoadjuvant Strategies for Triple-Negative and HER2-Positive Breast Cancer

Although the selection of a neoadjuvant regimen is covered in previous chapters, objective imaging response, clinical response, and pCR rates are of critical importance to the surgeon. Understanding tumor biology, and what to expect from various therapies is crucial to surgical planning. NAC is an especially attractive option for TNBC and HER2-positive tumors as pCR rates in both the breast and axilla are upwards of 40%. Rates of pCR are even higher with contemporary chemotherapy and targeted anti-HER2 therapy options. A meta-analysis of 9460 patients with TNBC after NAC from 27 studies found a pooled pCR rate of 29%, although pCR rates >40% were seen with longer NAC duration [17]. Standardized treatment regimens and newly investigated agents such as immunotherapy agents further increase the pCR rate. In the first analysis of the prospective clinical trial KEYNOTE 522, in which 602 TNBC patients were randomized to NAC with pembrolizumab or placebo, the pCR rate was 65% in the pembrolizumab-chemotherapy group and 51% in the placebo-chemotherapy group ($p < 0.01$) [18]. In HER2-positive breast cancer, the addition of targeted anti-HER2 agents significantly increased the pCR rates in neoadjuvant trials of trastuzumab and pertuzumab. In a randomized trial of chemotherapy with or without trastuzumab in a cohort of patients with HER2-positive locally advanced breast cancer, the addition of trastuzumab increased overall pCR rates from 19% to 38% ($p < 0.01$) and breast pCR rates 22–43% ($p < 0.01$) [19]. In the NeoSphere phase II randomized trial, pCR rates increased from 29% in the taxol + trastuzumab arm to 46% with dual anti-HER2 therapy (taxol + trastuzumab + pertuzumab; $p = 0.01$). Rates of pCR with dual anti-HER2 therapy were highest in patients with HR-negative disease at 63% compared to 26% in those with HR-positive disease [20]. The TRYPHENA phase II trial analyzed three different neoadjuvant regimens including trastuzumab and pertuzumab for HER2-positive patients with pCR as a secondary endpoint; pCR rates ranged from 57% to 66% [21]. A meta-analysis of 16 studies of NAC by subtype found a more than threefold association with pCR for HER2-positive tumors overall (3.6 times more likely in HR-positive/HER2-positive, $p < 0.01$ and 2.3 times more likely in HR-negative/HER2-positive tumors, $p = 0.01$) [22].

With high pCR rates in these patient subtypes, it is logical that these patients would be most likely to downstage to BCT. Interestingly, there is not always a clear correlation. In a surgical companion trial to the randomized CALGB 40603 trial, which assessed NAC with the addition of carboplatin with or without bevacizumab in TNBC, pCR was >40%, including pCR in 41–58% of patients who were initially considered BCT-ineligible. After NAC, 42% of patients initially deemed BCT-ineligible converted to BCT-eligible. However, less than half of these patients underwent attempted BCT [23]. In the TRYPHAENA trial testing trastuzumab and pertuzumab for HER2-positive tumors, pCR was upwards of 55%; however, only 17–27% of patients who were initially planned for mastectomy underwent BCT [21]. A meta-analysis assessing the association of pCR and BCT in 12,311 patients in 36 studies found no significant association between pCR and BCT ($p = 0.27$), including after adjustment for HER2 and clinical nodal statuses [24]. These studies suggest decisions for BCT are complex and are not dependent solely on response to NAC or achievement of pCR. Furthermore, a cultural component is suggested in the analysis of surgical outcomes in the multicenter international BrighTNess clinical trial of TNBC patients treated with NAC. Overall, 53% of BCT-ineligible patients converted to BCT-eligible after NAC; however, patients treated in Europe and Asia were more likely to undergo BCT than those treated in North America (odds ratio 2.66, 95% CI 1.84–3.84) [25], which may be explained in part by the lack of insurance coverage for breast reconstruction outside the USA.

Considerations regarding surgical choices are multifaceted, including in those patients with TNBC and HER2-positive subtypes. However, because of their high pCR rates with NAC, these are optimal target groups for further de-escalation of surgical management of breast cancer. Several prospective multicenter studies have examined the feasibility of using breast tumor-bed biopsy after NAC to select patients that have experienced a pCR and may be eligible for omission of surgical treatment of the breast. Overall, false negative rates were higher than acceptable, ranging from 18% to 50% depending on the type (vacuum-assisted or core) and size of the biopsy needle used [26–29]. The German RESPONDER trial reported an 18% false negative rate (FNR) with vacuum-assisted biopsy in 452 patients with <2 cm of residual disease and at least a partial imaging response reported; half of these false negatives were potentially avoidable with optimized biopsy and comprehensive imaging techniques [27]. An international trial of 166 patients at three centers in the USA, the UK, and Korea with a median pretreatment tumor size of 3.4 cm reported a pCR rate of 51% and an overall FNR of 19% with image-guided biopsy. In the subset of patients with <2 cm of residual imaging abnormality and at least five biopsy specimens by vacuum-assisted biopsy, the FNR decreased to 3% [29]. Though steps are being made towards omitting surgery in patients with pCR, further refinement of patient selection and biopsy technique is needed before these techniques can be applied broadly.

Efforts are also being made to define a subset of patients that can be considered for omission of axillary surgery after NAC. Of 290 patients at the MD Anderson Cancer Center with cT1-2N0 breast cancer as determined by negative axillary ultrasound examination at presentation, 100% had pathologically negative nodes at the time of axillary surgery after NAC [30]. Of 303 patients with cT1-3N0 disease treated with NAC in the Netherlands, 86% had pathologically negative nodes after NAC overall, including 98% of TNBC and 100% of HER2-positive patients [31]. Analysis of 30,821 patients with cT1-2N0-1 breast cancer treated with NAC from the National Cancer Database (NCDB) found nodal positivity rates of <2% in TNBC and HER2-positive patients with breast pCR [32]. While further prospective data and long-term follow-up are needed to establish oncologic safety, these data suggest an opportunity for omission of axillary surgery in well-selected patients.

Neoadjuvant Strategies for HR-Positive HER2-Negative Breast Cancer

In comparison to TNBC and HER2-positive breast cancer patients, those with HR-positive breast cancer experience modest pCR rates [33]. Further, though burden of residual disease after NAC is prognostic across all breast cancer subtypes

[34], pCR as a dichotomous variable does not correlate with improved survival among patients with Luminal A subtype [35]. Thus, less prognostic information is gained by measuring the in vivo response to NAC for HR-positive breast cancer patients than for other subtypes. Additionally, there is ample evidence that subsets of HR-positive breast cancer do not benefit from chemotherapy, as evidenced by lower risk scores based on genomic assays (such as OncotypeDX and Mammaprint), making the utility of NAC for HR-positive patients dubious.

There is ample evidence that tumor biology within the HR-positive cohort drives outcomes and adjuvant therapy choice. The prospective Trial Assigning Individualized Options for Treatment (TAILORx) trial enrolled 10,273 women with HR-positive HER2-negative node-negative breast cancer. Based on the recurrence score result from the OncotypeDX 21-gene assay, patients with a midrange score (11–25) were randomized to endocrine therapy alone versus endocrine plus chemotherapy. Among these 6711 women, endocrine therapy alone was non-inferior to endocrine plus chemotherapy in terms of invasive disease-free survival (hazard ratio 1.08; 95% confidence interval [CI], 0.94–1.24; $p = 0.26$) [36]. Similarly, the MINDACT study (EORTC 10041/BIG3-04) randomized HR-positive breast cancer patients with discordant clinical and genomic risk (as determined by the Mammaprint 70-gene signature) to treatment with or without chemotherapy, including patients with up to three positive lymph nodes. Among patients with high clinical risk but low genomic risk, there was no difference in distant disease-free survival based on treatment with chemotherapy (hazards ratio [HR] 0.78; 95% CI, 0.50–1.21; $p = 0.27$). One thousand five hundred and fifty (46%) of 3356 patients with high clinical risk had low genomic risk, and therefore if adjuvant therapy decisions were based on genomic risk alone, these 46% could be spared chemotherapy [37]. The OncotypeDX recurrence score was also validated for patients with node-positive disease in the West German Study Group PlanB prospective randomized trial. Patients with low scores (0–10) experienced excellent survival rates with endocrine therapy alone (94% disease-free and 99% overall survival at 5 years), including the 41% of these patients that were node-positive [38]. The prognostic value of OncotypeDX among node-positive patients was validated retrospectively among patients enrolled to two prospective randomized clinical trials. The phase III SWOG-8814 trial enrolled post-menopausal women with HR-positive node-positive breast cancer and found that the addition of chemotherapy to endocrine therapy improved survival. However, in subsequent analysis of 367 sufficient tissue specimens, no benefit was seen for patients with recurrence scores less than 18 [39]. Further analysis of node-positive patients from the SWOG-8814 trial revealed that OncotypeDX score was also prognostic for LRR [40]. In the TransATAC study, which randomized HR-positive breast cancer patients to tamoxifen versus anastrozole, 1231 tumor blocks were examined, 306 of which were from node-positive patients. Recurrence score was associated with time to distant recurrence in both node-negative and node-positive disease ($p < 0.01$ for both) [41]. Finally, the SWOG-1007 RxPONDER trial randomized patients with HR-positive breast cancer with 1–3 positive nodes and a recurrence score less than 25 to endocrine therapy with or without chemotherapy. Among the post-menopausal patient cohort ($N = 3350$) the 5-year invasive disease-free survival was 91.6% for those treated with chemotherapy and 91.9% for those treated with endocrine therapy alone (HR 0.97, 95% CI 0.78–1.22; $p = 0.82$) indicating that post-menopausal women with HR-positive pN1 breast cancer can safely forgo chemotherapy [42]. Alternative approaches have also been used, such as the Magee equation. The original equation showed that nuclear grade, mitotic count, estrogen receptor immunohistochemistry score, progesterone immunohistochemistry score, and HER2 as a dichotomous variable significantly correlated with recurrence score [43]. Future modifications of the equation, to include Ki-67 for example, further refined the equation and more accurately predicted recurrence scores, suggesting that common histopathologic characteristics could be used in place of the more expensive genomic tools [44].

In addition to guiding adjuvant systemic therapy, there is growing evidence that genomic assays can be used to guide neoadjuvant therapy decisions for HR-positive breast cancer patients. A prospective trial by Bear et al. demonstrated that OncotypeDX recurrence score could be used to triage patients to the appropriate neoadjuvant therapy. Patients with scores between 0 and10 were treated with neoadjuvant endocrine therapy (NET), between 11 and 25 were randomized to NAC versus NET, and over 25 were treated with NAC. Of the 33 patients with scores between 11 and 25, only five declined their treatment assignments suggesting that patients accept the recurrence score results to guide neoadjuvant therapy decisions [45]. An NCDB study of 989 HR-positive breast cancer patients treated with NAC revealed that a high OncotypeDX recurrence score was associated with increased pCR rate (odds ratio 4.87; 95% confidence interval 2.01–11.82), also suggesting that recurrence scores may be used to select appropriate patients for neoadjuvant regimens [46]. As in the adjuvant space, there are alternative resources to guide treatment decisions in the neoadjuvant space as well. For example, baseline and on-treatment Ki-67 staining levels have demonstrated prognostic significance and a Ki-67-based neoadjuvant treatment selection approach has been tested [47]. In the ALTERNATE trial, patients with an on-treatment Ki67 staining level >10% at week 4 or 12, determined by research biopsy, were switched off trial to NAC [48].

Based on this body of evidence, patients with HR-positive breast cancer who require tumor downsizing are likely overtreated with NAC, and alternative regimens should be considered. NET was initially investigated for elderly patients who were unfit for surgery [49]. Since, several landmark studies have demonstrated the efficacy of NET to downsize breast tumors and achieve BCT [50]. Three trials (P024, IMPACT, and PROACT) established the superiority of aromatase inhibitors over tamoxifen. The P024 trial randomized 337 postmenopausal women with HR-positive breast cancer ineligible for BCT to 4 months of letrozole versus tamoxifen. Objective response by palpation was superior for letrozole (55% vs. 36%, respectively, $p < 0.01$) as was the proportion of patients who were eligible for BCT (45% vs. 35%, $p = 0.02$) [51]. The IMPACT trial randomized 330 postmenopausal women with HR-positive breast cancer to 3 months of anastrozole, tamoxifen or a combination of the two. Objective response by caliper measurement was similar among the three groups (37%, 36%, and 39%, respectively); however, BCT eligibility after

NET favored anastrozole over tamoxifen in 124 up-front mastectomy-only candidates (46%, 22%, and 26%, respectively, $p = 0.03$) [52]. Lastly, PROACT randomized 551 postmenopausal women with HR-positive breast cancer to 3 months of anastrozole versus tamoxifen and allowed for concomitant NAC administration. Objective response by ultrasound was similar among both NET + NAC and NET-only groups. Among patients who were mastectomy-only candidates or inoperable at baseline, surgical feasibility improved more with anastrozole than tamoxifen, (43% vs. 31%, $p = 0.04$) [53]. Following these three trials demonstrating the ability of NET to downsize breast tumors and the superiority of aromatase inhibitors over tamoxifen, the ACOSOG Z1031 trial aimed to determine the best aromatase inhibitor for use in future trials by randomizing 377 postmenopausal women with HR-positive breast cancer to letrozole, anastrozole, or exemestane. Clinical response rates were similar between groups (75%, 69%, and 63%, respectively) and a striking 51% of all mastectomy-only candidates were able to undergo BCT [54].

Several trials have directly compared NAC to NET. Semiglazov et al. randomized 239 postmenopausal patients with clinical T2-4N0-2M0 HR-positive breast cancer who were not eligible for BCT to 3 months of NAC or NET (anastrozole or exemestane). Clinical response rates by palpation were similar in all groups: 63%, 62%, and 67%, respectively ($p > 0.5$). Twenty-four percent of patients underwent BCT after NAC compared to 33% after NET ($p = 0.06$). Also, pCR rates were low among NAC and NET groups: 6% and 3%, respectively ($p > 0.05$) [55]. Later, the Spanish Breast Cancer Group GEICAM 2006-03 trial randomized 95 patients with HR-positive luminal A tumors of at least 2 cm to 24 weeks of NAC or NET (with ovarian suppression if premenopausal). Clinical response rates were 66% after NAC and 48% after NET ($p = 0.08$). BCT rates were similar between groups at 47% after NAC and 56% after NET ($p = 0.24$). Among all 95 patients, only one experienced a pCR (in the NAC group) [56]. Table 11.1 summarizes breast response and BCT rates among selected NET trials. These data suggest NET can downsize breast tumors as well as NAC [57], although pCR is uncommon in this subtype with either regimen.

In large part due to the lack of pCR, the quest continues for an optimal neoadjuvant regimen for HR-positive breast cancer patients. Ongoing studies are examining the addition of CDK 4/6 inhibitors and other targeted therapies to NET [58]. Completed trials include the PALLET and LORELEI trials. PALLET randomized 307 postmenopausal women to neoadjuvant letrozole with or without the CDK 4/6 inhibitor palbociclib. Ki67 staining (a marker of cell proliferation) was significantly lower in the palbociclib group, but clinical tumor response by ultrasound was not different between groups (54.3% with palbociclib vs. 49.5% letrozole alone, $p = 0.20$) [59]. LORELEI randomized 334 patients to letrozole with or without taselisib, a small molecule inhibitor of PIK3CA. Objective response rates were higher in the taselisib group (50% vs. 39% letrozole alone, $p < 0.05$), but there was no difference in pCR rates between groups, (2% in the taselisib group vs. 1% letrozole alone) [60]. Although these agents seem to suppress cell proliferation, they do not appear to significantly improve clinical response or pCR rates.

An additional important consideration in surgical planning for HR-positive patients is that their tumors may exhibit extensive calcifications [61, 62]. These calcifications are unlikely to change after NAC or NET, as the span of calcifications on post-treatment mammogram and ultimate pathologic tumor size do not correlate well [63]. MRI may be a more accurate method of predicting pathologic tumor size [64, 66]; however, no one imaging modality is accurate enough to preclude complete excision of calcifications and a multimodal approach is best [65, 66].

Overall, NET is an effective and attractive option in patients with HR-positive tumors that would benefit from a neoadjuvant approach. Individualized decisions regarding treatment based on other clinical and tumor factors, with the possible guidance of genomic assays on the tumor biopsy, will help optimize treatment decisions and prevent overtreatment in these HR-positive breast cancer patients.

Axillary Management After NET

Initial treatment approach with either neoadjuvant systemic therapy (NST) or up-front surgery should be carefully selected by tumor subtype to minimize the performance of axillary lymph node dissection (ALND). In a study from Memorial Sloan Kettering Cancer Center, an NAC approach decreased the necessity for ALND among TNBC and HER2-positive breast cancer patients. Conversely, there were increased ALND rates following NAC for cT1-2N0 HR-positive breast cancer patients compared to those treated with up-front surgery, especially among BCT candidates [67]. Increased ALND rates among HR-positive breast cancer patients treated with NAC are due to the standard performance of ALND for any residual nodal disease after NST and low pCR rates in the HR-positive population [68]. If HR-positive patients with cT1-2N0 disease are taken to surgery as their initial treatment, they are eligible for ACOSOG Z0011, EORTC 10981-22023 AMAROS, and IBCSG 23-01 [69–71]. Taken together, these trials show that omitting ALND is safe for patients treated with surgery first who are found to have small volume nodal metastases. In contrast, if patients are treated with NST, they are no longer eligible for the application of these trial findings, and even small volume residual nodal metastases lead to ALND. Ongoing trials are investigating the omission of ALND in patients who are treated with NAC and are found to have residual nodal disease [72]; however, in lieu of treatment on a clinical trial, there is no existing strategy to decrease the burden of ALND among HR-positive breast cancer patients who are treated with NAC. As such, the best strategy currently available for HR-positive clinically node-negative (cN0) patients to avoid ALND is up-front surgery, although this presents a predicament if patients also have large breast tumors and NST is needed to achieve BCT. NET presents an alternative neoadjuvant strategy that may reconcile this clinical challenge.

Utilization of SLNB after NET to surgically stage the axilla is considered reasonable, but this is largely extrapolated from studies in cN0 and clinically node-positive (cN1) patients treated with NAC [73, 74]. Very few trials examining SLNB after systemic therapy have included patients treated with NET. A prospective multicenter trial from Sweden investigated SLNB feasibility after systemic therapy in 195 patients, one of which was treated with NET [75]. A prospective single-institution trial from Japan similarly investigated SLNB feasibility after systemic therapy, this time in 36 total patients, 16 treated with NET [76]. Two retrospective reviews have reported acceptable long-term outcomes of SLNB as the only axillary surgical staging procedure for cN0 and cN1 patients who have negative node pathology after systemic therapy. One of these trials did not specify the number of patients treated with NET, and the other included 56 (48 cN0 and 8 cN1-2) [77, 78]. Despite these limited data, it is standard to perform SLNB after NET in both cN0 and cN1 patient populations if the patient is cN0 after therapy.

According to NCCN guidelines, NET is considered NST and an ALND is indicated for patients with residual nodal disease on SLNB after NET [79]. Despite these recommendations, real world data indicate that completion ALND is performed less frequently for patients treated with NET who are found to have residual nodal disease than similar patients treated with NAC [80]. Moreover, there is growing evidence that axillary management after NET should not mirror axillary management after NAC.

First, axillary pCR rates appear to be even lower following NET than NAC. In a single institution study by Hammond et al., 30 of 39 cN1 patients treated with NET converted to cN0 after NET and 1 (3%) experienced a nodal pCR [81]. In a similar study by Montagna et al., 38 of 46 cN1 patients treated with NET converted to cN0 and 4 (11%) experienced a nodal pCR [82]. These findings are consistent with low axillary pCR rates after NET seen in analyses of the National Cancer Database (NCDB) [73, 80, 83, 84]. Although low axillary pCR rates after NET may seem like a drawback of this approach, an important distinction is that, in contrast to patients treated with NAC, patients treated with NET have only received a fraction of their optimal systemic therapy prior to definitive surgery.

Further, residual nodal disease of any size after NAC is independently associated with a poor prognosis across all breast cancer subtypes [85]. However, small volume residual nodal disease after NET does not carry the same prognostic significance. In a recent NCDB analysis of cT1-3N0-1 HR-positive breast cancer patients, the presence of small volume nodal disease (isolated tumor cells or micrometastases) after NET had no effect on overall survival. This mirrors what is seen in the up-front surgery population [86], and in this analysis, overall survival was similar for patients treated with up-front surgery and patients treated with NET matched by volume of nodal disease [87]. Additionally, analysis of a prospectively maintained single-institution database from the Dana-Farber Cancer Institute and a larger cohort from NCDB revealed that patients selected for NET have low volume nodal disease and the choice of axillary surgery (SLNB vs. ALND) in the larger NCDB cohort did not impact survival [88].

Synthesizing these data, it appears there is an opportunity to decrease ALND burden among HR-positive breast cancer patients by managing the axilla of patients with cN0 at diagnosis and treated with NET like that of patients who proceed to up-front surgery, as opposed to that of patients treated with NAC. Specifically, it may be reasonable to omit ALND for patients treated with NET who are found to have low volume nodal metastases, and extend ACOSOG Z0011, IBCSG 23-01, and AMAROS to the NET population. The omission of ALND among patients treated with NET needs to be tested in future clinical trials to determine appropriate patient selection and the long-term safety of this approach.

Conclusion

In summary, both NAC and NET are safe and effective strategies used to downsize breast tumors and achieve breast conservation, regardless of tumor subtype. It is important to recognize that factors aside from clinical and pathologic response, such as culture and patient preference, can influence choice of breast surgery. Standards for axillary surgery following NAC are well-delineated, but axillary surgery following NET is understudied and practice variation exists. Future research regarding surgery after NST is expected to focus on identifying exceptional responders for whom breast or axillary surgery may be omitted and testing the de-escalation of axillary surgery among patients treated with NET.

References

1. Fisher B, Brown A, Mamounas E, Wieand S, Robidoux A, Margolese RG, Cruz AB Jr, Fisher ER, Wickerham DL, Wolmark N, DeCillis A, Hoehn JL, Lees AW, Dimitrov NV. Effect of preoperative chemotherapy on local-regional disease in women with operable breast cancer: findings from National Surgical Adjuvant Breast and Bowel Project B-18. J Clin Oncol. 1997;15(7):2483–93. https://doi.org/10.1200/JCO.1997.15.7.2483. PMID: 9215816.
2. van der Hage JA, van de Velde CJ, Julien JP, Tubiana-Hulin M, Vandervelden C, Duchateau L. Preoperative chemotherapy in primary operable breast cancer: results from the European Organization for Research and Treatment of Cancer trial 10902. J Clin Oncol. 2001;19(22):4224–37. https://doi.org/10.1200/JCO.2001.19.22.4224. PMID: 11709566.
3. Early Breast Cancer Trialists' Collaborative Group (EBCTCG). Long-term outcomes for neoadjuvant versus adjuvant chemotherapy in early breast cancer: meta-analysis of individual patient data from ten randomised trials. Lancet Oncol. 2018;19(1):27–39. https://doi.org/10.1016/S1470-2045(17)30777-5. PMID: 29242041; PMCID: PMC5757427.
4. Volders JH, Negenborn VL, Spronk PE, Krekel NMA, Schoonmade LJ, Meijer S, Rubio IT, van den Tol MP. Breast-conserving surgery following neoadjuvant therapy-a systematic review on surgical outcomes. Breast Cancer Res Treat. 2018;168(1):1–12. https://doi.org/10.1007/s10549-017-4598-5. Erratum in: Breast Cancer Res Treat. 2018 Jan 11; PMID: 29214416; PMCID: PMC5847047.
5. Spronk PER, Volders JH, van den Tol P, Smorenburg CH, Vrancken Peeters MT. Breast conserving therapy after neoadjuvant chemotherapy; data from the Dutch Breast Cancer Audit. Eur J Surg Oncol. 2019;45(2):110–7. https://doi.org/10.1016/j.ejso.2018.09.027. PMID: 30348601.
6. Bossuyt V, Symmans WF. Standardizing of pathology in patients receiving neoadjuvant chemotherapy. Ann Surg Oncol. 2016;23(10):3153–61. https://doi.org/10.1245/s10434-016-5317-x. PMID: 27380637.

7. Baker GM, King TA, Schnitt SJ. Evaluation of breast and axillary lymph node specimens in breast cancer patients treated with neoadjuvant systemic therapy. Adv Anat Pathol. 2019;26(4):221–34. https://doi.org/10.1097/PAP.0000000000000237. PMID: 31149907.
8. Mamounas EP, Anderson SJ, Dignam JJ, Bear HD, Julian TB, Geyer CE Jr, Taghian A, Wickerham DL, Wolmark N. Predictors of locoregional recurrence after neoadjuvant chemotherapy: results from combined analysis of National Surgical Adjuvant Breast and Bowel Project B-18 and B-27. J Clin Oncol. 2012;30(32):3960–6. https://doi.org/10.1200/JCO.2011.40.8369. PMID: 23032615; PMCID: PMC3488269.
9. van Nes JG, Putter H, Julien JP, Tubiana-Hulin M, van de Vijver M, Bogaerts J, de Vos M, van de Velde CJ, Cooperating Investigators of the EORTC. Preoperative chemotherapy is safe in early breast cancer, even after 10 years of follow-up; clinical and translational results from the EORTC trial 10902. Breast Cancer Res Treat. 2009;115(1):101–13. https://doi.org/10.1007/s10549-008-0050-1. PMID: 18484198.
10. Valachis A, Mamounas EP, Mittendorf EA, Hayashi N, Ishitobi M, Natoli C, Fitzal F, Rubio IT, Tiezzi DG, Shin HC, Anderson SJ, Hunt KK, Matsuda N, Ohsumi S, Totomi A, Nilsson C. Risk factors for locoregional disease recurrence after breast-conserving therapy in patients with breast cancer treated with neoadjuvant chemotherapy: an international collaboration and individual patient meta-analysis. Cancer. 2018;124(14):2923–30. https://doi.org/10.1002/cncr.31518. PMID: 29723396.
11. Moran MS, Schnitt SJ, Giuliano AE, Harris JR, Khan SA, Horton J, Klimberg S, Chavez-MacGregor M, Freedman G, Houssami N, Johnson PL, Morrow M. Society of Surgical Oncology-American Society for Radiation Oncology consensus guideline on margins for breast-conserving surgery with whole-breast irradiation in stages I and II invasive breast cancer. Int J Radiat Oncol Biol Phys. 2014;88(3):553–64. https://doi.org/10.1016/j.ijrobp.2013.11.012. PMID: 24521674; PMCID: PMC4790083.
12. Wimmer K, Bolliger M, Bago-Horvath Z, Steger G, Kauer-Dorner D, Helfgott R, Gruber C, Moinfar F, Mittlböck M, Fitzal F. Impact of surgical margins in breast cancer after preoperative systemic chemotherapy on local recurrence and survival. Ann Surg Oncol. 2020;27(5):1700–7. https://doi.org/10.1245/s10434-019-08089-x. PMID: 31873929; PMCID: PMC7138765.
13. Choi J, Laws A, Hu J, Barry W, Golshan M, King T. Margins in breast-conserving surgery after neoadjuvant therapy. Ann Surg Oncol. 2018;25(12):3541–7. https://doi.org/10.1245/s10434-018-6702-4. Erratum in: Ann Surg Oncol. 2018 Aug 25. PMID: 30128902.
14. Houssami N, Macaskill P, von Minckwitz G, Marinovich ML, Mamounas E. Meta-analysis of the association of breast cancer subtype and pathologic complete response to neoadjuvant chemotherapy. Eur J Cancer. 2012;48(18):3342–54. https://doi.org/10.1016/j.ejca.2012.05.023. PMID: 22766518.
15. Boughey JC, McCall LM, Ballman KV, Mittendorf EA, Ahrendt GM, Wilke LG, Taback B, Leitch AM, Flippo-Morton T, Hunt KK. Tumor biology correlates with rates of breast-conserving surgery and pathologic complete response after neoadjuvant chemotherapy for breast cancer: findings from the ACOSOG Z1071 (Alliance) Prospective Multicenter Clinical Trial. Ann Surg. 2014;260(4):608–14. https://doi.org/10.1097/SLA.0000000000000924; discussion 614-6. PMID: 25203877; PMCID: PMC4159769.
16. Petruolo O, Sevilimedu V, Montagna G, Le T, Morrow M, Barrio AV. How often does modern neoadjuvant chemotherapy downstage patients to breast-conserving surgery? Ann Surg Oncol. 2020;28:287–94. https://doi.org/10.1245/s10434-020-08593-5.
17. Wu K, Yang Q, Liu Y, Wu A, Yang Z. Meta-analysis on the association between pathologic complete response and triple-negative breast cancer after neoadjuvant chemotherapy. World J Surg Oncol. 2014;12:95. https://doi.org/10.1186/1477-7819-12-95. PMID: 24731479; PMCID: PMC4011773.
18. Schmid P, Cortes J, Pusztai L, McArthur H, Kümmel S, Bergh J, Denkert C, Park YH, Hui R, Harbeck N, Takahashi M, Foukakis T, Fasching PA, Cardoso F, Untch M, Jia L, Karantza V, Zhao J, Aktan G, Dent R, O'Shaughnessy J, KEYNOTE-522 Investigators. Pembrolizumab for early triple-negative breast cancer. N Engl J Med. 2020;382(9):810–21. https://doi.org/10.1056/NEJMoa1910549. PMID: 32101663.

19. Gianni L, Eiermann W, Semiglazov V, Manikhas A, Lluch A, Tjulandin S, Zambetti M, Vazquez F, Byakhow M, Lichinitser M, Climent MA, Ciruelos E, Ojeda B, Mansutti M, Bozhok A, Baronio R, Feyereislova A, Barton C, Valagussa P, Baselga J. Neoadjuvant chemotherapy with trastuzumab followed by adjuvant trastuzumab versus neoadjuvant chemotherapy alone, in patients with HER2-positive locally advanced breast cancer (the NOAH trial): a randomised controlled superiority trial with a parallel HER2-negative cohort. Lancet. 2010;375(9712):377–84. https://doi.org/10.1016/S0140-6736(09)61964-4. PMID: 20113825.
20. Gianni L, Pienkowski T, Im YH, Roman L, Tseng LM, Liu MC, Lluch A, Staroslawska E, de la Haba-Rodriguez J, Im SA, Pedrini JL, Poirier B, Morandi P, Semiglazov V, Srimuninnimit V, Bianchi G, Szado T, Ratnayake J, Ross G, Valagussa P. Efficacy and safety of neoadjuvant pertuzumab and trastuzumab in women with locally advanced, inflammatory, or early HER2-positive breast cancer (NeoSphere): a randomised multicentre, open-label, phase 2 trial. Lancet Oncol. 2012;13(1):25–32. https://doi.org/10.1016/S1470-2045(11)70336-9. PMID: 22153890.
21. Schneeweiss A, Chia S, Hickish T, Harvey V, Eniu A, Hegg R, Tausch C, Seo JH, Tsai YF, Ratnayake J, McNally V, Ross G, Cortés J. Pertuzumab plus trastuzumab in combination with standard neoadjuvant anthracycline-containing and anthracycline-free chemotherapy regimens in patients with HER2-positive early breast cancer: a randomized phase II cardiac safety study (TRYPHAENA). Ann Oncol. 2013;24(9):2278–84. https://doi.org/10.1093/annonc/mdt182. PMID: 23704196.
22. Schettini F, Pascual T, Conte B, Chic N, Brasó-Maristany F, Galván P, Martínez O, Adamo B, Vidal M, Muñoz M, Fernández-Martinez A, Rognoni C, Griguolo G, Guarneri V, Conte PF, Locci M, Brase JC, Gonzalez-Farre B, Villagrasa P, De Placido S, Schiff R, Veeraraghavan J, Rimawi MF, Osborne CK, Pernas S, Perou CM, Carey LA. Prat a. HER2-enriched subtype and pathological complete response in HER2-positive breast cancer: a systematic review and meta-analysis. Cancer Treat Rev. 2020;84:101965. https://doi.org/10.1016/j.ctrv.2020.101965. PMID: 32000054; PMCID: PMC7230134.
23. Golshan M, Cirrincione CT, Sikov WM, Berry DA, Jasinski S, Weisberg TF, Somlo G, Hudis C, Winer E, Ollila DW. Alliance for Clinical Trials in Oncology. Impact of neoadjuvant chemotherapy in stage II-III triple negative breast cancer on eligibility for breast-conserving surgery and breast conservation rates: surgical results from CALGB 40603 (Alliance). Ann Surg. 2015;262(3):434–9. https://doi.org/10.1097/SLA.0000000000001417; discussion 438-9. PMID: 26222764; PMCID: PMC4710511.
24. Criscitiello C, Golshan M, Barry WT, Viale G, Wong S, Santangelo M, Curigliano G. Impact of neoadjuvant chemotherapy and pathological complete response on eligibility for breast-conserving surgery in patients with early breast cancer: a meta-analysis. Eur J Cancer. 2018;97:1–6. https://doi.org/10.1016/j.ejca.2018.03.023. PMID: 29734046.
25. Golshan M, Loibl S, Wong SM, Houber JB, O'Shaughnessy J, Rugo HS, Wolmark N, McKee MD, Maag D, Sullivan DM, Metzger-Filho O, Von Minckwitz G, Geyer CE Jr, Sikov WM, Untch M. Breast conservation after neoadjuvant chemotherapy for triple-negative breast cancer: surgical results from the BrighTNess Randomized Clinical Trial. JAMA Surg. 2020;155(3):e195410. https://doi.org/10.1001/jamasurg.2019.5410. PMID: 31913413; PMCID: PMC6990971.
26. Vrancken Peeters MJ, van Loevezijn A, van der Noordaa MEM, van Duijnhoven FH, Loo, CE, van Werkhoven E, van de Vijver KK, Wiersma T, Winter-Warnars HAO, Sonke GS, Blanken C, Zonnevels B. Towards omitting breast surgery in patients with a pathologic complete response after neoadjuvant systemic treatment: interim analysis of the MICRA trial (Minimally Invasive Complete Response Assessment). Paper presented at San Antonio Breast Cancer Symposium; 2019; San Antonio, TX. https://www.abstractsonline.com/pp8/#!/7946/presentation/2170
27. Heil J, Pfob A, Sinn HP, Rauch G, Bach P, Thomas B, Schaefgen B, Kuemmel S, Reimer T, Hahn M, Thill M, Blohmer JU, Hackmann J, Malter W, Bekes I, Friedrichs K, Wojcinski S, Joos S, Paepke S, Ditsch N, Rody A, Große R, van Mackelenbergh M, Reinisch M, Karsten M, Golatta M, RESPONDER Investigators. Diagnosing pathologic complete response in the breast

after neoadjuvant systemic treatment of breast cancer patients by minimal invasive biopsy: Oral presentation at the San Antonio breast cancer symposium on Friday, December 13, 2019, program number GS5-03. Ann Surg. 2020; https://doi.org/10.1097/SLA.0000000000004246. PMID: 32657944.
28. Basik M, Cecchini RS, De Los Santos JF, Umphrey HR, Julian TB, Mamounas EP, White J, Lucas PC, Balanoff C, Tan AR, Weber JJ, Edmonson DA, Brown-Glaberman UA, Diego EJ, Teshome M, Matsen CB, Seaward SA, Wapnir IL, Wager JL, Tjoe JA, Thompson AM, Wolmar N. Primary analysis of NRG-BR005, a phase II trial assessing accuracy of tumor bed biopsies in predicting pathologic complete response (pCR) in patients with clinical/radiologic complete response after neoadjuvant chemotherapy (NCT) to explore the feasibility of breast-conserving treatment without surgery. Paper presented at San Antonio Breast Cancer Symposium; 2019; San Antonio, TX. https://www.abstractsonline.com/pp8/#!/7946/presentation/2169
29. Tasoulis MK, Lee HB, Yang W, Pope R, Krishnamurthy S, Kim SY, Cho N, Teoh V, Rauch GM, Smith BD, Valero V, Mohammed K, Han W, MacNeill F, Kuerer HM. Accuracy of post-neoadjuvant chemotherapy image-guided breast biopsy to predict residual cancer. JAMA Surg. 2020;155(12):e204103. https://doi.org/10.1001/jamasurg.2020.4103. PMID: 33026457; PMCID: PMC7542519.
30. Tadros AB, Yang WT, Krishnamurthy S, Rauch GM, Smith BD, Valero V, Black DM, Lucci A Jr, Caudle AS, DeSnyder SM, Teshome M, Barcenas CH, Miggins M, Adrada BE, Moseley T, Hwang RF, Hunt KK, Kuerer HM. Identification of patients with documented pathologic complete response in the breast after neoadjuvant chemotherapy for omission of axillary surgery. JAMA Surg. 2017;152(7):665–70. https://doi.org/10.1001/jamasurg.2017.0562. Erratum in: JAMA Surg. 2017 Jul 1;152(7):708. PMID: 28423171; PMCID: PMC5547923.
31. van der Noordaa MEM, van Duijnhoven FH, Cuijpers FNE, van Werkhoven E, Wiersma TG, Elkhuizen PHM, Winter-Warnars G, Dezentje V, Sonke GS, Groen EJ, Stokkel M, Vrancken Peeters MTFD. Toward omitting sentinel lymph node biopsy after neoadjuvant chemotherapy in patients with clinically node-negative breast cancer. Br J Surg. 2020;186(2):527–34. https://doi.org/10.1002/bjs.12026. PMID: 33031572.
32. Barron AU, Hoskin TL, Day CN, Hwang ES, Kuerer HM, Boughey JC. Association of low nodal positivity rate among patients with ERBB2-positive or triple-negative breast cancer and breast pathologic complete response to neoadjuvant chemotherapy. JAMA Surg. 2018;153(12):1120–6. https://doi.org/10.1001/jamasurg.2018.2696. PMID: 30193375; PMCID: PMC6583006.
33. Esserman LJ, Berry DA, DeMichele A, et al. Pathologic complete response predicts recurrence-free survival more effectively by cancer subset: results from the I-SPY 1 TRIAL--CALGB 150007/150012, ACRIN 6657. J Clin Oncol. 2012;30(26):3242–9.
34. Symmans WF, Wei C, Gould R, Yu X, Zhang Y, Liu M, Walls A, Bousamra A, Ramineni M, Sinn B, Hunt K, Buchholz TA, Valero V, Buzdar AU, Yang W, Brewster AM, Moulder S, Pusztai L, Hatzis C, Hortobagyi GN. Long-term prognostic risk after neoadjuvant chemotherapy associated with residual cancer burden and breast cancer subtype. J Clin Oncol. 2017;35(10):1049–60. https://doi.org/10.1200/JCO.2015.63.1010. PMID: 28135148; PMCID: PMC5455352.
35. von Minckwitz G, Untch M, Blohmer JU, Costa SD, Eidtmann H, Fasching PA, Gerber B, Eiermann W, Hilfrich J, Huober J, Jackisch C, Kaufmann M, Konecny GE, Denkert C, Nekljudova V, Mehta K, Loibl S. Definition and impact of pathologic complete response on prognosis after neoadjuvant chemotherapy in various intrinsic breast cancer subtypes. J Clin Oncol. 2012;30(15):1796–804. https://doi.org/10.1200/JCO.2011.38.8595. PMID: 22508812.
36. Sparano JA, Gray RJ, Makower DF, Pritchard KI, Albain KS, Hayes DF, Geyer CE Jr, Dees EC, Goetz MP, Olson JA Jr, Lively T, Badve SS, Saphner TJ, Wagner LI, Whelan TJ, Ellis MJ, Paik S, Wood WC, Ravdin PM, Keane MM, Gomez Moreno HL, Reddy PS, Goggins TF, Mayer IA, Brufsky AM, Toppmeyer DL, Kaklamani VG, Berenberg JL, Abrams J, Sledge GW. Adjuvant chemotherapy guided by a 21-gene expression assay in breast cancer. N Engl J Med. 2018;379(2):111–21. https://doi.org/10.1056/NEJMoa1804710. PMID: 29860917; PMCID: PMC6172658.

37. Cardoso F, van't Veer LJ, Bogaerts J, Slaets L, Viale G, Delaloge S, Pierga JY, Brain E, Causeret S, de Lorenzi M, Glas AM, Golfinopoulos V, Goulioti T, Knox S, Matos E, Meulemans B, Neijenhuis PA, Nitz U, Passalacqua R, Ravdin P, Rubio IT, Saghatchian M, Smilde TJ, Sotiriou C, Stork L, Straehle C, Thomas G, Thompson AM, van der Hoeven JM, Vuylsteke P, Bernards R, Tryfonidis K, Rutgers E, Piccart M, MINDACT Investigators. 70-gene signature as an aid to treatment decisions in early-stage breast cancer. N Engl J Med. 2016;375(8):717–29. https://doi.org/10.1056/NEJMoa1602253. PMID: 27557300.
38. Nitz U, Gluz O, Christgen M, et al. Reducing chemotherapy use in clinically high-risk, genomically low-risk pN0 and pN1 early breast cancer patients: five-year data from the prospective, randomised phase 3 West German Study Group (WSG) PlanB trial [published correction appears in Breast Cancer Res Treat. 2019 Jan 10]. Breast Cancer Res Treat. 2017;165(3):573–83.
39. Albain KS, Barlow WE, Shak S, et al. Prognostic and predictive value of the 21-gene recurrence score assay in postmenopausal women with node-positive, oestrogen-receptor-positive breast cancer on chemotherapy: a retrospective analysis of a randomised trial. Lancet Oncol. 2010;11(1):55–65.
40. Woodward WA, Barlow WE, Jagsi R, et al. Association between 21-gene assay recurrence score and locoregional recurrence rates in patients with node-positive breast cancer. JAMA Oncol. 2020;6(4):505–11. https://doi.org/10.1001/jamaoncol.2019.5559.
41. Dowsett M, Cuzick J, Wale C, et al. Prediction of risk of distant recurrence using the 21-gene recurrence score in node-negative and node-positive postmenopausal patients with breast cancer treated with anastrozole or tamoxifen: a TransATAC study. J Clin Oncol. 2010;28(11):1829–34.
42. SABCS 2020 abstract citation. Kalinsky K, Barlow WE, Meric-Bernstam F, Gralow JR, Albain KS, Hayes D, Lin N, Pere EA, Goldstein LJ, Chia S, Dhesy-Thind S, Rastogi P, Alba E, Delaloge S, Martin M, Gil Gil M, Arce-Salinas C, Brain E, Park IH, Pierga JY, Hernandex Lluch A, Ramos Vasques M, Ruis Borrego M, Jung KH, Ferrero JM, Schott A, Shak S, Sharma P, Lew DL, Miao J, Tripathy D, Hortobagyi G, Pusztai L. First results from a phase III randomized clinical trial of standard adjuvant endocrine therapy ± chemotherapy in patients with 1–3 positive nodes, hormone receptor-positive and HER2-negative breast cancer with recurrence score ≤25: SWOG S1007 (RxPonder). Paper presented at San Antonio Breast Cancer Symposium; 2020; San Antonio, TX. https://www.abstractsonline.com/pp8/#!/9223/presentation/2794
43. Flanagan MB, Dabbs DJ, Brufsky AM, Beriwal S, Bhargava R. Histopathologic variables predict Oncotype DX recurrence score. Mod Pathol. 2008;21(10):1255–61. https://doi.org/10.1038/modpathol.2008.54. PMID: 18360352.
44. Bhargava R, Clark BZ, Carter GJ, Brufsky AM, Dabbs DJ. The healthcare value of the Magee Decision Algorithm™: use of Magee Equations™ and mitosis score to safely forgo molecular testing in breast cancer. Mod Pathol. 2020;33(8):1563–70. https://doi.org/10.1038/s41379-020-0521-4. PMID: 32203092; PMCID: PMC7384988.
45. Bear HD, Wan W, Robidoux A, Rubin P, Limentani S, White RL Jr, Granfortuna J, Hopkins JO, Oldham D, Rodriguez A, Sing AP. Using the 21-gene assay from core needle biopsies to choose neoadjuvant therapy for breast cancer: a multicenter trial. J Surg Oncol. 2017;115(8):917–23. https://doi.org/10.1002/jso.24610. Erratum in: J Surg Oncol. 2018 Sep;118(4):722. PMID: 28407247; PMCID: PMC5481477.
46. Pease AM, Riba LA, Gruner RA, Tung NM, James TA. Oncotype DX® recurrence score as a predictor of response to neoadjuvant chemotherapy. Ann Surg Oncol. 2019;26(2):366–71. https://doi.org/10.1245/s10434-018-07107-8. PMID: 30542840.
47. Dowsett M, Smith IE, Ebbs SR, et al. Prognostic value of Ki67 expression after short-term presurgical endocrine therapy for primary breast cancer. J Natl Cancer Inst. 2007;99(2):167–70.
48. Ma CX, Suman VJ, Leitch AM, Sanati S, Vij KR, Unetig GW, Hoog J, Watson M, Hahn OM, Guenther JM, Caudle AS, Dockter T, Korde LA, Weiss A, Hunt K, Hudis CA, Winter EP, Partridge AH, Carey LA, Ellis MJ. ALTERNATE: neoadjuvant endocrine theratment (NET)

approaches for clinical stage II or III estroget recetpro-positive HER2-negative breast cancer in postmenopausal women: Alliance A011106. J Clin Oncol. 2020;38(15 suppl):504.
49. Hind D, et al. Surgery versus primary endocrine therapy for elderly women with operable primary breast cancer. Cochrane Database Syst Rev. 2006;(1):CD004272.
50. Weiss A, King TA, Mittendorf EA. The landmark series: neoadjuvant endocrine therapy for breast cancer. Ann Surg Oncol. 2020;27(9):3393–401. https://doi.org/10.1245/s10434-020-08530-6. PMID: 32591951.
51. Eiermann W, Paepke S, Appfelstaedt J, et al. Preoperative treatment of postmenopausal breast cancer patients with letrozole: a randomized double-blind multicenter study. Ann Oncol. 2001;12(11):1527–32. https://doi.org/10.1023/a:1013128213451.
52. Smith IE, Dowsett M, Ebbs SR, et al. Neoadjuvant treatment of postmenopausal breast cancer with anastrozole, tamoxifen, or both in combination: the Immediate Preoperative Anastrozole, Tamoxifen, or Combined with Tamoxifen (IMPACT) multicenter double-blind randomized trial. J Clin Oncol. 2005;23(22):5108–16. https://doi.org/10.1200/JCO.2005.04.005.
53. Cataliotti L, Buzdar AU, Noguchi S, et al. Comparison of anastrozole versus tamoxifen as preoperative therapy in postmenopausal women with hormone receptor-positive breast cancer: the Pre-Operative "Arimidex" Compared to Tamoxifen (PROACT) trial. Cancer. 2006;106(10):2095–103. https://doi.org/10.1002/cncr.21872.
54. Ellis MJ, Suman VJ, Hoog J, et al. Randomized phase II neoadjuvant comparison between letrozole, anastrozole, and exemestane for postmenopausal women with estrogen receptor–rich stage 2 to 3 breast cancer: clinical and biomarker outcomes and predictive value of the baseline PAM50-based intrinsic subtype—ACOSOG Z1031. J Clin Oncol. 2011;29(17):2342–9. https://doi.org/10.1200/JCO.2010.31.6950.
55. Semiglazov VF, Semiglazov VV, Dashyan GA, et al. Phase 2 randomized trial of primary endocrine therapy versus chemotherapy in postmenopausal patients with estrogen receptor-positive breast cancer. Cancer. 2007;110(2):244–54.
56. Alba E, Calvo L, Albanell J, et al. Chemotherapy (CT) and hormonotherapy (HT) as neoadjuvant treatment in luminal breast cancer patients: results from the GEICAM/2006-03, a multicenter, randomized, phase-II study. Ann Oncol. 2012;23(12):3069–74.
57. Spring LM, Gupta A, Reynolds KL, et al. Neoadjuvant Endocrine Therapy for Estrogen Receptor–Positive Breast Cancer: A Systematic Review and Meta-analysis. JAMA Oncol. 2016;2(11):1477–86. https://doi.org/10.1001/jamaoncol.2016.1897.
58. A neoadjuvant study of abemaciclib (LY2835219) in postmenopausal women with hormone receptor positive, HER2 negative breast cancer (neoMONARCH). https://clinicaltrials.gov/ct2/show/NCT02441946. Accessed 6 Apr 2020.
59. Johnston S, Puhalla S, Wheatley D, et al. Randomized phase II study evaluating Palbociclib in addition to Letrozole as neoadjuvant therapy in estrogen receptor-positive early breast cancer: PALLET trial. J Clin Oncol. 2019;37(3):178–89.
60. Saura C, Hlauschek D, Oliveira M, et al. Neoadjuvant letrozole plus taselisib versus letrozole plus placebo in postmenopausal women with oestrogen receptor-positive, HER2-negative, early-stage breast cancer (LORELEI): a multicentre, randomised, double-blind, placebo-controlled, phase 2 trial. Lancet Oncol. 2019;20(9):1226–38.
61. Nyante SJ, Lee SS, Benefield TS, Hoots TN, Henderson LM. The association between mammographic calcifications and breast cancer prognostic factors in a population-based registry cohort. Cancer. 2017;123(2):219–27. https://doi.org/10.1002/cncr.30281.
62. Zheng K, Tan J-X, Li F, et al. Relationship between mammographic calcifications and the clinicopathologic characteristics of breast cancer in Western China: a retrospective multicenter study of 7317 female patients. Breast Cancer Res Treat. 2017;166(2):569–82. https://doi.org/10.1007/s10549-017-4406-2.
63. Li J, Chen C, Gu Y, et al. The role of mammographic calcification in the neoadjuvant therapy of breast cancer imaging evaluation. PLoS One. 2014;9(2):e88853. https://doi.org/10.1371/journal.pone.0088853.

64. Weiss A, Lee KC, Romero Y, et al. Calcifications on mammogram do not correlate with tumor size after neoadjuvant chemotherapy. Ann Surg Oncol. 2014;21(10):3310–6. https://doi.org/10.1245/s10434-014-3914-0.
65. Feliciano Y, Mamtani A, Morrow M, Stempel MM, Patil S, Jochelson MS. Do calcifications seen on mammography after neoadjuvant chemotherapy for breast cancer always need to be excised? Ann Surg Oncol. 2017;24(6):1492–8. https://doi.org/10.1245/s10434-016-5741-y.
66. Jochelson MS, Lampen-Sachar K, Gibbons G, et al. Do MRI and mammography reliably identify candidates for breast conservation after neoadjuvant chemotherapy? Ann Surg Oncol. 2015;22(5):1490–5. https://doi.org/10.1245/s10434-015-4502-7.
67. Pilewskie M, Zabor EC, Mamtani A, Barrio AV, Stempel M, Morrow M. The optimal treatment plan to avoid axillary lymph node dissection in early-stage breast cancer patients differs by surgical strategy and tumor subtype. Ann Surg Oncol. 2017;24(12):3527–33. https://doi.org/10.1245/s10434-017-6016-y. PMID: 28762114; PMCID: PMC5697709.
68. Mamtani A, Barrio AV, King TA, Van Zee KJ, Plitas G, Pilewskie M, El-Tamer M, Gemignani ML, Heerdt AS, Sclafani LM, Sacchini V, Cody HS 3rd, Patil S, Morrow M. How often does neoadjuvant chemotherapy avoid axillary dissection in patients with histologically confirmed nodal metastases? Results of a prospective study. Ann Surg Oncol. 2016;23(11):3467–74. https://doi.org/10.1245/s10434-016-5246-8. PMID: 27160528; PMCID: PMC5070651.
69. Giuliano AE, Ballman KV, McCall L, Beitsch PD, Brennan MB, Kelemen PR, Ollila DW, Hansen NM, Whitworth PW, Blumencranz PW, Leitch AM, Saha S, Hunt KK, Morrow M. Effect of axillary dissection vs no axillary dissection on 10-year overall survival among women with invasive breast cancer and sentinel node metastasis: the ACOSOG Z0011 (Alliance) randomized clinical trial. JAMA. 2017;318(10):918–26. https://doi.org/10.1001/jama.2017.11470. PMID: 28898379; PMCID: PMC5672806.
70. Donker M, van Tienhoven G, Straver ME, Meijnen P, van de Velde CJ, Mansel RE, Cataliotti L, Westenberg AH, Klinkenbijl JH, Orzalesi L, Bouma WH, van der Mijle HC, Nieuwenhuijzen GA, Veltkamp SC, Slaets L, Duez NJ, de Graaf PW, van Dalen T, Marinelli A, Rijna H, Snoj M, Bundred NJ, Merkus JW, Belkacemi Y, Petignat P, Schinagl DA, Coens C, Messina CG, Bogaerts J, Rutgers EJ. Radiotherapy or surgery of the axilla after a positive sentinel node in breast cancer (EORTC 10981-22023 AMAROS): a randomised, multicentre, open-label, phase 3 non-inferiority trial. Lancet Oncol. 2014;15(12):1303–10. https://doi.org/10.1016/S1470-2045(14)70460-7. PMID: 25439688; PMCID: PMC4291166.
71. Galimberti V, Cole BF, Viale G, Veronesi P, Vicini E, Intra M, Mazzarol G, Massarut S, Zgajnar J, Taffurelli M, Littlejohn D, Knauer M, Tondini C, Di Leo A, Colleoni M, Regan MM, Coates AS, Gelber RD, Goldhirsch A, International Breast Cancer Study Group Trial 23-01. Axillary dissection versus no axillary dissection in patients with breast cancer and sentinel-node micrometastases (IBCSG 23-01): 10-year follow-up of a randomised, controlled phase 3 trial. Lancet Oncol. 2018;19(10):1385–93. https://doi.org/10.1016/S1470-2045(18)30380-2. PMID: 30196031.
72. Clinicaltrials.gov. Comparison of axillary lymph node dissection with axillary radiation for patients with node-positive breast cancer treated with chemotherapy: NCT01901094. https://clinicaltrials.gov/ct2/show/NCT01901094
73. Hunt KK, Yi M, Mittendorf EA, et al. Sentinel lymph node surgery after neoadjuvant chemotherapy is accurate and reduces the need for axillary dissection in breast cancer patients. Ann Surg. 2009;250(4):558–66. https://doi.org/10.1097/SLA.0b013e3181b8fd5ent.
74. Boughey JC, Suman VJ, Mittendorf EA, Ahrendt GM, Wilke LG, Taback B, Leitch AM, Kuerer HM, Bowling M, Flippo-Morton TS, Byrd DR, Ollila DW, Julian TB, McLaughlin SA, McCall L, Symmans WF, Le-Petross HT, Haffty BG, Buchholz TA, Nelson H, Hunt KK, Alliance for Clinical Trials in Oncology. Sentinel lymph node surgery after neoadjuvant chemotherapy in patients with node-positive breast cancer: the ACOSOG Z1071 (Alliance) clinical trial. JAMA. 2013;310(14):1455–61. https://doi.org/10.1001/jama.2013.278932. PMID: 24101169; PMCID: PMC4075763.

75. Zetterlund LH, Frisell J, Zouzos A, et al. Swedish prospective multicenter trial evaluating sentinel lymph node biopsy after neoadjuvant systemic therapy in clinically node-positive breast cancer. Breast Cancer Res Treat. 2017;163(1):103–10. https://doi.org/10.1007/s10549-017-4164-1.
76. Fu J-F, Chen H-L, Yang J, et al. Feasibility and accuracy of sentinel lymph node biopsy in clinically node-positive breast cancer after neoadjuvant chemotherapy: a meta-analysis. PLoS One. 2014;9(9):e105316. https://doi.org/10.1371/journal.pone.0105316.
77. Chang JM, Kosiorek HE, Wasif N, et al. The success of sentinel lymph node biopsy after neoadjuvant therapy: a single institution review. Am J Surg. 2017;214(6):1096–101. https://doi.org/10.1016/j.amjsurg.2017.08.024.
78. Galimberti V, Ribeiro Fontana SK, Maisonneuve P, et al. Sentinel node biopsy after neoadjuvant treatment in breast cancer: five-year follow-up of patients with clinically node-negative or node-positive disease before treatment. Eur J Surg Oncol. 2016;42(3):361–8. https://doi.org/10.1016/j.ejso.2015.11.019.
79. National Comprehensive Cancer Network. NCCN clinical guidelines in oncology: breast cancer v6.2020. https://www.nccn.org/professionals/physician_gls/pdf/breast_blocks.pdf. Accessed 29 Nov 2020.
80. Weiss A, Wong S, Golshan M, Freedman RA, Metzger O, Bellon J, Mittendorf EA, King TA. Patterns of axillary management in stages 2 and 3 hormone receptor-positive breast cancer by initial treatment approach. Ann Surg Oncol. 2019;26(13):4326–36. https://doi.org/10.1245/s10434-019-07785-y. PMID: 31562601.
81. Hammond JB, Parnall TH, Scott DW, Kosiorek HE, Pockaj BA, Ernst BJ, Northfelt DW, McCullough AE, Ocal IT, Cronin PA. Gauging the efficacy of neoadjuvant endocrine therapy in breast cancer patients with known axillary disease. J Surg Oncol. 2020;122(4):619–22. https://doi.org/10.1002/jso.26047. PMID: 32506815.
82. Montagna G, Sevilimedu V, Fornier M, Jhaveri K, Morrow M, Pilewskie ML. How effective is neoadjuvant endocrine therapy (NET) in downstaging the axilla and achieving breast-conserving surgery? Ann Surg Oncol. 2020;27(12):4702–10. https://doi.org/10.1245/s10434-020-08888-7. PMID: 32839900; PMCID: PMC7554166.
83. Thornton MJ, Williamson HV, Westbrook KE, et al. Neoadjuvant endocrine therapy versus neoadjuvant chemotherapy in node-positive invasive lobular carcinoma. Ann Surg Oncol. 2019;26(10):3166–77. https://doi.org/10.1245/s10434-019-07564-9.
84. Stafford A, Williams A, Edmiston K, Cocilovo C, Cohen R, Bruce S, Yoon-Flannery K, De La Cruz L. Axillary response in patients undergoing neoadjuvant endocrine treatment for node-positive breast cancer: systematic literature review and NCDB analysis. Ann Surg Oncol. 2020;27(12):4669–77. https://doi.org/10.1245/s10434-020-08905-9. PMID: 32909130; PMCID: PMC7480656.
85. Wong SM, Almana N, Choi J, Hu J, Gagnon H, Natsuhara K, Shen AH, DeSantis S, Dominici L, Golshan M, Weiss A, Bellon J, Mittendorf EA, King TA. Prognostic significance of residual axillary nodal micrometastases and isolated tumor cells after neoadjuvant chemotherapy for breast cancer. Ann Surg Oncol. 2019;26(11):3502–9. https://doi.org/10.1245/s10434-019-07517-2. PMID: 31228134.
86. Giuliano AE, Hawes D, Ballman KV, et al. Association of occult metastases in sentinel lymph nodes and bone marrow with survival among women with early-stage invasive breast cancer. JAMA. 2011;306(4):385–93.
87. Kantor O, Wong S, Weiss A, Metzger O, Mittendorf EA, King TA. Prognostic significance of residual nodal disease after neoadjuvant endocrine therapy for hormone receptor-positive breast cancer. NPJ Breast Cancer. 2020;6:35. https://doi.org/10.1038/s41523-020-00177-6. PMID: 32821803; PMCID: PMC7426953.
88. Kantor O, Wakeman M, Weiss A, Wong S, Laws A, Grossmith S, Mittendorf EA, King TA. Axillary management after neoadjuvant endocrine therapy for hormone receptor-positive breast cancer. Ann Surg Oncol. 2020;28(3):1358–67. https://doi.org/10.1245/s10434-020-09073-6. PMID: 32869154.

89. Rastogi P, Anderson SJ, Bear HD, Geyer CE, Kahlenberg MS, Robidoux A, Margolese RG, Hoehn JL, Vogel VG, Dakhil SR, Tamkus D, King KM, Pajon ER, Wright MJ, Robert J, Paik S, Mamounas EP, Wolmark N. Preoperative chemotherapy: updates of National Surgical Adjuvant Breast and Bowel Project Protocols B-18 and B-27. J Clin Oncol. 2008;26(5):778–85. https://doi.org/10.1200/JCO.2007.15.0235. Erratum in: J Clin Oncol. 2008 Jun 1;26(16):2793. PMID: 18258986.
90. Ellis MJ, Suman VJ, Hoog J, Goncalves R, Sanati S, Creighton CJ, DeSchryver K, Crouch E, Brink A, Watson M, Luo J, Tao Y, Barnes M, Dowsett M, Budd GT, Winer E, Silverman P, Esserman L, Carey L, Ma CX, Unzeitig G, Pluard T, Whitworth P, Babiera G, Guenther JM, Dayao Z, Ota D, Leitch M, Olson JA Jr, Allred DC, Hunt K. Ki67 proliferation index as a tool for chemotherapy decisions during and after neoadjuvant aromatase inhibitor treatment of breast cancer: results from the American College of Surgeons Oncology Group Z1031 Trial (Alliance). J Clin Oncol. 2017;35(10):1061–9. https://doi.org/10.1200/JCO.2016.69.4406. PMID: 28045625; PMCID: PMC5455353.

Part V
The Role of Radiation Therapy in Patients Receiving Neoadjuvant Systemic Therapy

Chapter 12
Regional Nodal Irradiation Considerations in Patients Receiving Neoadjuvant Systemic Therapy

Jose G. Bazan and Julia R. White

Introduction

Rationale for Neoadjuvant Systemic Therapy

Neoadjuvant systemic therapy (NST) is a common treatment approach for patients with operable breast cancer particularly in the setting of triple-negative breast cancer (TNBC), HER2+ disease, and/or clinically node-positive disease (cN1). The commonly cited advantages of NST includes that it (1) Increases the rate of breast-conserving surgery [1, 2]. (2) Allows for real-time assessment of the efficacy of the chemotherapy agents used [3]. and (3) Lends itself to testing the efficacy of new agents in clinical trials [3]. In addition to these long-held reasons for use of NST, the prognostic value of disease response to NST has emerged as an important indication, particularly for patients with triple negative breast cancer (TNBC) and HER2+ positive breast cancer [4]. In patients with TNBC that do not achieve a pathologic complete response to NST, a large randomized trial demonstrated that these patients benefit in terms of disease-free and overall survival from adjuvant capecitabine [5]. There currently are multiple other randomized studies investigating the role of adjuvant systemic therapy in patients with TNBC that have residual disease after NST [6–8]. In addition, for patients with HER2+ breast cancer that do not achieve a pathologic complete response to NST, adjuvant ado-trastuzumab emtansine has been shown to significantly improve similar outcomes in the adjuvant setting [9].

J. G. Bazan (✉) · J. R. White
Department of Radiation Oncology, The Ohio State University Comprehensive Cancer Center – Arthur G. James Cancer Hospital and Solove Research Institute, Stefanie Spielman Comprehensive Breast Center, Columbus, OH, USA
e-mail: jose.bazan2@osumc.edu; Julia.White@OSUMC.edu

A. Soran, F. Nakhlis (eds.), *Management of the Breast and Axilla in the Neoadjuvant Setting*, https://doi.org/10.1007/978-3-030-88020-0_12

Therefore, NST is increasingly used in these breast cancer subtypes given the importance of identifying patients without a good response who can benefit from adjuvant systemic therapies.

Impact of Neoadjuvant Systemic Therapy on Adjuvant Radiation Recommendations

One of the potential disadvantages of NST is that it complicates radiotherapy decision-making in patients that present with axillary nodal metastases that then become pathologically node-negative after NST. In patients treated with lumpectomy, the question becomes whether to treat the breast and regional lymphatics versus the breast only. In patients that undergo mastectomy, the decision becomes whether or not to deliver radiation therapy that encompasses the chest wall and regional nodes or whether to omit radiation altogether. In patients that receive NST, it is unclear if risk of recurrence is driven by the disease burden prior to initiation of NST, the residual disease burden after NST, or the disease response to NST, particularly in the axillary lymph nodes. Historically, the likelihood of nodal radiation therapy to reduce breast-cancer mortality (BCM) has mostly been assessed in terms related to the absolute risk of locoregional recurrence (LRR) [10]. Further complicating matters is that the high-risk breast cancer subtypes (TNBC and HER2+) are the most likely to have the greatest response to NST [4], yet are known to have higher risk of LRR overall. Pathologic complete response rates (pCR), defined as absence of invasive disease in the breast and the axillary lymph nodes, can be >50% in these subtypes, and achievement of a pCR is strongly prognostic for overall survival [4]. On the other hand, patients with hormone-sensitive (ER+/PR+/HER2−) breast cancer achieve much lower rates of pCR, yet seem to have a more favorable prognosis for LRR compared to other subtypes demonstrating that factors that drive recurrence risk are highly dependent upon breast cancer subtype as well. Furthermore, it is not clear that those factors that are prognostic for a favorable LRR outcome after NST are predictive for absence of radiation therapy benefit—particularly as much of the outcome data generated so far reflect radiation therapy use.

What Is Regional Nodal Irradiation?

Regional nodal irradiation (RNI) can be delivered post-mastectomy or post-lumpectomy. After mastectomy and axillary surgery, the term post-mastectomy radiation therapy refers to treatment of the chest wall and regional draining lymph nodes. After lumpectomy and axillary surgery, RNI refers to the treatment of the breast and regional lymph nodes.

The current standard for RNI is inclusion of the axillary nodes, the supraclavicular nodes, and the internal mammary nodes most commonly in the first three intercostal spaces (Fig. 12.1). The axillary nodes that are treated with radiation encompass

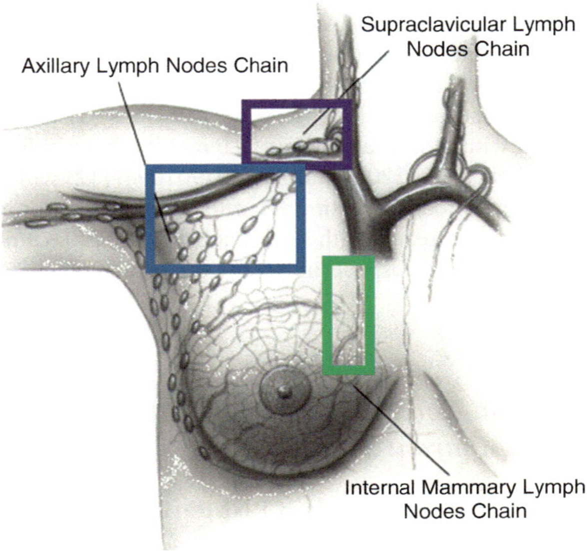

Fig. 12.1 Schematic depicting regional nodal irradiation. The supraclavicular lymph node chain is depicted by the purple box, axillary lymph nodes in blue, and the internal mammary nodes in the first three intercostal spaces in green

the region that did not get removed with sentinel lymph node biopsy or dissection ("undissected" or "retained axilla"). All randomized trials and meta-analyses that have demonstrated a reduction in distant metastases and breast cancer mortality from radiation therapy has targeted the axillary, supraclavicular, and internal mammary nodes.

After an axillary lymph node dissection, the axillary radiation target volume is generally the medial level II and the level III axillary nodal regions. After a sentinel lymph node biopsy, the axillary target volume is the level I–III axillary lymph node regions. The internal mammary nodal (IMN) target volume generally encompasses the first three intercostal spaces. The supraclavicular (SCL) target volume targets the nodal space in the low neck from just below the caudal edge of the cricoid cartilage to the confluence of the internal jugular, brachiocephalic, and subclavian veins. Subtotal RNI to the SCL plus or minus the axilla results in reduction in LRR, but has not consistently effected distant disease rates.

What Is the Role of RNI After NST?

Here, we set to help answer this question based on the currently available data. Review of the expanding indications for RNI after initial surgery serve as an important basis for understating radiation benefit that has been informed by high-level randomized data and meta-analyses. To date, there is no randomized trial data to provide evidence for RNI use after NST. Instead, we will examine the available retrospective literature on patients treated with NST followed by surgery with or without RNI to understand the current practice trends. Two ongoing phase III clinical trials will provide needed evidence for RNI post-NST. The NRG Oncology 9353/National Surgical Adjuvant Breast and Bowel Project (NSABP) B51/Radiation Therapy Oncology Group (RTOG) 1304 (NCT01872975) [11]—the first phase III trial in North America that is studying the effects of RNI in patients with clinical anatomic stage II–IIIA (cT1-3 cN1) axillary lymph-node positive breast cancer treated with NST that convert to lymph node negative at the time of surgery. The ALLIANCE A011202 Trial (NCT01901094) [12] will determine if RNI alone without axillary node dissection is sufficient treatment for axillary lymph-node positive breast cancer treated with NST that becomes cN0 but remains positive at SNB. The optimal technical aspects of RNI treatment planning and delivery will also be briefly discussed.

Regional Nodal Irradiation Efficacy Established in the Adjuvant Setting

Early Randomized Trials of RNI/PMRT, and Initial Treatment Guidelines

To understand RNI post-NST, it is important to understand its role when surgery is followed by adjuvant systemic therapy. Three practice-changing phase III randomized trials that were reported in the late 1990s/early 2000s set the standard for RNI use after mastectomy: Vancouver, British Columbia, Danish Breast Cancer Group (DBCG) 82b and DBCG 82c [13–15]. These trials randomized over 3500 patients, with pathologically involved axillary nodes (pN+) to RNI vs. no RNI after mastectomy and adjuvant systemic therapy of cyclophosphamide- methotrexate-5-flurouracil for premenopausal women and tamoxifen for those that were postmenopausal. Roughly half of the trial populations were N2 (4 or more positive nodes) and the remainder N1 (1–3 positive nodes). RNI included treatment of the Scl, Axilla, and IM nodes in each trial, and resulted in significant reductions in LRR and improved overall survival. Several consensus statements from large Oncology Societies were released shortly thereafter advocating for the routine use of RNI in patients with ≥4 nodes (pN2) or for 1 or more nodes with a tumor size >5 cm (pT3pN1 or Stage IIIA) disease [16–18]. Radiation was recommended to the chest wall, SCL, and axillary nodes. Considerable debate ensued about when to irradiate those with N1 disease and about the necessity of targeting the IM nodes.

Meta-Analyses

In 2005, the Early Breast Cancer Trialists' Collaborative Group (EBCTCG) published a meta-analysis of 36 trials that studied the impact of RNI on LRR and BCM [10]. Patients with pN0 disease had low absolute 10-year LRR rates (2.3% with RNI vs. 6.3% without RNI) and no significant difference in breast cancer mortality (27.7% with RNI vs. 31.3% without RNI). In contrast, for patients with pN+

disease, RNI resulted in significantly lower rates of LRR (5.8% vs. 22.8%) at 5 years and breast cancer mortality (54.7% vs. 60.1%) at 15 years. In addition, this meta-analysis stratified patients into three groups based on absolute reduction in 5-year LRR risk (<10%, 10–20%, >20%). Only patients that had a 5-year absolute reduction in LRR of 10% or more derived a reduced risk of BCM at 15 years [10]. Given that RNI tends to reduce LRR risk by a relative factor of two thirds, this analysis suggested that the individual absolute 5-year LRR has to be ≥10–15% for RNI to result in a breast cancer survival benefit. This appeared to support the existing treatment guidelines recommending PMRT/RNI in those with N2 axillary or stage IIIA disease.

Among the criticisms of this meta-analysis was the fact that not all trials had adjuvant chemotherapy and the radiation was inconsistent across the trials studied: sometimes all nodal sites were irradiated, other times just the SCL was targeted and often the chest wall was excluded. In addition, there was skepticism about the meta-analysis outcomes as the axillary surgery varied widely across the 36 trials included.

Updated Meta-Analysis, Modern Randomized Trials, and New Guidelines

The EBCTCG meta-analysis was updated in 2014 [19], including 8135 women in 22 randomized trials. To address prior criticisms, this meta-analysis included only those PMRT trials that used systemic therapy, had axillary node dissections that included 10 or more nodes removed, and delivered radiation to the chest wall and axillary, SCL, and IM nodes. For the 3131 women with node positive disease and axillary dissection, the addition of radiation significantly reduced LRR and overall recurrence at 10 years resulting in an absolute reduction of 8.1% in breast cancer mortality at 20 years. For a subset of 1314 women with 1–3 positive nodes who had axillary dissection RNI significantly reduced local and all recurrences at 10 years resulting in an absolute reduction of 7.9% in breast cancer mortality (42.3% vs. 50.2%) at 20 years. In a smaller subgroup of 318 patients with only 1+ node, RNI reduced 10-year LRR which resulted in a non-significant reduction in BCM (31.7% vs. 38.2%). Finally, this updated analysis confirmed the earlier finding that patients with pN0 disease derive no benefit from RNI in 10-year LRR (3.0% with RNI vs. 1.6% without RNI) or 10-year BCM (18.4% with RNI vs. 18.3% without RNI). While the radiation and surgical methods were more consistent with modern practice in the trials included in this meta-analysis, it still reflected higher than expected local, regional, and all recurrences likely attributable to the use of outdated systemic therapy regimens.

In 2015, two more modern randomized trials were published that further clarified the benefit of RNI on breast cancer outcomes in patients with N1 disease [20–22]. The European Organization for Research and Treatment of Cancer (EORTC 22922/10925) trial included patients treated with mastectomy (24%) and BCS, while the National Cancer Institute of Canada (NCIC) MA.20 trial was restricted to BCS patients only. In the NCIC MA.20 trial, patients were randomized to whole-breast irradiation or whole breast+RNI (axillary, SCL, and internal mammary nodes). In this study, RNI resulted in a modestly improved LRR (3.2% vs. 5.2%, $p = 0.02$), a larger effect in improving distant disease-free survival (86.3% vs. 82.4%, $p = 0.03$) and disease-free survival (89.7% vs. 84%, $p = 0.003$) and trended toward improved overall survival (92.7% vs. 90.7%, $p = 0.07$). In the EORTC 22922/10925 trial, >4000 patients with pathologic stage I–III (pN+ or pN0/medial tumors) were randomized to radiation of the internal-mammary nodes/medial supraclavicular fossa that included upper level II–III axilla (IM-MS) versus no IM-MS radiation. IM-MS radiation had a small non-significant effect on LRR, but resulted in improved distant disease free survival (78% vs. 75%, $p = 0.02$), disease-free survival (72.1% vs. 69.1%, $p = 0.04$) and overall survival (82.3% vs. 80.7%, $p = 0.06$). The 15-year long term results of the EORTC 22922 trial demonstrate that RNI significantly reduces any breast cancer recurrence and breast cancer mortality although the specific impacts on disease-free survival and distant-metastasis free survival were no longer statistically significant, which the authors attributed to missing data [22]. These trials were remarkable for larger reductions in distant metastasis than on LRR, calling into question the practice of using risk of LRR as a major factor in treatment decisions. In addition, these trials led to an updated combined guideline from the American Society of Clinical Oncology, American Society of Radiation Oncology, and the Society of Surgical Oncology stating that the available evidence supports PMRT/RNI in patients with 1–3 positive axillary nodes with T1–2 tumors and acknowledged that effective RNI includes the chest wall/breast, SCL, axillary, and IM nodes [23].

Summary

The randomized trials and meta-analyses lead to several important conclusions regarding RNI after surgery with adjuvant systemic therapy. First, patients with pN0 disease tend to derive little to no benefit from RNI after mastectomy. Second, PMRT/RNI benefits most patients with 1–3 positive axillary nodes with T1–2 tumors as well as those with N2 axillary disease and/or larger tumors (T3), and effective RNI includes the chest wall/breast, SCL, axillary, and IM nodes. Last, there are still unanswered questions about RNI benefits for patients with pN0/medial quadrant tumors, as these patients were included in EORTC 22922/10925.

THE Role of RNI After NST

In contrast to when surgery is followed by adjuvant chemotherapy, there currently are no prospective, randomized data to help guide the use of RNI after NST. In 2008, a consensus statement based on best available retrospective single institution data was released regarding the role of locoregional treatments after NST [24]. In this statement, it was recommended that RNI should be considered for patients with clinical stage III breast cancer or for patients with pathologically involved lymph nodes after NST. Nonetheless, due to the lack of prospective data, there remains wide variation in radiotherapy practice patterns after NST. In a recent analysis on patterns of locoregional management following NST on the American College of Surgeons Oncology Group (ACOSOG) Z1071 trial, the investigators found underutilization of RNI in patients with residual lymph node-positive disease, particularly in patients that underwent breast reconstruction, and no consistency in the lymph node regions irradiated [25]. These data underscore the importance of randomized trials to help define a standard of care, such as is being conducted on NRG Oncology 9353/NSABP B51/RTOG 1304 and ALLIANCE A011202 trials.

Historical Perspective on RNI After Mastectomy in Patients that Receive NST

The University of Texas MD Anderson Cancer Center (MDACC) investigators published a series of retrospective studies in the early 2000's that set to identify prognostic factors for LRR in patients treated with NST followed by mastectomy without RNI and with RNI. These early data helped form the early basis for RNI decision making, including the 2008 consensus statement guideline.

In 2002, Buchholz et al. [26] reported results of 150 patients (44% clinical stage I/II, 23% stage IIIA, 25% stage IIIB, 7% stage IV) with non-inflammatory breast cancer treated on institutional protocols from 1974 to 1998 with NST without RNI. The 5-year LRR rates were ≤5% in patients with clinical stage I–IIA disease, 16–17% in patients with clinical stage IIB/IIIA disease and 50–79% in clinical stage IIIB/IV disease. Patients with clinical T1-2 disease and ypN0 disease had 5-year LRR rate of 5%. On multivariate analysis, factors associated with increased risk of LRR included clinical stage IIIB/IV disease, ypN2 disease, and no receipt of tamoxifen. In addition, patients with unacceptably high 5-year rates of LRR (≥15%) included those with ≥clinical stage IIB disease, ypN+ disease regardless of initial tumor size, and residual invasive disease >2 cm.

In 2004, Huang et al. [27] reported the outcomes of 542 patients treated with NST, mastectomy and RNI to 134 patients treated with NST, mastectomy, and no RNI. Patients in the RNI cohort had more advanced clinical stage (83% stage IIIA–IV vs. 50%). More patients in the RNI cohort achieved pCR compared to those that did not receive RNI (14% vs. 6%). LRR at the10-year period was significantly reduced with RNI (11% vs. 22%), and this translated into improved OS. When looking at only the patients with clinical stage III/IV disease that achieved pCR (35 RNI patients and 11 no RNI patients), RNI significantly reduced LRR (3% vs. 33%). RNI also reduced LRR rates in patients with cT3–T4 tumors, clinical stage IIB disease, residual disease >2 cm, and ypN2 disease. RNI improved breast cancer-specific survival in patients with cT4 disease, clinical stage IIIB/IV disease, cN2-N3, and ypN2 disease.

The role of RNI in patients that have achieved a pCR was reported by McGuire et al. [28] This series included 106 patients with clinical stage II (34%)/III (66%) disease treated from 1982 to 2002 with NST and mastectomy with ($N = 72$) or without ($N = 34$) RNI. At a median follow-up of just over 5 years, 10-year LRR was similar between the two cohorts (5% RNI vs. 10% no RNI, $p = 0.40$). In particular, for patients with clinical stage I/II disease ($N = 32$) and pCR, the 10-year LRR = 0%. In contrast, for the 74 patients that presented with initial clinical stage III disease, the 10-year LRR was significantly reduced with RNI (7% vs. 33%, $p = 0.04$), and survival was also improved with RNI (77% vs. 33%, $p = 0.002$).

Investigators at the MDACC have also retrospectively examined very young patients and those with cT3N0 disease undergoing NST. Garg et al. analyzed the effect of RNI in 107 young patients (<35 years old) with stage IIA–IIIC breast cancer treated with NST followed by mastectomy [29]. Approximately 80% received RNI, significantly higher in patients with clinical stage III disease (84%) compared to clinical stage II disease (42%). The pCR rate was 19% in patients that received RNI and 15% in those that did not receive RNI. RNI was associated with improved local-regional control (88% vs. 63%) and OS (67% vs. 48%) in this group of young patients. Nagar et al. reported outcomes of 162 patients with clinical T3N0 disease treated from 1985 to 2004 with NST, mastectomy and RNI ($N = 119$) or no RNI ($N = 43$) [30]. The 5-year LRR was 9% for the entire population, and significantly higher in patients that did not receive RNI (24% vs. 4%, $p < 0.0001$). In the 39 patients with ypN0 disease, the 5-year LRR was also numerically higher in patients that did not receive RNI, though this did not reach statistical significance (2% with RNI vs. 14% without RNI, $p = 0.06$). Patients in the non-irradiated group that had ypN+ disease had a 5-year LRR rate of 53% compared to 5% in the group that received RNI.

The MD Anderson series of retrospective data was very influential in establishing the benefit of PMRT/RNI in those with advanced disease after NST whether there was pCR or not and identified the need to further study patients with earlier disease (cT1-2, N1) for benefit of RNI.

LRR After NST in Clinical Trials Evaluating Chemotherapy Regimens: The Impact of Response

The Collaborative Trials in Neoadjuvant Breast Cancer (CTNeoBC) working group performed a pooled analysis of 11,959 patients on various clinical trials and set to determine the optimal definition of pCR and to examine impact of pCR on outcomes [4]. The best definition of pCR is absence of invasive disease in the breast and in the lymph nodes (ypT0/Tis ypN0). With this definition, pCR results in a significant reduction in the risk of death (HR = 0.36). Further, the authors found that the impact of pCR on reducing the risk of death was greatest in patients with triple-negative breast cancer (HR = 0.16) and in patients with HR-/HER2+ disease treated with anti-HER2-directed therapy (HR = 0.08) [4]. Subsequently, LRR after NST and relative to patient response to therapy has been studied in retrospective analyses of large randomized controlled systemic therapy trials.

An important analysis by Mamounas et al. in 2012, that combined data from the NSABP B18 and NSABP B27 clinical trials, underscores the importance of nodal response to NST, and more specifically, the downstaging from cN1 to ypN0 disease and its influence on LRR incidence [31]. These trials, mandated that patients who underwent NST followed by mastectomy did not receive RNI and those who had BCS received breast radiation only. Most of the patients enrolled had early-stage disease: 55% cT1-2N0, 20% cT1-2N1, 16% cT3N0, and 9% cT3N1. LRR incidence was 12.6% among 1947 patients treated with mastectomy (9.0% local; 3.6% regional) and 10.3% among 1100 patients treated with lumpectomy plus breast XRT (8.1% local; 2.2% regional). On multivariate analysis, several factors were associated with LRR, including age <50, pre-NST clinical tumor size, pre-NST clinically positive nodes, and breast and nodal response to NST. Clinically node-negative patients with ypN0 and tumors <5 cm in size disease had low rates of 10-year LRR, regardless of the presence of residual invasive disease in the breast after mastectomy or BCS (cumulative incidence of LRR between 6% and 9%). In the mastectomy cohort, 32 patients that had cN1 disease and had a pCR (breast and no nodes) post-NST, no LRR events were seen at 10 years. In the larger subset of 121 mastectomy patients with cN1 disease that achieved ypN0 disease, but with residual disease in the breast, 10-year LRR rates were fairly low, regardless of initial tumor size (10.8% for cT1-2 tumors and 9.2% for cT3 tumors). Similar trends were seen for those who had BCS after NST. When pCR was present in the nodes and breast, LRR were lowest (~6–7% LRR at 10 years) and remained acceptable in those that had some residual disease in the breast (~8–9%). In contrast, the presence of residual nodal disease (ypN+) resulted in high LRR 10-year incidence in patients that presented with cN1 disease who underwent mastectomy (~19.5%) or BCS (~18.5%).

A similar analysis examining factors predictive of LRR following NST was performed by Gillon et al. the EORTC10994 /BIG 1-00 study that compared two chemotherapy regimens completed prior to surgery [32]. A total of 1153 were included in the analysis, of which 44% had clinical T3-T4 tumors and 54% were clinical node positive. Mastectomy was performed after NST in 53.4% and 46.6% had BCS with breast radiation. The extent of RNI used in this trial was not specified. With a median follow-up of 4.4 years, the cumulative incidence of LRR was 4.9%. On multivariate analysis, two factors were identified as predictors of LRR as a first event after NST: pathological response and breast cancer subtype, ($p < 0.0001$ for both factors). Patients with the highest risk of LRR were those that had any size residual tumor in the breast (ypT+) and ypN+ with 4 or greater residual nodes which was 9.5% in comparison to an LRR of 2.3% in those that were ypN0. Patients with a Luminal A-like subtype had a very low rate of LRR at 1.6% compared to 8.9% for triple negative breast cancer.

A pooled analysis from the German Breast Group (GBG) by Krug et al. examined LRR post-mastectomy following NST in three prospective randomized trials: GeparTrio, GeparQuattro, and GeparQuinto [33]. From a pool of 6139 patients treated on these trials, 1569 had undergone mastectomy and 817 had radiation data.

Radiation was delivered to 617 and included the chest wall, SCL, and upper axilla typically. About half the patients were cT3-4, 61% were clinical node positive, 51% were hormone sensitive, 25% HER2 positive and 15% triple negative. The 5-year cumulative incidence of LRR was 15.2% without PMRT/RNI and 11.2% for those irradiated. On multivariate analysis, RT was associated with a lower risk of LRR (hazard ratio 0.51, 95% CI 0.27–1.0; $p = 0.05$). This benefit from radiation was confined to cT3-4 and CN+ disease and those that were ypN0. In the subgroup of patients who converted from CN+ to ypN0, PMRT/RNI was associated with a lower risk of LRR (HR 0.19, 95% CI 0.04–0.97; $p = 0.05$). Finally, estrogen receptor, progesterone receptor, and clinical nodal status was also prognostic for LRR on multivariate analysis.

LRR from PMRT/RNI Post-NST in Single Institution and Registry Retrospective Analyses

Single Institutions

Several retrospective series from single institutions have examined the rates of post-mastectomy LRR with and without RNI in patients with clinical stage II–III breast cancer and ypN0 disease after NST. In 2012, Le Scodan et al. [34] reported the outcomes of 134 patients with clinical stage II–III breast cancer treated with NST and mastectomy with ypN0 disease. Nearly 2/3 of the patients had clinical stage II disease at presentation and 58% received RNI. Radiation was delivered to the chest wall, supraclavicular lymph nodes, and internal mammary nodes. With a median follow-up of 91 months, the 5-year LRR rate was 4% in patients that received RNI versus 7.5% in those that did not receive RNI ($p = 0.12$). There was no significant difference in the 10-year overall survival leading to the conclusion that omission of RNI in this group of patients does not increase the risk of LRR or death.

Similarly, Shim et al. [35] reported results of 151 patients with clinical stage II (60%) or III (40%) breast cancer treated from 1998 to 2009 with NST and mastectomy all with ypN0 disease. Approximately 70% of the cohort received RNI. Radiation was delivered to the chest wall, SCL, and axillary nodes consistently with only 37% receiving IM node irradiation. With nearly 5 years of median follow-up, the LRR rates were not different based on use of RNI (2% RNI vs. 8% no RNI, $p = 0.15$). No difference in 5-year overall survival was found based on use of RNI. While the absolute number of patients in both of these studies is small, both support the notion that 5-year LRR is sufficiently low in patients with clinical stage II–III breast cancer and ypN0 disease.

Most recently, Wang et al. assessed the impact of RNI after mastectomy in 142 patients with cT1-2 cN1 breast cancer treated with NST, mastectomy and all had ypN0 disease [36]. More than 75% received RNI ($N = 110$), while the remainder did not receive radiation therapy after mastectomy. Radiation was delivered to the chest wall and SCL nodes. With a median follow-up of 66 months, RNI was associated with a significant improvement in recurrence-free survival in the entire cohort and on a propensity-score matched subset analysis. However, in the subgroup of 48 patients that had a pathologic complete response in the breast, RNI was not statistically significantly associated with an improvement in recurrence-free survival.

In one of the largest retrospective studies to date, Huang et al. evaluated a total of 1813 patients with clinical stage II–III (cT1-4 cN1-2) breast cancer from 12 institutions treated from 2000 to 2014 with preoperative systemic therapy followed by mastectomy with or without RNI [37]. RNI consisted of the SCL nodal region, while coverage of the IMN was not recommended. Approximately 70% of patients in total received RNI with increasing rates based on pathologic nodal status (47% of ypN0 patients up to 87% of ypN2-3 patients). In addition, most patients received an anthracycline-based chemotherapy regimen, but only 35% of the 560 patients with HER2 positive disease received anti-HER2 therapy. The authors found that RNI improved outcomes, including OS, for patients with ypN2-3 disease, but for patients with ypN0 or ypN1 disease suggesting that RNI may be omitted in these lower-risk patients.

Likewise, numerous single institutions have examined the incidence of LRR after BCS following NST. Daveau et al. reported on 248 breast cancer patients with cN0-2 disease treated with NST followed by BCS with ypN0 disease [38]. It should be noted that >66% of the population had cN0 disease at onset ($N = 164$) and 63.7% ($N = 158$) received RNI. Radiation was delivered to the breast and SCL nodes and included IMN irradiation in 25%. Median follow-up was 88 months. There was no significant difference in 5-year local-regional recurrence-free survival (89.4% with RNI vs. 86.2% no RNI, $p = 0.68$) or 5-year OS (88.7% RNI vs. 92% no RNI) based on receipt of RNI. However, it is difficult to draw meaningful conclusions from this study since the majority of patients had cN0 and ypN0 disease.

In 2012, Bae et al. reported on 98 patients with cT3-4 disease or cN+ disease treated with NST followed by surgery and radiation therapy with ypN0-1 disease [39]. Of these, 45% ($N = 44$) underwent BCS followed by radiation to the breast and SCL nodal region. No IMN irradiation was delivered to these patients. While the numbers of patients in each subgroup were small and with a median follow-up of 5 years, there was no difference in local-regional recurrence-free survival or disease-free survival in patients with ypN0 disease.

In 2014, Noh et al. detailed results of a multicenter retrospective study (Korean Radiation Oncology Group 12-05) of 260 patients with clinical stage II–III breast cancer treated with NST followed by BSC and radiation therapy to the breast [40]. All patients had ypN0 disease and 136 (52.3%) received RNI, which consisted of SCL nodal irradiation in all of these patients and IMN irradiation in only 14 patients (10.2% of the RNI population). Median follow-up was 66.2 months. There was no significant difference in 5-year local-regional recurrence-free survival (95.3% with RNI vs. 95.9% no RNI) or disease-free survival based on RNI (90.9% with RNI vs. 90.2% no RNI).

Registry Analyses

Within the past 4 years, several studies have examined the question of RNI after NST using the NCDB, often with conflicting results. In 2016, Rusthoven et al. [41] analyzed the National Cancer Database (NCDB) to determine the impact of RNI on overall survival in patients with cT1-3cN1 breast cancer treated with neoadjuvant chemotherapy and mastectomy from 2003 to 2011. It should be noted that the NCDB does not collect recurrence data. Median follow-up was 39 months. In 5032 patients with cT1-3cN1 breast cancer that underwent BCS post NST, roughly 50% had breast and RNI and 50% had breast-only irradiation. There was no significant benefit to RNI in BCS patients with ypN0 or ypN+ based on receipt of RNI. In total, 10,283 mastectomy patients were identified (3040 with ypN0 disease and 7243 with ypN+ disease). In contrast, the authors found that RNI post-mastectomy was associated with a 27% reduction in the risk of death for ypN0 disease and a 23% reduction in the risk of death in patients with ypN+ disease. ER negative disease was found to be a poor prognostic factor for OS. The impact of RNI was greatest in patients with ypN2-3 disease (HR = 0.68), but was also significantly improved in patients with ypN1 disease (HR = 0.84) and ypN0 disease (HR = 0.74). While there are many limitations to NCDB analysis, this study is provocative in that it questions the safety of avoiding RNI in patients with cT1-3cN1 disease that becomes ypN0 after NST and mastectomy.

Almost contemporaneously, Liu et al. published a similar NCDB analysis focused on 1560 patients with cN1 (stage II–III) breast cancer treated from 1998 to 2009 with NST and mastectomy all of whom were ypN0 [42]. In this cohort, 53% received RNI. Unlike the analysis by Rusthoven et al., RNI was not associated with a significant improvement in overall survival (HR = 0.82, $p = 0.12$). While the two cohorts of patients are not uniform, there is substantial overlap (2003–2009) of the patient population in both studies yet the results are disparate.

In 2016, Kantor et al. evaluated 8321 patients with clinically node-positive (cN1-2) breast cancer treated from 2004 to 2008 with NST followed by mastectomy with or without radiation therapy from the NCDB [43]. Nearly 2/3 had cN1 nodal involvement and >60% had cT3-T4 tumors. At a median follow-up of 69 months for the entire cohort, RNI was associated with a significant overall survival benefit. However, in patients that converted to ypN0 at the time of surgery, RNI was not associated with an overall survival benefit in either patients with cN1 disease (5-year OS 87.3% with RNI vs. 86.0% without RNI, $p = 0.43$) nor patients with cN2 disease (5-year OS 92.9% with RNI vs. 90.1% without RNI, $p = 0.21$). While HER2 status was unknown for these patients, those that had ER−/PR− disease did benefit from RNI regardless of nodal response (HR = 0.65, 95% CI 0.48–0.88 for ypN0; HR = 0.72, 95% CI 0.64–0.81 for ypN+).

Last, Ohri et al. used the NCDB to identify all patients with non-metastatic breast cancer treated from 2004 to 2013 with NST followed by mastectomy with ypN+ disease and set to determine the impact of RNI on survival in these patients [44].

The study included 29,270 patients and >60% received RNI. The authors found that RNI did not impact OS in patients with ypN1 or ypN2 disease, but that RNI resulted in improved survival in patients with ypN3 disease (5-yr OS 66% vs. 63%, $p = 0.042$). On multivariate analysis, RNI was associated with survival benefit also only in the ypN3 patients. Analysis of results by breast cancer subtype was not reported.

Overall, it must be emphasized that the NCDB collects outcomes data only on survival. Other important outcomes such as local-regional recurrence, distant recurrence, and breast cancer mortality are not available. With OS as the only endpoint available, an important lesson from the EBCTCG meta-analyses is that reductions in LRR at 5 years take at least 10–15 years to impact breast-cancer mortality. Therefore, longer follow-up periods are needed before the true effect of RNI on survival should be studied in these databases. In addition, HER2 status has only been collected in the NCDB since 2010 and the use of anti-HER2 therapy only since 2013. Furthermore, the NCDB does not capture which lymph node regions (SCL, IMN, Axilla) are targeted by RNI. Therefore, any survival differences reported in these studies could likely reflect imbalance in unmeasured confounding variables.

The Impact of Breast Cancer Subtype

In the analysis of the EORTC10994/BIG 1-00 study breast cancer subtype was an important predictor of LRR [32]. Many other older studies are hampered by collection of data and treatment delivery in a time before the importance of biologic subtype was fully recognized and before the advent of modern anti-HER2 therapy. Only recently have some studies been able to provide a more detailed analysis of LRR by breast cancer subtype in an era of effective systemic therapy, including anti-HER2 therapy. In 2014, Mamounas et al. presented LRR results of the Collaborative Trials in Neoadjuvant Breast Cancer (CTNeoBC) by breast cancer subtype and by surgery [45]. Of the 11,955 patients in the original cohort, subtype data and covariate data was available in 5252 patients, of which 2041 (39%) underwent mastectomy. Radiotherapy details were not available on all patients, but it is estimated that approximately 1/3 of these patients received RNI. The 5-year LRR for all mastectomy patients was 10.4%, but varied greatly by response to NST (3.3% pCR, 8.2% ypT1-3ypN0 and 13.1% ypN+). Compared to patients with ER+/HER2−, grade 1–2 disease, all other breast cancer subtypes had significantly higher risk for LRR with hazard ratios >3 for patients with HR-/HER2+ disease and triple negative disease. Of note, patients with HR+/HER2−, grade 1–2 disease had extremely low rates of LRR regardless of response to chemotherapy (0% pCR, 7.3% ypT1-3ypN0, 5.3% ypN+).

Summary: When Is RNI Recommended and When Is It Safe to Omit RNI After NST

The data presented above are consistent with a few key principles. First, patients with locally advanced breast cancer (≥clinical stage IIIB) are at high risk of LRR regardless of response to NST. Patients with ypN+ disease represent another high-risk group and consensus is to recommend RNI in this situation. Importantly, nodal response to preoperative systemic therapy appears to be an important prognostic factor as first mentioned in the seminal study by Mamounas et al. [31], in which no patient received RNI after BCS or mastectomy and then largely confirmed in several other retrospective series. Table 12.1 summarizes these key studies that evaluated breast cancer outcomes with and without RNI based on nodal response to NAC. However, omission of RNI based on nodal response remains a hypothesis that is currently being investigated in a prospective, phase III clinical trial discussed below. Last, the EORTC 10994/BIG 1-00 [32] and CTNeoBC analysis [45] demonstrated that breast cancer subtype is also predictive of LRR after NST and luminal A-like breast cancer appears to have a low 5-year LRR risk that is less related to response in the breast or nodes.

In the absence of mature data from randomized, prospective trials, we therefore recommend that RNI should be delivered as a standard of care for any patient with upfront biopsy-proven clinically node-positive disease (cN1-3) and/or any residual disease in the regional lymphatics after completion of NST (ypN0(i+)-ypN3), regardless of breast cancer subtype. We reserve omission of RNI for patients with early-stage, clinically node-negative disease and ypN0 disease. These patients are at very low risk of LRR, and routine use of RNI is not warranted in these cases.

Table 12.1 Summary of local-regional recurrence rates in retrospective studies evaluating the role of regional nodal irradiation after preoperative systemic therapy based on nodal complete response

Study	No. of patients	Follow-up (months)	Clinical stage	% ypN0	LRR (RNI vs. no RNI)	*p*-value
McGuire [27]	106	62	I–II 33% III 67%	100%	5% vs. 10% (7% vs. 33% in Stage III)	0.40 (0.04 for stage III)
Le Scodan [30]	134	91	II 63% III 37%	100%	4% vs. 12%	0.12
Shim [31]	151	57	II 60% III 40%	100%	2% vs. 8%	0.15
Wang [32]	142	72	II 100%	100%	5.5% vs. 9.9%	0.15
Huang [33]	490	72.9	II 53% III 47%	100%	5% vs. 9%	0.07

Abbreviations: *ypN0* no residual nodal disease, *LRR* local-regional recurrence, *RNI* regional nodal irradiation

Special Situations: Sentinel Lymph Node Biopsy After NST and Neoadjuvant Anti-Endocrine Therapy

In addition to the complexity of RNI decision-making after NST due to the lack of prospective, randomized data, the increasing use of neoadjuvant anti-endocrine therapy (NET) in postmenopausal patients with estrogen-receptor (ER+) or progesterone-receptor (PR+) positive disease and changes in the surgical management of the axilla complicate matters further. Here, we briefly review these trends and assess the impact on RNI use.

Neoadjuvant Anti-Endocrine Therapy

Owing to lower rates of pCR seen after NST in patients with ER+/PR+ disease compared to patients with triple-negative or HER2+/ER−/PR− disease, several trials have investigated the role of NET in these patients. Pathologic complete response rates with NET are low at ≤1%, so other endpoints of tumor response are often reported. In the major randomized trials, the endpoints reported have included clinical response rates on exam, radiological response rates, and rates of breast conserving surgery [46–48]. However, a more consistent secondary endpoint measured has been Ki67 response. On multivariate analysis of the P024 trial (compared 4 months of neoadjuvant letrozole to tamoxifen) [46], Ki67 response, pathological tumor size (T1-2 vs. T3-4), pathological nodal status, and ER status of the tumor were prognostic for relapse and death after relapse [47]. This led to the development of the preoperative endocrine prognostic index (PEPI). The PEPI score has been validated in the IMPACT trial [48]. In an analysis of patients on the P024 trial, no relapses were seen in the 29 patients that fell into the PEPI 0 category (pT1-2, pN0, Ki67 ≤ 2.7%, and maintained ER expression). The authors conclude that for breast cancer patients with pathological stage 1 or 0 disease after NET and a PEPI score 0, the risk of relapse is extremely low, and these are therefore unlikely to benefit from adjuvant chemotherapy [47]. This patient population is also likely to have no benefit from RNI. Future prospective RNI trials after NET should focus on the safety of the omission of RNI in patients with pathologic T1-2, node-negative tumors with PEPI score 0.

The validation of the modified PEPI score 0 (all factors with the exception of ER status) as a marker for low risk of recurrence is one of the primary endpoints of the ongoing phase III trial Alliance A011106 (Alternate approaches for clinical stage II or III estrogen receptor positive breast cancer neoadjuvant treatment in postmenopausal patients) [49]. This trial evaluated the role of neoadjuvant fulvestrant, anastrozole, or both in the neoadjuvant setting with a required biopsy at week 4 and optional biopsy at week 12 to test for endocrine resistance (Ki67 > 10%). The primary endpoint was to assess the endocrine-sensitive disease rate (ESDR), defined as the number of patients with modified PEPI 0/number of eligible patients initiating neoadjuvant endocrine therapy with a hypothesis that treatment with fulvestrant or fulvestrant+anastrzole would increase the ESDR relative to anastrozole alone. Preliminary results demonstrated that neither fulvestrant (ESDR 22.7%) nor fulvestrant+anastrozole (ESDR 20.5%) significantly improved the ESDR relative to anastrozole alone (ESDR 18.6%) [50]. Mature results for recurrence-free survival are pending at this time. Nonetheless, the nearly 20% of patients that achieve a modified PEPI score of 0 represent a subset in which omission of RNI may be considered after completion of neoadjuvant endocrine therapy.

Surgical Management of the Axilla After NST

In the up-front surgical setting, sentinel lymph node biopsy (SNB) has replaced axillary lymph node dissection (ALND) for patients with clinically negative axilla (cN0) without sentinel lymph node (SLN) metastases [51] and for patients with early stage breast cancer with involvement of 1–2 SLN [52]. Most patients that present with cN+ axilla and receive NST will undergo ALND. However, the role of SNB after NST continues to evolve in these patients and in patients that present with initially cN0 axilla. The concern with SNB after NST is that this approach may result in higher false-negative rates (FNR) than those seen with SNB in the upfront setting. The Sentinel Neoadjuvant (SENTINA) trial [53] and ACOSOG Z1071 [54] trials both demonstrated that SNB technique is critical in achieving low FNR. In the group of patients on the SENTINA trial that presented with cN+ disease that became ypN0 after SNB and ALND, the FNR of the SNB was 24% if only 1 SLN was removed and 18% if only 2 SLNs were removed. However, the FNR was <5% with removal of 3 SLNs and <10% with use of a dual tracer technique. Similarly, the ACOSOG Z1071 study found that the FNR of SNB in patients that present with cN+ disease is ≤10% with removal of >2 SLNs or with use of dual tracer.

Axillary Management After NET

In patients receiving NET, surgical management of the axilla has not been well studied. Recently, Kantor et al. used the NCDB to examine the prognostic significance of residual nodal disease after NET in a cohort of 4496 patients with cT1-3 cN0-1 hormone-receptor positive, HER2 negative breast cancer treated from 2010 to 2016 [55]. Nearly half of the patients underwent sentinel lymph node biopsy, 32% axillary lymph node dissection, and the axillary surgery was unknown in 18%.

In the patients with cN0 disease, final nodal status was ypN0 in 65%, ypN0(i+) in 3%, ypN1mi in 6% and ypN1a in 26%. Patients with cN1 status achieved ypN0 in 10%, ypN0 (i+) in 1%, ypN1mi in 3% and ypN1 in 86%. There were no differences in overall survival rates between patients with ypN0 disease, ypN0(i+) or ypN1mi after NET. In addition, the authors matched patients with any residual nodal disease to patients treated with up-front surgery and found no differences in OS rates by nodal stage. Based on this, the authors conclude that since NET patient outcomes reflect those treated with up-front surgery, de-escalation of axillary surgery could be considered in these patients [55]. Whether the same logic can be applied regarding adjuvant radiation therapy in these patients is worthy of future investigation as well.

Prospective, Randomized Evaluation of Regional Nodal Irradiation in Patients with Clinically Node-Positive Disease Treated with Preoperative Systemic Therapy

Prospective, randomized data are needed to optimize locoregional therapy in patients that present with cN+ disease and receive NST. This group of patients is now the subject of two ongoing cooperative group trials addressing locoregional management based on pathologic response in the lymph nodes. As summarized previously, whether patients that present with cT1-3 cN1 (stage IIA–IIIA) breast cancer and achieve ypN0 disease after NST benefit from RNI is a current matter of debate and the subject of the NSABP B51/Radiation Therapy Oncology Group (RTOG) 1304 phase III clinical trial [11]. In this study, patients with cT1-3 cN1 (node-positive disease must be documented by core-needle biopsy or fine-needle aspirate prior to initiation of NST) treated with NST that convert to ypN0 disease (regardless of presence of residual disease in the breast) at the time of surgery are randomized to RNI vs. no RNI after mastectomy or BCS. The target volumes in RNI are defined as the chest wall and the undissected axilla, internal mammary nodes in the first three intercostal spaces, and the supraclavicular fossa. The primary endpoint of the study is to determine if RNI/RNI results in a significant reduction in invasive breast cancer recurrence-free interval (defined as time from randomization until invasive local, regional, or distant recurrence, or death from breast cancer).

The ALLIANCE A011202 trial has the same enrollment criteria as NSABP B51/RTOG 1304, but requires SNB at the time of surgery [12]. Patients that are ypN+ on SNB are randomized to completion ALND+RNI versus RNI alone. In addition, patients on the Alliance A011106 trial that develop endocrine resistance at week 4 or week 12 (Ki67 > 10%) will then go on to receive preoperative chemotherapy. These patients with cN+ disease that convert to ypN0 will also be eligible for NSABP B51/RTOG 1304. Together, these two landmark studies will have a significant impact on the local-regional management of clinically node-positive breast cancer treated with NST.

Clinical Evaluation of the Regional Lymphatics Prior to Initiation of Preoperative Systemic Therapy

Prior to initiation of preoperative systemic therapy, we recommend a thorough evaluation to determine the presence or absence of nodal disease in the axilla, SCL, and IM regions. In a detailed review of imaging of the axilla prior to preoperative chemotherapy, we recommend that all patients receiving preoperative systemic therapy, including endocrine therapy, should undergo ultrasound of the axilla with biopsy of any suspicious-appearing lymph nodes [55]. Imaging features that most accurately distinguish malignant from benign-appearing lymph nodes include loss of a fatty hilum, eccentrically widened cortex, and a longitudinal/transverse greatest dimension ratio <2 [56]. Compared to ultrasound alone, imaging along with biopsy of a suspicious lymph node improves the specificity from a range of 44–97% to a range of 97–100% and the positive predictive value from a range of 45–95% to a range of 93–100% [57].

In addition to the evaluation of the axillary nodes with ultrasound ± biopsy, we also recommend that patients undergo 3-dimensional cross-sectional imaging to evaluate the lymph nodes in the supraclavicular, infraclavicular, and internal mammary nodal regions. Any lymph node involvement outside of the level I/II axillary nodal region is an indication for RNI, as these lymph nodes are not commonly resected. At our institution, all patients receiving preoperative systemic therapy undergo a CT scan of the thorax with contrast with a field of view that extends cranially to encompass the supraclavicular fossa superiorly to the caudal aspect of the cricoid cartilage. Ideally, the contrast dye should be injected on the contralateral side to the breast cancer so as not to obscure adequate visualization of the supraclavicular, infraclavicular and subpectoral lymph nodes. Magnetic resonance imaging may be helpful in identifying suspicious internal mammary and/or axillary nodes, but the field of view often does not fully encompass the supraclavicular nodal region. In patients that undergo systemic staging, 18-fluoro-deoxy-glucose (FDG)-positron emission (PET) can be helpful in detecting occult nodal metastases to extra-axillary nodal regions. In one study of over 300 breast cancer patients set to receive preoperative systemic therapy, FDG-PET detected internal mammary nodal metastases in 26 patients (8%) and peri-clavicular nodal metastases in 32 patients (10%) [58]. Overall, this resulted in a change in the radiotherapy plan for 50 patients in the study (16%). There is a gap in knowledge regarding standards for imaging prior to NST and given the ability of CT chest (and/or FDG-PET if full staging is warranted) to detect potential occult lymph node metastases outside of the level I/II axillary region, we strongly recommend that all patients undergo at least one of these studies prior to initiation of preoperative systemic therapy to help accurately stage the extent of disease.

Radiotherapy Technique

Our approach to treatment-planning for RNI has been detailed previously [59, 60]. We use an adaptive planning algorithm to determine the best treatment technique, which varies based on individual patient anatomy (Fig. 12.2). At the time of simulation, all patients undergo computed tomography (CT)-based simulation with a free-breath scan and deep-inspiration breath hold (DIBH) to enable respiratory gating, if necessary, to meet normal tissue constraints. While DIBH is commonly used for RNI for left-sided breast cancers in order to achieve dose constraints to the heart and ipsilateral lung, DIBH may be useful in right-sided cases to help lower the ipsilateral lung and liver dose [61].

After simulation, target volumes are contoured using the guidelines and recommendations from the RTOG Breast Contouring Atlas and the RTOG 1304/NSABP B51 protocol [62]. Our clinical target volumes (CTV) created include: breast CTV or chest wall CTV, lumpectomy CTV or mastectomy scar CTV, axilla CTV, supraclavicular (SCL) CTV, and internal mammary node (IMN) CTV. The axilla CTV contains the retained axillary nodes, which is generally the level III and medial level II axillary nodes after an axillary lymph node dissection and levels I–III after a sentinel lymph node biopsy. We treat the internal mammary nodes in the first three intercostal spaces in all cases, given that the phase III RNI studies that led to reduction in breast cancer mortality included the IMNs [13–15, 20, 21] and the preponderance of evidence demonstrating improved outcomes with irradiation of the internal mammary nodes [63, 64]. Margins are then added to create the appropriate planning target volumes (PTV). In select cases (for example, patients presenting with gross SCL nodal involvement), a nodal boost CTV/PTV is also created. For each case, the following normal tissues are also routinely contoured: heart, ipsilateral lung, contralateral lung, esophagus, thyroid, and contralateral breast.

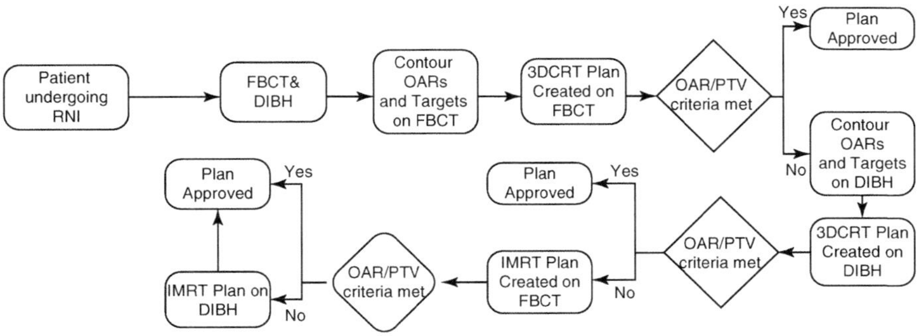

Fig. 12.2 Adaptive treatment planning algorithm for regional nodal irradiation. *Abbreviations*: 3DCRT 3D conformal radiation therapy, DIBH deep inspiration breath hold, FBCT free-breath computed tomography, IMRT intensity-modulated radiation therapy, OAR organ-at-risk, PTV planning target volume

3D conformal (3DCRT) radiation plans are then created to optimize dose to the PTVs and spare normal tissues as much as possible. Our institutional standard is to use a mono-isocentric technique to treat the chest wall/breast and regional lymph nodes. The breast/chest wall and IMC PTV are most commonly treated with tangential fields using the field-in-field technique to improve dose homogeneity. Depending upon the chest wall geometry, matching photon and medial electron fields are sometimes used to treat the CW PTV and IMC PTV. The SCL PTV/axilla PTV are treated together in a separate plan with an opposed obliques or rotational technique most heavily weighted from the anterior beam. In cases in which a 3D conformal radiotherapy plan either results in inadequate dose to the PTVs or in excess dose to organs-at-risk, inverse planned intensity modulated radiation therapy (IMRT) plans are then created, first on the free-breathing CT then on the DIBH, if needed. In these cases, all PTVs are generally treated in a single plan using 5–9 beams.

With this adaptive treatment-planning algorithm, we have found that treatment with 3DCRT or IMRT results in equivalent rate of disease control and similar rates of acute toxicity [60], with the exception of acute symptomatic esophagitis, which tends to be higher in patients treated with IMRT compared to 3DCRT [59, 65]. Based on our experience, we have found esophageal dose-volume esophageal parameters that are associated with higher rates of toxicity, and we have now implemented constraints to the esophagus to potentially help limit esophageal toxicity, particularly in patients receiving IMRT [65].

Our standard prescription dose is 50 Gy in 25 fractions. We reserve hypofractionation for patients treated on ongoing protocols, such as ALLIANCE A221505 [66], or for elderly patients (≥70 years old). Most patients receive a boost to the lumpectomy cavity after BCS. Use of a mastectomy scar boost is not routinely delivered, but is strongly considered for patients with significant residual disease after completion of NST. In plan evaluation, we aim to achieve the planning objectives to the target volumes and constraints to the OARs set forth in Table 12.2, which are adapted from the NSABP B51/RTOG 1304 protocol.

Table 12.2 Planning objectives for regional nodal irradiation with conventional fractionation (2 Gy per day to 50 Gy) at The Ohio State University Department of Radiation Oncology

Structure	Ideal	Acceptable
Breast or chest wall PTV		
Coverage	V47.5 Gy ≥ 95%	V47.5 Gy ≥ 90%
Hot spots	V54 Gy ≤ 50%	V56 Gy ≤ 50%
Cumulative dose (with boost)	V-Total dose ≤ 30%	V-Total dose ≤ 35%
Lumpectomy or scar PTV	V50 Gy ≥ 95%	V47.5 Gy ≥ 95%
Internal mammary node PTV	V47.5 Gy ≥ 95%	V40 Gy ≥ 90%
Supraclavicular PTV	V47.5 Gy ≥ 95%	V47.5 Gy ≥ 90%
Axilla PTV	V47.5 Gy ≥ 95%	V47.5 Gy ≥ 90%
Heart		
LEFT		

Table 12.2 (continued)

Structure	Ideal	Acceptable
Mean dose	≤4 Gy	≤5 Gy
Maximum dose	≤45 Gy	≤50 Gy
Other	V25 Gy ≤ 5%	V30 Gy ≤ 5%
RIGHT		
Mean dose	≤2 Gy	≤4 Gy
Maximum dose	≤30 Gy	≤45 Gy
Ipsilateral Lung		
V20	≤30%	≤35%
V10	≤50%	≤60%
V5	≤65%	≤75%
Total Lungs	Mean dose ≤ 10 Gy	Mean dose ≤ 11 Gy
Contralateral lung	As low as possible	V5 Gy ≤ 15%
Esophagus		
Mean Dose	≤10 Gy	≤11 Gy
V10 Gy	≤30%	≤35%
V20 Gy	≤15%	≤20%
Contralateral breast	V3 Gy ≤ 5%	V4.1 Gy ≤ 5%
Liver	As low as possible	Mean dose ≤ 10 Gy

PTV planning target volume, *Vx* volume of structure that receives × Gy or more

Conclusion

In summary, review of the best available evidence suggests that RNI should be recommended for patients with residual nodal disease at the time of surgery and patients that present with clinically involved axillary or extra-axillary nodal disease prior to initiation of preoperative systemic therapy. Patients with clinically node-negative disease and pathologically node-negative disease are at low risk of breast cancer recurrence, and RNI can safely be omitted in these patients. However, clinically node-negative should include evaluation of the SCL, infraclavicular, and internal mammary nodal basins with either CT chest with contrast or FDG-PET to ensure that there are no occult metastases in these nodal basins prior to starting systemic therapy. For patients that present with clinically lymph node-positive disease that convert to pathologically node negative, there is conflicting and therefore insufficient evidence to recommend RNI omission at this time. We await the results of RTOG 1304/NSABP B51, which will provide a definitive answer to the role of RNI in this situation. Patients that remain ypN+ on SNB should receive RNI (with or without ALND) and consider enrollment on the ongoing ALLIANCE A011202 phase III trial.

References

1. Bear HD, Anderson S, Smith RE, et al. Sequential preoperative or postoperative docetaxel added to preoperative doxorubicin plus cyclophosphamide for operable breast cancer:National Surgical Adjuvant Breast and Bowel Project Protocol B-27. J Clin Oncol. 2006;24:2019–27.
2. Fisher B, Bryant J, Wolmark N, et al. Effect of preoperative chemotherapy on the outcome of women with operable breast cancer. J Clin Oncol. 1998;16:2672–85.
3. Kaufmann M, von Minckwitz G, Mamounas EP, et al. Recommendations from an international consensus conference on the current status and future of neoadjuvant systemic therapy in primary breast cancer. Ann Surg Oncol. 2012;19:1508–16.
4. Cortazar P, Zhang L, Untch M, et al. Pathological complete response and long-term clinical benefit in breast cancer: the CTNeoBC pooled analysis. Lancet. 2014;384:164–72.
5. Masuda N, Lee SJ, Ohtani S, et al. Adjuvant capecitabine for breast cancer after preoperative chemotherapy. N Engl J Med. 2017;376:2147–59.
6. NCT02445391: platinum based chemotherapy or capecitabine in treating patients with residual triple-negative basal-like breast cancer following neoadjuvant chemotherapy.
7. NCT02954874: testing MK-3475 (pembrolizumab) as adjuvant therapy for triple receptor-negative breast cancer.
8. NCT04052555: testing the addition of an anti-cancer drug, M6620, to the usual treatment (radiation therapy) for chemotherapy-resistant triple-negative and estrogen and/or progesterone receptor positive, HER2 negative breast cancer.
9. von Minckwitz G, Huang CS, Mano MS, et al. Trastuzumab emtansine for residual invasive HER2-positive breast cancer. N Engl J Med. 2019;380:617–28.
10. Clarke M, Collins R, Darby S, et al. Effects of radiotherapy and of differences in the extent of surgery for early breast cancer on local recurrence and 15-year survival: an overview of the randomised trials. Lancet. 2005;366:2087–106.
11. NCT01872975: standard or comprehensive radiation therapy in treating patients with early-stage breast cancer previously treated with chemotherapy and surgery.
12. NCT01901094: comparison of axillary lymph node dissection with axillary radiation for patients with node-positive breast cancer treated with chemotherapy.
13. Overgaard M, Hansen PS, Overgaard J, et al. Postoperative radiotherapy in high-risk premenopausal women with breast cancer who receive adjuvant chemotherapy. Danish Breast Cancer Cooperative Group 82b Trial. N Engl J Med. 1997;337:949–55.
14. Overgaard M, Jensen MB, Overgaard J, et al. Postoperative radiotherapy in high-risk postmenopausal breast-cancer patients given adjuvant tamoxifen: Danish Breast Cancer Cooperative Group DBCG 82c randomised trial. Lancet. 1999;353:1641–8.
15. Ragaz J, Olivotto IA, Spinelli JJ, et al. Locoregional radiation therapy in patients with high-risk breast cancer receiving adjuvant chemotherapy: 20-year results of the British Columbia randomized trial. J Natl Cancer Inst. 2005;97:116–26.
16. Harris JR, Halpin-Murphy P, McNeese M, et al. Consensus statement on postmastectomy radiation therapy. Int J Radiat Oncol Biol Phys. 1999;44:989–90.
17. Recht A, Edge SB, Solin LJ, et al. Postmastectomy radiotherapy: clinical practice guidelines of the American Society of Clinical Oncology. J Clin Oncol. 2001;19:1539–69.
18. Taylor ME, Haffty BG, Rabinovitch R, et al. ACR appropriateness criteria on postmastectomy radiotherapy expert panel on radiation oncology-breast. Int J Radiat Oncol Biol Phys. 2009;73:997–1002.
19. EBCTCG, McGale P, Taylor C, et al. Effect of radiotherapy after mastectomy and axillary surgery on 10-year recurrence and 20-year breast cancer mortality: meta-analysis of individual patient data for 8135 women in 22 randomised trials. Lancet. 2014;383:2127–35.
20. Poortmans PM, Struikmans H, Bartelink H. Regional nodal irradiation in early-stage breast cancer. N Engl J Med. 2015;373:1879–80.
21. Whelan TJ, Olivotto IA, Levine MN. Regional nodal irradiation in early-stage breast cancer. N Engl J Med. 2015;373:1878–9.

22. Poortmans PM, Weltens C, Fortpied C, et al. Internal mammary and medial supraclavicular lymph node chain irradiation in stage I-III breast cancer (EORTC 22922/10925): 15-year results of a randomised, phase 3 trial. Lancet Oncol. 2020;21(12):1602–10.
23. Recht A, Comen E, Fine R, et al. Postmastectomy radiotherapy: an American society of clinical oncology, American society for radiation oncology, and society of surgical oncology focused guideline update. PRO. 2016;6:219–34.
24. Buchholz TA, Lehman CD, Harris JR, et al. Statement of the science concerning locoregional treatments after preoperative chemotherapy for breast cancer: a National Cancer Institute conference. J Clin Oncol. 2008;26:791–7.
25. Haffty BG, McCall LM, Ballman KV, et al. Patterns of local-regional management following neoadjuvant chemotherapy in breast cancer: results from ACOSOG Z1071 (Alliance). Int J Radiat Oncol Biol Phys. 2016;94:493–502.
26. Buchholz TA, Tucker SL, Masullo L, et al. Predictors of local-regional recurrence after neoadjuvant chemotherapy and mastectomy without radiation. J Clin Oncol. 2002;20:17–23.
27. Huang EH, Tucker SL, Strom EA, et al. Postmastectomy radiation improves local-regional control and survival for selected patients with locally advanced breast cancer treated with neoadjuvant chemotherapy and mastectomy. J Clin Oncol. 2004;22:4691–9.
28. McGuire SE, Gonzalez-Angulo AM, Huang EH, et al. Postmastectomy radiation improves the outcome of patients with locally advanced breast cancer who achieve a pathologic complete response to neoadjuvant chemotherapy. Int J Radiat Oncol Biol Phys. 2007;68:1004–9.
29. Garg AK, Oh JL, Oswald MJ, et al. Effect of postmastectomy radiotherapy in patients <35 years old with stage II-III breast cancer treated with doxorubicin-based neoadjuvant chemotherapy and mastectomy. Int J Radiat Oncol Biol Phys. 2007;69:1478–83.
30. Nagar H, Mittendorf EA, Strom EA, et al. Local-regional recurrence with and without radiation therapy after neoadjuvant chemotherapy and mastectomy for clinically staged T3N0 breast cancer. Int J Radiat Oncol Biol Phys. 2011;81:782–7.
31. Mamounas EP, Anderson SJ, Dignam JJ, et al. Predictors of locoregional recurrence after neoadjuvant chemotherapy: results from combined analysis of National Surgical Adjuvant Breast and Bowel Project B-18 and B-27. J Clin Oncol. 2012;30:3960–6.
32. Gillon P, Touati N, Breton-Callu C, et al. Factors predictive of locoregional recurrence following neoadjuvant chemotherapy in patients with large operable or locally advanced breast cancer: an analysis of the EORTC 10994/BIG 1-00 study. Eur J Cancer. 2017;79:226–34.
33. Krug D, Lederer B, Seither F, et al. Post-mastectomy radiotherapy after neoadjuvant chemotherapy in breast cancer: a pooled retrospective analysis of three prospective randomized trials. Ann Surg Oncol. 2019;26:3892–901.
34. Le Scodan R, Selz J, Stevens D, et al. Radiotherapy for stage II and stage III breast cancer patients with negative lymph nodes after preoperative chemotherapy and mastectomy. Int J Radiat Oncol Biol Phys. 2012;82:e1–7.
35. Shim SJ, Park W, Huh SJ, et al. The role of postmastectomy radiation therapy after neoadjuvant chemotherapy in clinical stage II-III breast cancer patients with pN0: a multicenter, retrospective study (KROG 12-05). Int J Radiat Oncol Biol Phys. 2014;88:65–72.
36. Wang Q, Zhao J, Han X, et al. Is there a role for post-mastectomy radiotherapy for T1-2N1 breast cancers with node-positive pathology after patients become node-negative pathology following neoadjuvant chemotherapy? Front Oncol. 2020;10:892.
37. Huang Z, Zhu L, Huang XB, et al. Postmastectomy radiation therapy based on pathologic nodal status in clinical node-positive stage II to III breast cancer treated with neoadjuvant chemotherapy. Int J Radiat Oncol Biol Phys. 2020;108:1030–9.
38. Daveau C, Stevens D, Brain E, et al. Is regional lymph node irradiation necessary in stage II to III breast cancer patients with negative pathologic node status after neoadjuvant chemotherapy? Int J Radiat Oncol Biol Phys. 2010;78:337–42.
39. Bae SH, Park W, Huh SJ, et al. Radiation treatment in pathologic n0-n1 patients treated with neoadjuvant chemotherapy followed by surgery for locally advanced breast cancer. J Breast Cancer. 2012;15:329–36.

40. Noh JM, Park W, Suh CO, et al. Is elective nodal irradiation beneficial in patients with pathologically negative lymph nodes after neoadjuvant chemotherapy and breast-conserving surgery for clinical stage II-III breast cancer? A multicentre retrospective study (KROG 12-05). Br J Cancer. 2014;110:1420–6.
41. Rusthoven CG, Rabinovitch RA, Jones BL, et al. The impact of postmastectomy and regional nodal radiation after neoadjuvant chemotherapy for clinically lymph node-positive breast cancer: a National Cancer Database (NCDB) analysis. Ann Oncol. 2016;27:818–27.
42. Liu J, Mao K, Jiang S, et al. The role of postmastectomy radiotherapy in clinically node-positive, stage II-III breast cancer patients with pathological negative nodes after neoadjuvant chemotherapy: an analysis from the NCDB. Oncotarget. 2016;7:24848–59.
43. Kantor O, Pesce C, Singh P, et al. Post-mastectomy radiation therapy and overall survival after neoadjuvant chemotherapy. J Surg Oncol. 2017;115:668–76.
44. Ohri N, Moshier E, Ho A, et al. Postmastectomy radiation in breast cancer patients with pathologically positive lymph nodes after neoadjuvant chemotherapy: usage rates and survival trends. Int J Radiat Oncol Biol Phys. 2017;99:549–59.
45. Mamounas EP, Cortazar P, Zhang L, et al. Locoregional recurrence (LRR) after neoadjuvant chemotherapy (NAC): pooled-analysis results from the collaborative trials in neoadjuvant breast cancer (CTNeoBC). J Clin Oncol. 2014;32:61.
46. Eiermann W, Paepke S, Appfelstaedt J, et al. Preoperative treatment of postmenopausal breast cancer patients with letrozole: a randomized double-blind multicenter study. Ann Oncol. 2001;12:1527–32.
47. Ellis MJ, Tao Y, Luo J, et al. Outcome prediction for estrogen receptor-positive breast cancer based on postneoadjuvant endocrine therapy tumor characteristics. J Natl Cancer Inst. 2008;100:1380–8.
48. Smith IE, Dowsett M, Ebbs SR, et al. Neoadjuvant treatment of postmenopausal breast cancer with anastrozole, tamoxifen, or both in combination: the Immediate Preoperative Anastrozole, Tamoxifen, or Combined with Tamoxifen (IMPACT) multicenter double-blind randomized trial. J Clin Oncol. 2005;23:5108–16.
49. NCT01953588: fulvestrant and/or anastrozole in treating postmenopausal patients with stage II-III breast cancer undergoing surgery.
50. Ma CX, Suman VJ, Leitch AM, et al. ALTERNATE: neoadjuvant endocrine treatment (NET) approaches for clinical stage II or Ill estrogen receptor-positive HER2-negative breast cancer (ER+HER2-BC) in postmenopausal (PM) women: alliance A011106. J Clin Oncol. 2020;38:504.
51. Krag DN, Anderson SJ, Julian TB, et al. Sentinel-lymph-node resection compared with conventional axillary-lymph-node dissection in clinically node-negative patients with breast cancer: overall survival findings from the NSABP B-32 randomised phase 3 trial. Lancet Oncol. 2010;11:927–33.
52. Giuliano AE, Hunt KK, Ballman KV, et al. Axillary dissection vs no axillary dissection in women with invasive breast cancer and sentinel node metastasis: a randomized clinical trial. JAMA. 2011;305:569–75.
53. Kuehn T, Bauerfeind I, Fehm T, et al. Sentinel-lymph-node biopsy in patients with breast cancer before and after neoadjuvant chemotherapy (SENTINA): a prospective, multicentre cohort study. Lancet Oncol. 2013;14:609–18.
54. Boughey JC, Suman VJ, Mittendorf EA, et al. Sentinel lymph node surgery after neoadjuvant chemotherapy in patients with node-positive breast cancer: the ACOSOG Z1071 (Alliance) clinical trial. JAMA. 2013;310:1455–61.
55. Kantor O, Wong S, Weiss A, et al. Prognostic significance of residual nodal disease after neoadjuvant endocrine therapy for hormone receptor-positive breast cancer. NPJ Breast Cancer. 2020;6:35.
56. Bazan JG, White J. Imaging of the axilla before preoperative chemotherapy: implications for postmastectomy radiation. Cancer. 2015;121:1187–94.

57. Vassallo P, Wernecke K, Roos N, et al. Differentiation of benign from malignant superficial lymphadenopathy: the role of high-resolution US. Radiology. 1992;183:215–20.
58. Koolen BB, Valdes Olmos RA, Elkhuizen PH, et al. Locoregional lymph node involvement on 18F-FDG PET/CT in breast cancer patients scheduled for neoadjuvant chemotherapy. Breast Cancer Res Treat. 2012;135:231–40.
59. Bazan J, DiCostanzo D, Kuhn K, et al. Likelihood of unacceptable normal tissue doses in breast cancer patients undergoing regional nodal irradiation in routine clinical practice. Pract Radiat Oncol. 2017;7:154–60.
60. Bazan JG, Healy E, Beyer S, et al. Clinical effectiveness of an adaptive treatment planning algorithm for intensity modulated radiation therapy versus 3D conformal radiation therapy for node-positive breast cancer patients undergoing regional nodal irradiation/postmastectomy radiation therapy. Int J Radiat Oncol Biol Phys. 2020;108:1159–71.
61. Pandeli C, Smyth LML, David S, et al. Dose reduction to organs at risk with deep-inspiration breath-hold during right breast radiotherapy: a treatment planning study. Radiat Oncol. 2019;14:223.
62. White JR, Arthur D, et al. Breast cancer atlas for radiation therapy planning: consenus definitions 2011. https://www.nrgoncology.org/Portals/0/Scientific%20Program/CIRO/Atlases/BreastCancerAtlas_corr.pdf?ver=2018-04-18-144201-270. Access on November 15, 2020.
63. Kim KH, Noh JM, Kim YB, et al. Does internal mammary node irradiation affect treatment outcome in clinical stage II-III breast cancer patients receiving neoadjuv ant chemotherapy? Breast Cancer Res Treat. 2015;152:589–99.
64. Thorsen LB, Offersen BV, Dano H, et al. DBCG-IMN: a population-based cohort study on the effect of internal mammary node irradiation in early node-positive breast cancer. J Clin Oncol. 2016;34:314–20.
65. Yaney A, Ayan AS, Pan X, et al. Dosimetric parameters associated with radiation-induced esophagitis in breast cancer patients undergoing regional nodal irradiation. Radiother Oncol. 2020;155:167–73.
66. NCT03414970: hypofractionated radiation therapy after mastectomy in preventing recurrence in patients with stage IIa-IIIa breast cancer.

Part VI
Pathology, Guidelines and Ongoing Clinical Trials

Chapter 13
Pathology of Neoadjuvant Systemic Therapy Response

Beth Z. Clark

Introduction

Neoadjuvant systemic therapy is administered following a diagnosis of invasive breast cancer for a variety of indications, including downstaging of locally advanced disease or to facilitate breast-conserving surgery. Response to neoadjuvant chemotherapy can also be used as an in situ test for chemosensitivity and is accepted as an endpoint in trials of effectiveness of novel agents [1]. The decisions to administer neoadjuvant systemic therapy and specific agents chosen are determined by clinical stage, tumor grade, phenotype, and sometimes by genomic assays or other tools such as the Magee Equations™ [2]. Tumor grade and phenotype can be determined on percutaneous core biopsy specimens, allowing for pre-operative decisions regarding systemic therapy. In addition to information provided in standard pathologic examination, such as margin status and tumor size, the pathologist must provide additional information regarding response to neoadjuvant systemic therapy, for prognostic purposes and to guide further treatment. Pathologists must be informed that neoadjuvant systemic therapy has been administered in order to provide an accurate, informative pathology report.

Review of Pathology of Invasive Breast Carcinoma

For purposes of understanding diagnosis and management of invasive breast carcinoma, the most important histopathologic features include tumor type, tumor grade, and tumor genotype/phenotype. Invasive carcinoma in the breast is defined as

B. Z. Clark (✉)
UPMC Magee-Women's Hospital, Pittsburgh, PA, USA
e-mail: clarkbz@upmc.edu

A. Soran, F. Nakhlis (eds.), *Management of the Breast and Axilla in the Neoadjuvant Setting*, https://doi.org/10.1007/978-3-030-88020-0_13

neoplastic cells that have infiltrated beyond the basement membrane of ducts and lobules of the breast parenchyma. Occasionally, the growth pattern makes it difficult to distinguish invasive carcinoma from in situ carcinoma, in which neoplastic cells are confined within ducts and lobules of the breast parenchyma. Myoepithelial cells can be identified on routine hematoxylin and eosin (H&E) stains as small, hyperchromatic angulated cells at the periphery of ducts and lobules (Fig. 13.1). In situ carcinoma can be identified by a peripheral rim of myoepithelial cells, which are highlighted by immunohistochemical stains for myoepithelial cells, such as p63 and smooth muscle myosin heavy chain, among others.

Invasive ductal carcinoma and invasive lobular carcinoma account for >90% of invasive breast carcinomas, while other types, such as metaplastic carcinoma and adenoid cystic carcinoma, are much less common. Some types of invasive carcinoma, such as tubular carcinoma, cribriform carcinoma, and pure low-grade mucinous carcinoma, have an excellent prognosis. These tumors are typically strongly ER+/PR+/Her-2/neu (HER2), with a low proliferative index, while metaplastic carcinoma, low-grade adenosquamous carcinoma, and adenoid cystic carcinoma are typically ER-/PR-/HER2-.

Tumor grade is most commonly reported by the Elston-Ellis modification of the Scarff-Bloom-Richardson grading system, also called the Nottingham system or Nottingham grade [3]. The Nottingham Grade is divided into grades 1, 2, and 3 based on pathologic features of the invasive carcinoma: tubule formation, nuclear pleomorphism, and mitotic activity. Each feature is graded from 1 to 3, and the total score determines the grade. The total score is referred to as the Nottingham score and ranges from 3 to 9. Grade 1 has a total score 3–5, grade 2 has a total score 6–7, and grade 3 – 8–9. Pure invasive lobular carcinoma, by definition, does not form tubular structures, and therefore the minimum Nottingham score is 5.

The four most important biomarkers used in determination of tumor phenotype are estrogen receptor (ER), progesterone receptor (PR), Her-2/neu (HER2), and the proliferation marker Ki67. ER, PR, and Ki67 are usually performed by

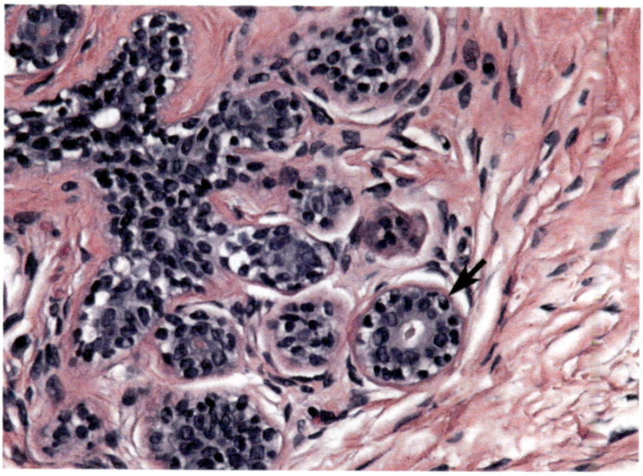

Fig. 13.1 Benign breast lobule with luminal epithelial and peripheral myoepithelial cells. Myoepithelial cells are smaller and more hyperchromatic than epithelial cells (arrow)

immunohistochemistry, while HER2 can be determined by immunohistochemistry or fluorescence in situ hybridization (FISH). These assays can be performed on core biopsy specimens in order to aid in management of breast carcinoma prior to definitive surgical therapy, with adherence to guidelines set forth by the American Society of Clinical Oncology and College of American Pathologists (ASCO/CAP) [4, 5]. These guidelines provide detailed requirements for tissue fixation, use of FDA-cleared assays, and recommendations for reporting. Semiquantitative reporting of ER and PR expression is required, with information about the intensity and percentage of tumor cells showing expression of the receptor. Common ways to report ER and PR include the Allred score and the histologic score or "H-score" methods. The Allred Score ranges from 0 to 8, with proportion of positive tumor cells graded from 0 to 5 and average intensity ranging from 0 to 3 [6]. The H-score ranges from 0 to 300, and is calculated by multiplying the proportion of cells staining at each intensity ranging from 0 to 3+, with the sum of all intensities representing the H-score [7, 8]. For example, an invasive carcinoma with 10% negative, 20% 1+, 30% 2+ and 40% 3+ staining has an H-score of $(10 \times 0) + (20 \times 1) + (30 \times 2) + (40 \times 3) = 200$. Recently, it was recommended that cases with a low percentage of ER or PR positive tumor cells (between 1% and 10%) by immunohistochemistry be reported as low positive, with documentation of the presence of internal and external positive controls, due to limited data on endocrine therapy benefit for cancers with low ER expression [4]. Criteria for HER2 gene amplification and HER2 overexpression by immunohistochemistry have evolved as testing has been refined and standardized. Many laboratories perform HER2 FISH as the first-line test for HER2 amplification, while other laboratories perform HER2 immunohistochemistry with reflex to FISH for equivocal (2+) cases. When IHC is performed, a score of 0 or 1+ is a negative result, and a score of 3+ is a positive result. The most recent update for HER2 testing defined five groups of HER2 FISH results based on the absolute HER2 gene copy number and the ratio of HER2 gene copies to the centromere for chromosome 17, on which the Erb-B2 gene is located [5] (Fig. 13.2). Ki67 is a proliferation marker that marks tumor cells in all phases of the cell cycle except for the G_0 phase. There are no universally accepted cut-offs for Ki67 proliferation index, and the marker is usually reported as a continuous variable from 0% to 100%.

In 2000, Perou et al. published a study of gene expression patterns in 65 breast cancers from 42 patients, revealing molecular portraits that formed the basis for our current understanding of breast cancer as a heterogeneous disease, with luminal, Erb-B2 (HER2-enriched), and basal clusters [9]. A similar study of a larger group of tumors published in 2001 by Sorlie et al. elucidated subtypes of the luminal cluster [10]. Molecular subtypes were shown to have significant differences in pCR rates in a small study by Rouzier et al. with the highest pCR rates seen in Erb-B2+ and basal subtypes [11]. The immunoprofile of ER, PR, HER2, and Ki67 are often used as surrogates for the molecular phenotypes, as it is not feasible to perform molecular analysis on all invasive breast carcinomas at the time of diagnosis. The tumor phenotype, combined with the clinical stage and imaging findings, contributes significantly to the decision to administer neoadjuvant systemic therapy, and the degree of expected response varies by tumor phenotype. Strongly ER-positive tumors have the lowest response rates, while tumors with low estrogen receptor expression (H-score < 100) have rates comparable to ER- tumors [12]. Pathologic complete response rates are highest in hormone receptor (HR)-negative tumors, with the highest response rates seen in HR-/HER2+ tumors, followed by HR-/HER2- tumors and HR+/HER2+ tumors, while pCR rates are lowest in HR+/HER2- tumors [13–16] (Fig. 13.3). It is most difficult to predict the likelihood of significant

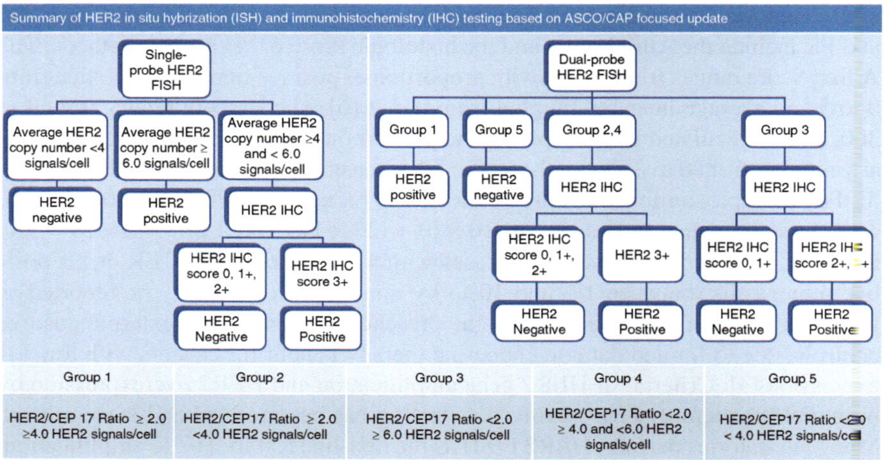

Fig. 13.2 Summary of Her-2/neu in situ ybridization (ISH) criteria, adapted from Wolff et al. [5] Dual-probe ISH uses probes for both Her-2/neu gene and for centromere of chromosome 17. Single-probe ISH uses a probe for Her-2/neu gene only

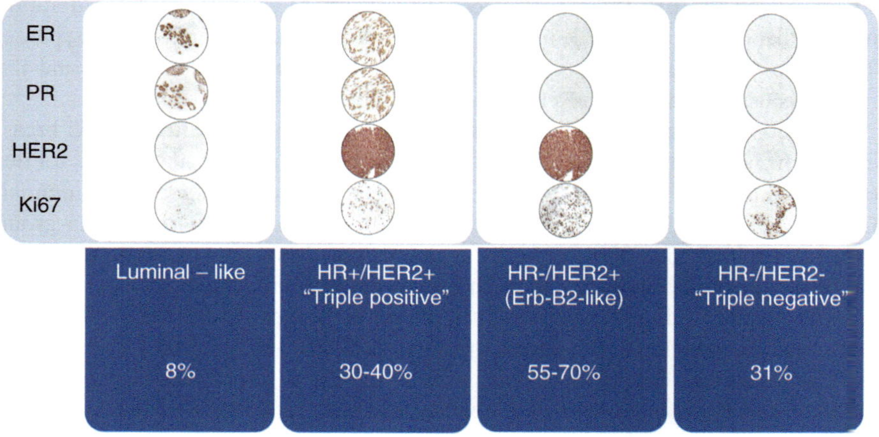

Fig. 13.3 Response rates to neoadjuvant chemotherapy by tumor phenotype. (References [13–16], UPMC Magee-Women's Hospital internal data)

response to neoadjuvant chemotherapy in invasive carcinoma with a "Luminal B"-like phenotype (ER +, PR +/−, HER2-, Ki67 moderate or high). Tumor phenotype is not the only factor predicting pCR in breast cancer. Tumors with Nottingham grade 3 and the presence of tumor and stromal lymphocytic infiltrates also have higher rates of pCR [17]. Metaplastic carcinomas, which are typically HR- and HER2-, also appear to have lower pCR rates than triple-negative breast carcinomas of non-metaplastic type [18].

Several tools are available to assist with prediction of response in ER+/HER2- tumors, including the Magee Equations™ and genomic assays for HR+ tumors. Magee Equation 3, which uses semiquantitative ER and PR expression expressed as H-score, HER2 status, and Ki67 proliferative index, as determined by biomarker studies performed on the diagnostic percutaneous core biopsy, can help to predict the likelihood of pCR with neoadjuvant chemotherapy in ER positive invasive breast carcinoma. The Magee Equations™ were originally devised to predict the Oncotype DX recurrence score, and Magee Equation scores in the low, intermediate, and high categories were shown to have pCR rates of 0%, 4%, and 36%, respectively [19]. A recent multi-institutional study of 166 cases showed similar findings, while also including pCR rates using an additional cut-off of 25. In this study, pCR rates using Magee Equation 3 (ME3) were 0%, 0%, 14%, and 40% for ME3 scores <18, 18–25, >25 to <31, and 31 or higher, respectively [20]. Magee Equations can be calculated by entering the ER, PR, HER2, and Ki67 data, along with Nottingham Score and tumor size if available, into the URL https://path.upmc.edu/onlineTools/mageeequations.html.

IHC4 is an immunohistochemical score that also utilizes routinely performed immunohistochemical markers and has been reported to provide prognostic information similar to that obtained from the 21-gene genomic assay [21]. The IHC4 score is calculated using the following equation: $IHC4 = 94.7 \times \{-0.100\, ER_{10} - 0.079\, PgR_{10} + 0.586\, HER2 + 0.240 \ln (1 + 10 \times Ki67)\}$. ER_{10} is obtained by dividing the ER H-score by 30 and PgR_{10} is obtained by dividing the percentage of positive cells by 10. Ki67 is expressed as the percentage of positively staining malignant cells. In a retrospective study of 113 patients with ER+ (22 HER2+, 91 HER2-) breast cancer treated with neoadjuvant chemotherapy, Ki67 and IHC4 were both positively associated with pCR and near pCR (RCB-1) when values for Ki67 and IHC4 were divided among quartiles [22]. The absence of an established cut-off value for a high IHC4 score, however, limits its use for decision-making currently. Oncotype DX recurrence score and Prosigna risk of recurrence (ROR) score genomic have also been reported to provide predictive information in response to neoadjuvant chemotherapy in ER+/HER2- breast carcinoma [23, 24].

The advent of standard percutaneous image-guided core biopsy and breast imaging modalities, such as MRI, set the stage for effective neoadjuvant systemic therapies. Percutaneous core biopsy of breast carcinoma allows for accurate pre-operative grading and classification of tumors, as well as phenotypic analysis through biomarker studies. Numerous studies have shown good concordance between biomarker status of core biopsy and surgical resection material [25–32].

The majority of patients will receive definitive surgical management following the administration of neoadjuvant systemic therapy. Exceptions may include rare patients in whom locoregional disease is deemed unresectable and rare patients who develop metastatic disease during neoadjuvant treatment. Clinical trials are ongoing to determine the safety of omission of local surgery in patients with exceptional responses to neoadjuvant chemotherapy [33]. In these cases, percutaneous core biopsies of the tumor bed are performed upon completion of neoadjuvant chemotherapy to evaluate for evidence of residual in situ or invasive carcinoma. If no residual tumor is identified on these specimens, surgery may be omitted. When evaluating these specimens, the surgical pathologist must be aware of the indication for the biopsy, and special protocols may be utilized to thoroughly evaluate the core biopsy tissue, including examination of multiple deeper levels through the tissue block.

Important Clinical Data

Because a patient's response to neoadjuvant systemic therapy has important implications for prognosis and further treatment recommendations, careful clinical-pathologic correlation is crucial for optimal histopathologic evaluation. Some pathologic features of systemic therapy response, such as a fibroelastotic tumor bed, may only be definitively identified when the clinical context is known. At the time of surgery, therefore, the specimen requisition should include the number and location of lesions, pre-therapy tumor size, pre-therapy lymph node evaluation, and type of neoadjuvant systemic therapy given. The pathologist and pathologist assistant must correlate the information given by the surgeon and results of pre- and post-therapy imaging studies to ensure that the tumor bed and all lesions of concern have been located and sampled for histologic examination.

Gross Examination of Post-therapy Surgical Specimens

Pathologic examination of post-therapy breast surgical specimens differs from non-neoadjuvant therapy specimens in important ways, particularly for specimens in which the response has been marked or complete, while tumors with minimal or moderate response to neoadjuvant therapy may show gross features similar to non-neoadjuvant cases. More tissue sampling may be required after neoadjuvant systemic therapy in order to properly evaluate for residual tumor. Careful correlation with imaging findings is important for locating lesions. Specimen radiographs may be used to locate biopsy clips or foci of calcifications. On gross examination, it can be difficult to locate findings noted on imaging studies, particularly MRI findings that have not been previously biopsied with placement of a biopsy marker clip. Cases with a marked or complete response to therapy may show only a fibrotic tumor bed, typically streak-like white or tan, which may be soft or rubbery (Fig. 13.4). Gross measurement of tumor size after a significant response to therapy may be inaccurate, and the pathologist must correlate the gross examination findings with histologic examination for proper assignment of post-therapy AJCC ("y") tumor stage. Because the gross examination findings may be subtle, placement of a biopsy marker clip prior to beginning neoadjuvant therapy is very helpful in localizing the tumor bed during pathologic examination. Measurement of the distance of gross residual tumor and the tumor bed to surgical margins should also be recorded. Accurate measurement of the tumor bed area is needed for calculation of the Residual Cancer Burden (RCB) [34].

Provenzano et al. published recommendations for standardization of pathologic evaluation and reporting of post-neoadjuvant specimens from reviews of clinical trial protocols in 2015 [35]. Recommendations were made for sampling in cases with no residual gross disease, and emphasized that the tumor bed/biopsy clip must be documented in order to confirm a pathologic complete response.

At our institution, partial/segmental mastectomy specimens are inked with six colors (medial, lateral, superior, inferior, anterior, and posterior) and sectioned into numbered tissue slices with systematic submission of tissue blocks. This method can be helpful in measurement of residual carcinoma involving the tumor bed that is not grossly measurable (Fig. 13.5). This can be accomplished by counting the number of tissue slices involved by invasive carcinoma and using the average slice thickness to calculate the maximum dimension of residual carcinoma. If residual tumor is not identified grossly, the tumor bed should be entirely submitted for histologic examination in order to document the presence of pathologic complete response with certainty.

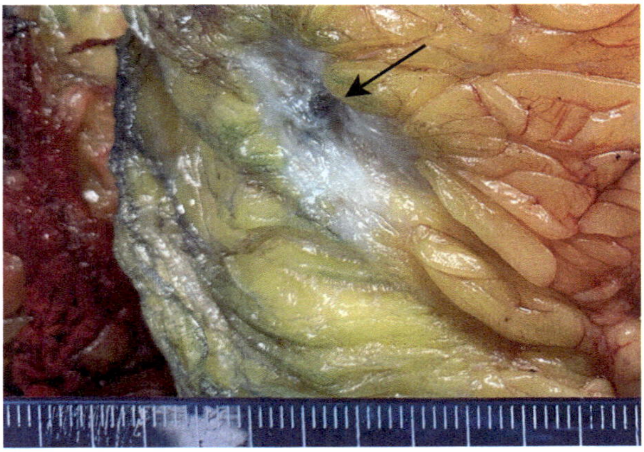

Fig. 13.4 Gross features of tumor bed following pathologic complete response (pCR) to neoadjuvant chemotherapy. Tumor bed consists of rubbery, white fibrosis with central biopsy clip (arrow) in the background of fatty breast tissue

Histopathologic Features in the Breast Following Neoadjuvant Therapy

Changes in benign breast tissue are generally subtle. Benign breast ductal epithelium may show scattered nuclear enlargement. Lobules may appear involuted and/or show thickening of the basement membrane (Fig. 13.6). Squamous metaplastic change of the breast epithelium may be identified. Scattered lymphocyte or histiocyte aggregates may be identified outside of the tumor bed area.

In the pre-therapy tumor area, or tumor bed, changes occur both within the stroma and in residual tumor cells, if present. Within the stroma, the most common finding is fibroelastosis, in which loose collagenous tissue with focal elastosis is identified at the site of the tumor. This fibroelastosis may be admixed with residual

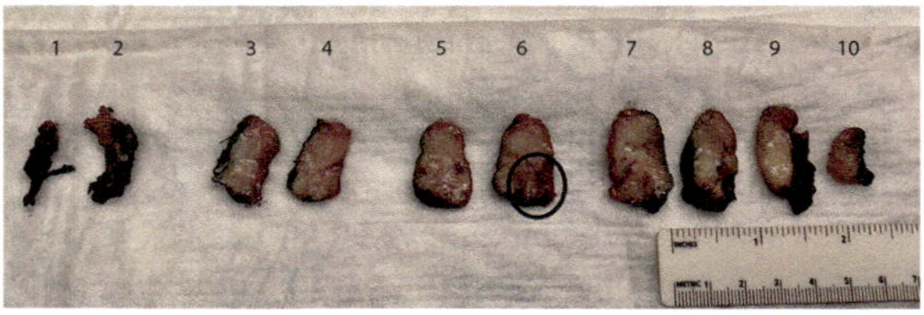

Fig. 13.5 Sectioning of partial/segmental mastectomy into numbered tissue slices and measurement of slice thickness can facilitate measurement of residual carcinoma when it is difficult to appreciate grossly. Residual carcinoma identified in slice 6 (circle)

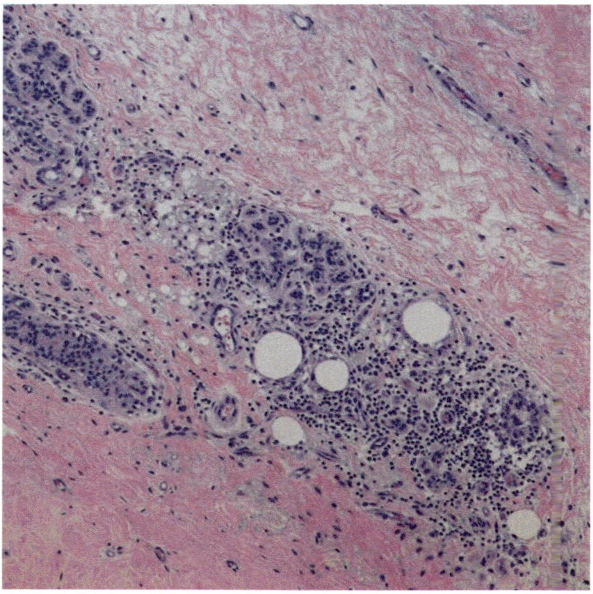

Fig. 13.6 Histologic changes of neoadjuvant chemotherapy in benign breast parenchyma include thickening of the basement membrane around ducts and lobules, along with perilobular lymphocytes and macrophages

tumor, or may be the only histologic finding in the tumor bed when there has been a pathologic complete response (Fig. 13.7). Typically, these areas of fibroelastosis are devoid of normal breast parenchyma but may include residual in situ carcinoma. Dense fibrosis occasionally represents the predominant change, and may include sclerotic, keloidal-type collagen. Macrophage aggregates, hemosiderin-laden macrophages, cholesterol clefts, and lymphocyte aggregates are also commonly identified in the tumor bed area (Fig. 13.8). The biopsy clip site is also a helpful landmark to document that the tumor bed has been examined when the histologic changes are subtle and no tumor remains, provided that there has not been migration of the biopsy clip. The biopsy clip site consists of a space within the tissue surrounded by palisading histiocytes (Fig. 13.9). The response may include symmetrical shrinkage of the tumor, with stromal changes identified at the periphery, or the stromal changes

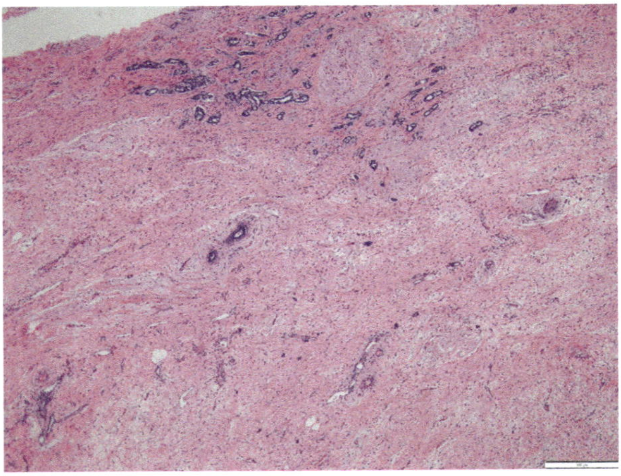

Fig. 13.7 Fibroelastotic tumor bed with scattered foci of residual invasive carcinoma

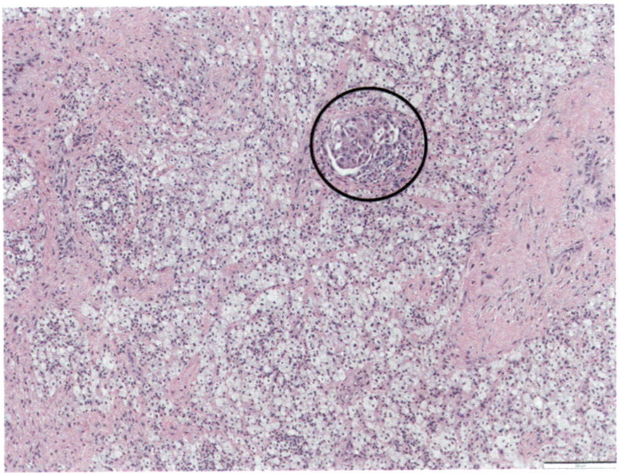

Fig. 13.8 Tumor bed with abundant macrophages and a rare cluster of residual tumor cells (circle)

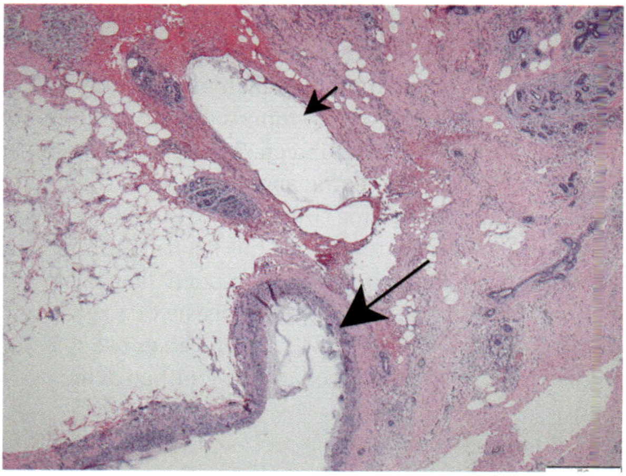

Fig. 13.9 Biopsy clip site consists of a space within the tissue surrounded by palisaded histiocytes (large arrow). The radioactive seed site appears as a space within the tissue that is usually surrounded by blood and acute inflammation due to the proximity of seed placement to the surgical procedure (small arrow)

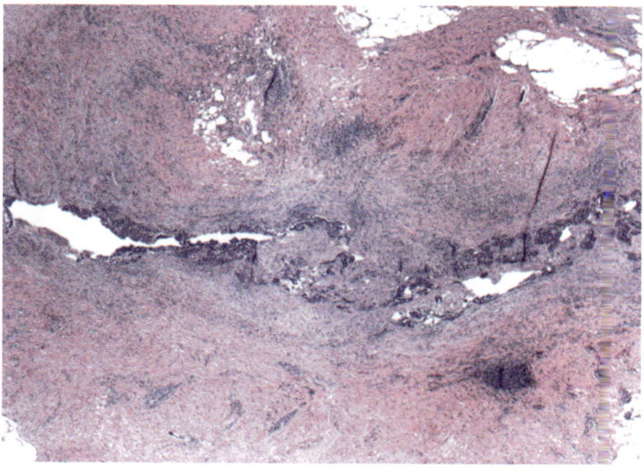

Fig. 13.10 Symmetrical shrinkage of invasive ductal carcinoma with partial response to neoadjuvant chemotherapy. Fibrosis, lymphocyte aggregates, and hemosiderin-laden macrophages surround residual carcinoma

may be admixed with residual tumor cells (Fig. 13.10). Decrease in cellularity may be minimal or marked and is associated with a concomitant increase in the stromal component of the pre-therapy tumor area. Evaluation of residual tumor cellularity or change in tumor cellularity is required for some methods of assessment of response to chemotherapy (see below). This assessment is most difficult in cases with uneven response within individual tumors or in tumor multifocality.

Cytologic changes to tumor cells may include increased pleomorphism, particularly in individual cells, more prominent nucleoli, bizarre nuclei and smudging, apoptotic debris, and decreased mitotic activity (Fig. 13.11). We have also uncommonly observed "differentiation" of tumor cells, in which a tumor showing high-grade features (lack of tubule formation with large, pleomorphic nuclei) on the pre-therapy biopsy displays glandular differentiation and smaller, more uniform nuclear features (Fig. 13.12). It is unclear whether this phenomenon is the result of histologic changes in the tumor cells as a result of therapy, or differential response

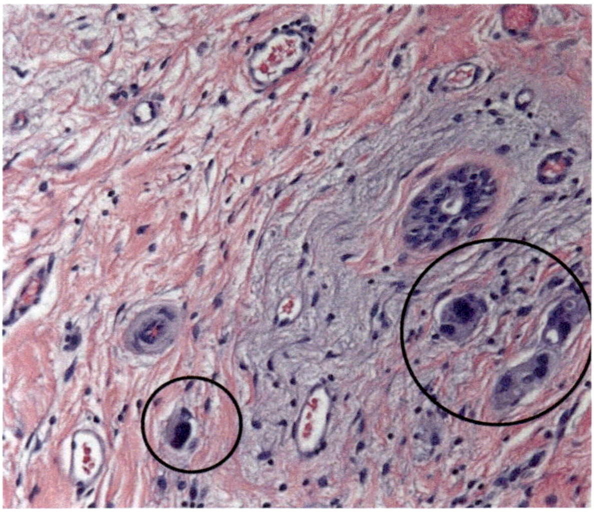

Fig. 13.11 Fibroelastotic tumor bed with scattered residual tumor cells. Tumor cells show large, smudged nuclei with abundant cytoplasm

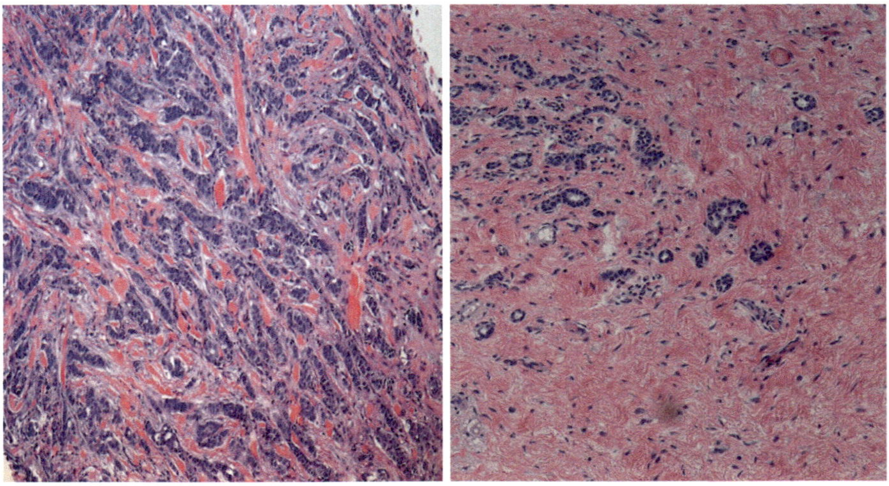

Fig. 13.12 Change in tumor grade after neoadjuvant chemotherapy. Pre-therapy core biopsy (left) shows invasive carcinoma with no tubule formation, nuclear grade 3. Post-therapy core biopsy shows tubule formation and nuclear grade 1–2

in tumors with both high-grade and unsampled low-grade areas. Diaz et al. reported that low mitotic count (defined as less than 13 mitotic figures per 10 high power fields) following neoadjuvant systemic chemotherapy has been with a lower risk of distant metastasis [36].

In rare cases, extensive lymphovascular space invasion may be the predominant finding, and should not be confused with residual ductal carcinoma in situ (Fig. 13.13). Immunohistochemical stains may be helpful in difficult cases. Residual

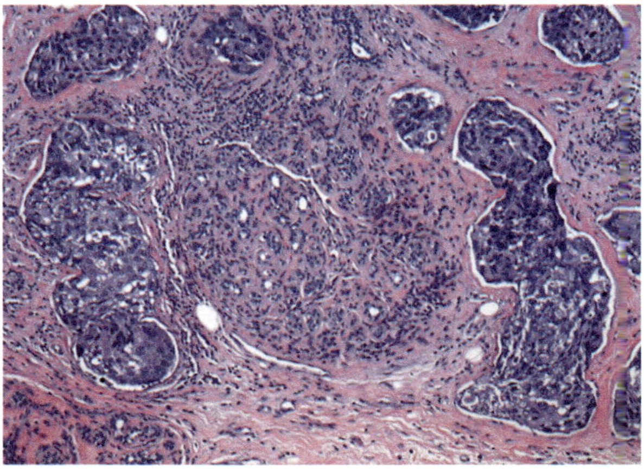

Fig. 13.13 Residual carcinoma as extensive lymphovascular space invasion. The large tumor emboli should not be mistaken for ductal carcinoma in situ. Slit-like spaces around tumor emboli provide the clue to a diagnosis of lymphovascular space invasion

in situ carcinoma may show similar cytologic changes to those seen in invasive tumor cells, including increased nuclear pleomorphism and few mitotic figures. Although in situ carcinoma does not respond as frequently to neoadjuvant chemotherapy, regression of ductal structures is a frequent finding, and may appear as calcifications with surrounding desmoplastic stromal response. Immunohistochemical stains for myoepithelial markers may also be useful to distinguish residual clusters of invasive carcinoma from in situ carcinoma. This distinction is very important for staging and determination of pathologic complete response vs. residual disease, particularly when the adjuvant systemic therapy regimen may be changed as a result of residual disease, such as trastuzumab-emtansine (TDM-1) for HER2+ breast cancer or adjuvant capecitabine for HER2- breast cancer [37, 38].

Pathologic Evaluation of Response to Neoadjuvant Chemotherapy

Following neoadjuvant chemotherapy, assessment of response and residual disease include three important elements: presence or absence of residual carcinoma (documentation of pathologic complete response (pCR) or residual disease), post-neoadjuvant therapy pathologic staging, and some quantitative measure of response to chemotherapy. The definition of pathologic complete response includes the absence of invasive carcinoma involving the breast and sampled lymph nodes. The presence of residual in situ carcinoma has been somewhat controversial, with several studies reporting that there is no difference in survival when the only residual disease is non-invasive [39–41]. Von Minckwitz et al., however, reported that disease-free survival was significantly superior with no residual DCIS [42].

The prognostic value of a pCR is well-documented, and thorough sampling and histologic examination of the tumor bed are essential in cases with a significant response to therapy [39]. National Surgical Adjuvant Breast and Bowel Project (NSABP) trials B-18 and B-27, which demonstrated equivalence between preoperative and postoperative chemotherapy in invasive breast carcinoma, with primary endpoints of disease-free survival and overall survival, used pCR and pINV (residual disease in the breast) as the primary means of assessment of response [43, 44]. Pathologic complete response in NSABP B-18 was also associated with improved rates of breast conserving surgery [45]. This distinction, as detailed above, is made through a combination of gross examination with careful sampling, and histologic examination of the residual tumor and/or tumor bed, with immunohistochemistry when indicated to distinguish invasive from in situ carcinoma.

In the American Joint Committee on Cancer (AJCC) 8th Edition staging manual, staging is divided into clinical or "c" staging, derived from physical examination and imaging findings, and pathologic or "p" staging, derived from pathologic examination of biopsy material and surgical resection specimens [46]. The "y" prefix is added to denote that the examination follows neoadjuvant systemic therapy (hormonal or chemotherapy), and the neoadjuvant pathologic tumor (T) and nodal (N) stages have the same measurement cutoffs used in cases of primary surgical management. These cutoff measurements are defined as the largest "continuous" focus of residual invasive cancer, not including treatment-related fibrosis. In practice, the largest continuous measurement of invasive carcinoma can be difficult to ascertain in cases with uneven response, and this determination can be aided by systematic tissue submission as outlined in the section above on Gross Examination. The AJCC 6th Ed. post-neoadjuvant therapy staging system was shown to have prognostic value in 132 patients with residual disease [47]. Characterization of the response to treatment is also recommended, separate from the AJCC Staging, which can simply be reported complete response, partial response, and no response noted, based on change in tumor size and presence or absence of therapy-related changes observed histologically.

Rarely, lymphovascular space invasion is identified in the absence of invasive carcinoma involving the breast parenchyma or lymph nodes. The post-therapy pathologic stage is reported as ypT0N0 in this circumstance, but should not be reported as a pathologic complete response, as the finding of pure intralymphatic carcinoma following neoadjuvant chemotherapy has been associated with a poor clinical outcome [48].

Aside from post-neoadjuvant AJCC staging, the most commonly reported method for quantification of residual carcinoma following neoadjuvant chemotherapy is the Residual Cancer Burden (RCB) method, which identifies prognostic subgroups independently of and within the AJCC staging system [15]. This method was developed at MD Anderson using cases from neoadjuvant trials and was first published in 2007, and uses pathologic parameters that are independently associated with a higher risk of distant relapse, including the primary tumor dimension expressed as the largest bi-dimensional measurement of the tumor bed, cellularity of the tumor bed corrected for the proportion of in situ carcinoma, and the axillary nodal burden expressed as the number of residual positive lymph nodes and the size of the largest lymph node metastasis. Residual cancer burden (RCB) is reported as the RCB index, a continuous variable, with 0 representing a pathologic complete response, and as four risk groups, the RCB categories. RCB 0 represents a pCR, and RCB-I represents a near-PCR, with RCB-II and RCB-III representing increasing burdens of residual disease. The RCB method does not require comparison with the pre-therapy core biopsy, which may not be available at the time of histologic examination of the surgical resection specimen. A more recent long-term follow-up study confirmed prognostic value of RCB in phenotypic subsets of HR+/HER2-, HER2+, and HR-/HER2- invasive breast carcinomas [49].

A study by Sheri et al. from 2015 concluded that the addition of post-treatment Ki67, dubbed the Residual Proliferative Cancer Burden, or RPCB, provided significantly more prognostic information than either Ki67 or RCB alone [50]. The RCB method has been found to be produce reproducible results in a study of 100 cases examined by five pathologists [51]. In this study, overall concordance correlation coefficient for RCB index was 0.931 (95% CI = 0.908–0.949). Kappa statistic for RCB categories was 0.583 (95% CI = 0.539–0.626), representing good agreement, with the lowest agreement observed for RCB-I.

At our institution, prior to the widespread adoption of the Residual Cancer Burden method, the Magee Method was used to provide a measure of the decrease in tumor volume following neoadjuvant therapy. In this method, the percentage tumor volume reduction is calculated by estimating the change in cellularity between the pre-therapy core biopsy and the post-therapy tumor bed, using the following formula: % tumor volume reduction = ([pre-therapy size – revised tumor size]/pre-therapy size) × 100, where the revised tumor size = gross size of fibrotic tumor bed × % cellularity in comparison to the pre-therapy biopsy [14]. This method requires an accurate pre-therapy clinical tumor size, and availability of the pre-therapy (diagnostic) core biopsy to determine the change in cellularity, and is therefore not easily applied in all settings.

Other methods to quantify response to neoadjuvant therapy have also been described. The Miller-Payne grading system requires comparison with the pre-therapy core biopsy to stratify patients into five groups based on change in cellularity, and this system was reported to be an independent predictor of survival in multivariate analysis [52]. The Residual Disease in Breast and Nodes (RDBN) method incorporates the tumor grade, lymph node stage, and tumor grade [53]. CPS + EG combines post-therapy AJCC 6th Ed. stage with ER status and grade [54]. These methods are less frequently used, as Residual Cancer Burden (RCB) has been the preferred method for clinical trials in recent years.

Lymph Node Assessment After Neoadjuvant Therapy

Lymph node evaluation after neoadjuvant chemotherapy is complicated by two competing goals: accurate assessment of lymph node status and the need to reduce morbidity through minimization of axillary lymph node surgery. When a lymph node has been histologically confirmed to harbor metastatic disease prior to neoadjuvant therapy, it is important to retrieve the node following therapy to assess response. Pathologic examination of sampled lymph nodes after neoadjuvant therapy is important for accurate post-therapy staging and for confirmation that previously involved lymph nodes have been retrieved. Sentinel lymph node biopsy using conventional methods may not always result in retrieval of the previously involved node. Among patients enrolled in ACOSOG Z1071, the false negative rate of sentinel lymph node biopsy was 6.8% when the clipped node was one of the sentinel lymph nodes identified, and 13.4% when no clip was placed [55]. Higher yield of previously involved lymph nodes can be achieved through the use of radiologic correlation, placement of a clip at the time of percutaneous core biopsy, radioactive seed-localization of previously involved nodes prior to definitive surgery, and histologic examination. This procedure has been referred to as selective axillary lymph node dissection, and is usually combined with sentinel lymph node biopsy when axillary lymph node dissection is not strictly indicated [56, 57]. A recent study by Caudle et al. demonstrated that radioactive seed localization of a previously biopsied, clipped lymph node decreases the false-negative rate of axillary lymph node evaluation after neoadjuvant therapy [56]. The clipped node was not retrieved via sentinel lymph node biopsy in 23% (31/134) of cases in this study, and in six cases, the sentinel lymph nodes were negative, but the clipped lymph node was positive, illustrating the importance of evaluation of these lymph nodes for accurate post-therapy staging. Fine-needle aspiration biopsy of the clipped lymph node has been reported to be unreliable for assessment of residual disease following neoadjuvant therapy [58].

Intraoperative frozen section assessment of these lymph nodes can be performed, and if residual disease remains, axillary lymph node dissection may be performed at the time of surgery, if indicated. Frozen section analysis of a previously biopsied, previously involved lymph node may be more difficult due to the presence of biopsy site changes, minimal residual disease, and therapy-related changes (Fig. 13.14).

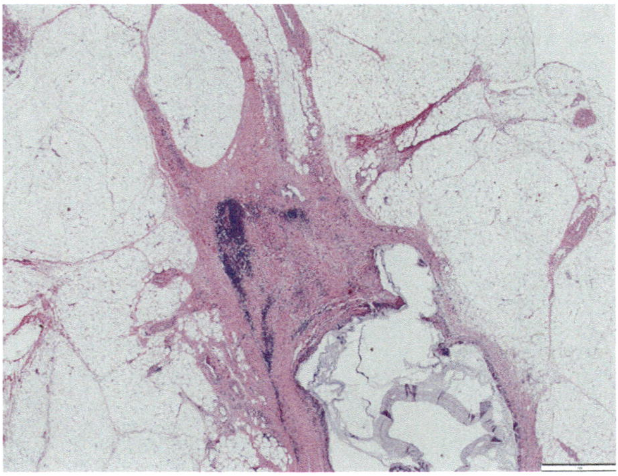

Fig. 13.14 Lymph node with pathologic complete response to neoadjuvant chemotherapy, with biopsy clip site (lower right), scant residual lymphoid tissue (center left), and fibroelastosis (center)

The presence of biopsy site changes, including scar-like fibrosis and the palisading histiocytes that have surrounded the biopsy clip (the "biopsy clip site"), also confirm that the previously biopsied lymph node has been retrieved. If a clip is not placed, or fine-needle aspiration biopsy has been performed, the histologic features of prior biopsy may be less pronounced.

Histologic features indicating response to neoadjuvant therapy include fibroelastosis, dense fibrosis, and/or macrophage aggregates, and are generally similar to the therapy-related changes observed in the breast (Fig. 13.15). Patients with residual metastatic tumor with evidence of treatment effect have been reported to have better disease-free survival and lower relapse rates than patients who have positive nodes without evidence of such changes [59].

Post-treatment pathologic nodal status was a strong predictor of overall and disease-free survival in both NSABP B-18 and B-27 [44]. Pathologic detection of a small volume of residual nodal disease after neoadjuvant chemotherapy has been shown to be associated with a poorer prognosis. Residual "mini"-micrometastases (<1 mm) and micrometastases (<2 mm) were associated with a poorer prognosis following neoadjuvant chemotherapy in NSABP B-18 [60]. More recently, in a large study, including cases from Dana-Farber/Brigham and Women's Cancer Center and the National Cancer Database, Wong et al. showed that low-volume residual nodal disease (isolated tumor cells and micrometastases) after neoadjuvant chemotherapy is associated with poorer disease-free and overall survival relative to those who are node negative [61]. This finding was most pronounced in patients with triple-negative and HER2+ disease. These findings emphasize the importance of both the procedure used to procure axillary lymph nodes and the thoroughness of the pathologic examination.

Understanding the correlation between the response to chemotherapy in the breast and axillary lymph nodes can help to optimize axillary management, and this knowledge can also help pathologists to refine protocols for lymph-node evaluation in neoadjuvant cases. Tadros et al. studied 527 consecutive patients with HER2+ or

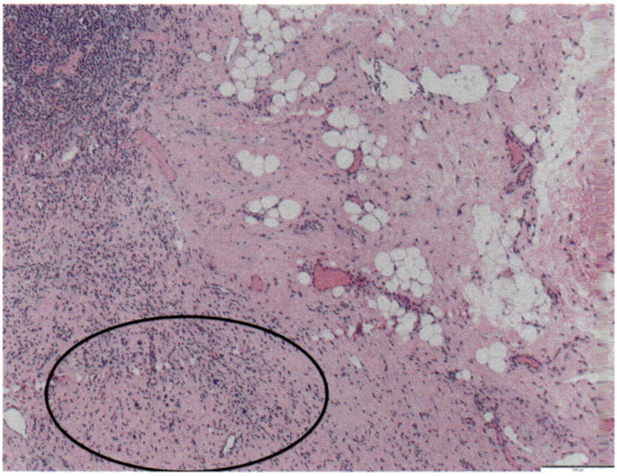

Fig. 13.15 Sentinel lymph node with rare residual tumor cells in single-cell arrangement in a background of therapy-related fibrosis

triple-negative breast cancer who received neoadjuvant chemotherapy in order to ascertain the risk of residual nodal disease [62]. Among patients with cN0 disease prior to chemotherapy and breast pCR, 100% had no evidence of axillary nodal metastasis, but among 237 patients with biopsy-proven N1 disease prior to chemotherapy, 10.4% of patients with breast pCR had residual nodal disease and 57.5% of patients without breast pCR had residual nodal disease. In a more recent study, breast pCR was strongly correlated with ypN0 in cN0 patients, especially in HER2+ and triple-negative breast carcinomas, while odds of ypN0 decreased in clinical T3 stage, cN1, and ER+/HER2- subtype and increased with breast pCR [63]. Zhao et al. also found nodal pCR rates to be highest in HER2+ tumors (58.6% with targeted therapy), intermediate in triple negative tumors (53.2%), and lowest in the HR+/HER2- subtype (21.2%) among 525 patients with clinically node-positive disease prior to neoadjuvant therapy [64]. In cases with a substantial but not complete response in the breast, this knowledge can help the pathologist to consider additional studies, such as immunohistochemistry for cytokeratin AE1/AE3, when residual nodal disease is not readily apparent on routine stains.

Neoadjuvant Hormonal Therapy

While the Residual Cancer Burden (RCB) has emerged as the most widely used method for assessment of breast carcinoma following neoadjuvant chemotherapy, pathologic assessment of response to neoadjuvant hormonal therapy is less well-established. The indications for neoadjuvant hormonal therapy are different from those of neoadjuvant chemotherapy, and a pCR is neither generally expected nor often the goal. Neoadjuvant hormonal therapy can improve rates of breast conservation, but pCR is uncommon and is not an effective surrogate of clinical outcome [65]. The most commonly used agents are aromatase inhibitors, although trials are ongoing for numerous agents in the neoadjuvant setting, such as cyclin-dependent kinase (CDK) 4/6 inhibitors [66].

Histologic features of response to neoadjuvant aromatase inhibitors or tamoxifen may be similar to those seen following neoadjuvant chemotherapy, but intratumoral fibrosis is more commonly observed than broad zones of fibroelastosis devoid of tumor cells. Tumor cells do not generally show scattered pleomorphism and smudgy nuclei seen after neoadjuvant chemotherapy, but cell size may decrease, particularly in classical invasive lobular carcinoma.

Histopathologic methods of assessment of response to neoadjuvant hormonal therapy have not yet been standardized. The Magee Method, described above, can be used to calculate an estimate of tumor volume reduction, which may be helpful to clinicians in assessment of response. The preoperative endocrine prognostic index (PEPI) score utilizes pathologic features of tumors, including ER status via Allred score, node status, tumor grade, and Ki67 proliferation index (using a cut-point of 2.7%) following neoadjuvant endocrine therapy to assess endocrine sensitivity [67]. In patients with PEPI = 0 (T1 or T2, N0, Ki67 $<$ 2.7%, ER Allred $>$2), relapse risk over 5 years was 3.6% without chemotherapy in the American College of Surgeons Oncology Group Z1031 Trial [68]. In that same trial, Ki67 proliferative index >10% following a short course of neoadjuvant endocrine therapy was used to determine a switch to chemotherapy. The Ki67 assessment scheme used in the study included counting several high-power fields if the whole slide estimate was between 2.7% and 10%, to a total of at least 100 cells. Other studies have also shown the prognostic significance of decrease in Ki67 proliferative index in the setting of neo-adjuvant endocrine therapy [69–71]. From a pathologic standpoint, standardization of assessment of Ki67 proliferative index remains a challenge. As decrease in Ki67 proliferative index becomes increasingly important in clinical trials of endocrine agents and in clinical use, standard counting approaches and image analysis will be invaluable to the practicing surgical pathologist.

Conclusion

The use of neoadjuvant systemic therapy in breast carcinoma presents opportunities and challenges in surgical pathology diagnosis and evaluation of resection specimens. Pathologic evaluation contributes to tumor phenotype determination and assessment of response to treatment and is crucial for multidisciplinary care of complex breast cancer cases. The most complete and accurate assessment of response to neoadjuvant therapy relies on access to detailed clinical history, imaging studies, and type of neoadjuvant therapy given.

References

1. Administration. USFaD. Guidance for industry: pathological complete response in neoadjuvant treatment of high-risk early-stage breast cancer: use as an endpoint to support accelerated approval. 2020. Available from: http://www.fda.gov/downloads/Drugs/GuidanceComplianceRegulatoryInformation/Guidances/UCM305501.pdf.
2. Klein ME, Dabbs DJ, Shuai Y, Brufsky AM, Jankowitz R, Puhalla SL, et al. Prediction of the Oncotype DX recurrence score: use of pathology-generated equations derived by linear regression analysis. Mod Pathol. 2013;26(5):658–64.
3. Elston CW, Ellis IO. Pathological prognostic factors in breast cancer. I. The value of histological grade in breast cancer: experience from a large study with long-term follow-up. Histopathology. 1991;19(5):403–10.
4. Allison KH, Hammond MEH, Dowsett M, McKernin SE, Carey LA, Fitzgibbons PL, et al. Estrogen and progesterone receptor testing in breast cancer: ASCO/CAP guideline update. J Clin Oncol. 2020;38(12):1346–66.
5. Wolff AC, Hammond MEH, Allison KH, Harvey BE, Mangu PB, Bartlett JMS, et al. Human epidermal growth factor receptor 2 testing in breast cancer: American Society of Clinical Oncology/College of American Pathologists Clinical Practice Guideline focused update. J Clin Oncol. 2018;36(20):2105–22.
6. Allred DC, Harvey JM, Berardo M, Clark GM. Prognostic and predictive factors in breast cancer by immunohistochemical analysis. Mod Pathol. 1998;11(2):155–68.

7. Flanagan MB, Dabbs DJ, Brufsky AM, Beriwal S, Bhargava R. Histopathologic variables predict Oncotype DX recurrence score. Mod Pathol. 2008;21(10):1255–61.
8. McCarty KS Jr, Miller LS, Cox EB, Konrath J, McCarty KS Sr. Estrogen receptor analyses. Correlation of biochemical and immunohistochemical methods using monoclonal antireceptor antibodies. Arch Pathol Lab Med. 1985;109(8):716–21.
9. Perou CM, Sorlie T, Eisen MB, van de Rijn M, Jeffrey SS, Rees CA, et al. Molecular portraits of human breast tumours. Nature. 2000;406(6797):747–52.
10. Sorlie T, Perou CM, Tibshirani R, Aas T, Geisler S, Johnsen H, et al. Gene expression patterns of breast carcinomas distinguish tumor subclasses with clinical implications. Proc Natl Acad Sci U S A. 2001;98(19):10869–74.
11. Rouzier R, Perou CM, Symmans WF, Ibrahim N, Cristofanilli M, Anderson K, et al. Breast cancer molecular subtypes respond differently to preoperative chemotherapy. Clin Cancer Res. 2005;11(16):5678–85.
12. Landmann A, Farrugia DJ, Zhu L, Diego EJ, Johnson RR, Soran A, et al. Low Estrogen Receptor (ER)-positive breast cancer and neoadjuvant systemic chemotherapy: is response similar to typical ER-positive or ER-negative disease? Am J Clin Pathol. 2018;150(1):34–42.
13. Bhargava R, Beriwal S, Dabbs DJ, Ozbek U, Soran A, Johnson RR, et al. Immunohistochemical surrogate markers of breast cancer molecular classes predicts response to neoadjuvant chemotherapy: a single institutional experience with 359 cases. Cancer. 2010;116(6):1431–9.
14. Bhargava R, Dabbs DJ, Beriwal S, Yildiz IA, Badve P, Soran A, et al. Semiquantitative hormone receptor level influences response to trastuzumab-containing neoadjuvant chemotherapy in HER2-positive breast cancer. Mod Pathol. 2011;24(3):367–74.
15. Boughey JC, McCall LM, Ballman KV, Mittendorf EA, Ahrendt GM, Wilke LG, et al. Tumor biology correlates with rates of breast-conserving surgery and pathologic complete response after neoadjuvant chemotherapy for breast cancer: findings from the ACOSOG Z1071 (Alliance) Prospective Multicenter Clinical Trial. Ann Surg. 2014;260(4):608–14. discussion 14–6
16. Houssami N, Macaskill P, von Minckwitz G, Marinovich ML, Mamounas E. Meta-analysis of the association of breast cancer subtype and pathologic complete response to neoadjuvant chemotherapy. Eur J Cancer. 2012;48(18):3342–54.
17. Li XB, Krishnamurti U, Bhattarai S, Klimov S, Reid MD, O'Regan R, et al. Biomarkers predicting pathologic complete response to neoadjuvant chemotherapy in breast cancer. Am J Clin Pathol. 2016;145(6):871–8.
18. Han M, Salamat A, Zhu L, Zhang H, Clark BZ, Dabbs DJ, et al. Metaplastic breast carcinoma: a clinical-pathologic study of 97 cases with subset analysis of response to neoadjuvant chemotherapy. Mod Pathol. 2019;32(6):807–16.
19. Bhargava R, Dabbs DJ. Magee equations and oncotype DX((R))-a perspective. Breast Cancer Res Treat. 2017;164(1):245–6.
20. Bhargava R, Esposito N, O'Connor S, Li Z, Turner B, Moisini I, et al. Magee equations and response to neoadjuvant chemotherapy in ER+/HER2- breast cancer: a multi-institutional study. Mod Pathol. 2020;34(1):77–84. Epub ahead of print
21. Cuzick J, Dowsett M, Pineda S, Wale C, Salter J, Quinn E, et al. Prognostic value of a combined estrogen receptor, progesterone receptor, Ki-67, and human epidermal growth factor receptor 2 immunohistochemical score and comparison with the Genomic Health recurrence score in early breast cancer. J Clin Oncol. 2011;29(32):4273–8.
22. Sheri A, Smith IE, Hills M, Jones RL, Johnston SR, Dowsett M. Relationship between IHC4 score and response to neo-adjuvant chemotherapy in estrogen receptor-positive breast cancer. Breast Cancer Res Treat. 2017;164(2):395–400.
23. Gianni L, Zambetti M, Clark K, Baker J, Cronin M, Wu J, et al. Gene expression profiles in paraffin-embedded core biopsy tissue predict response to chemotherapy in women with locally advanced breast cancer. J Clin Oncol. 2005;23(29):7265–77.

24. Prat A, Galvan P, Jimenez B, Buckingham W, Jeiranian HA, Schaper C, et al. Prediction of response to neoadjuvant chemotherapy using core needle biopsy samples with the Prosigna assay. Clin Cancer Res. 2016;22(3):560–6.
25. Abdsaleh S, Warnberg F, Azavedo E, Lindgren PG, Amini RM. Comparison of core needle biopsy and surgical specimens in malignant breast lesions regarding histological features and hormone receptor expression. Histopathology. 2008;52(6):773–5.
26. Chen X, Yuan Y, Gu Z, Shen K. Accuracy of estrogen receptor, progesterone receptor, and HER2 status between core needle and open excision biopsy in breast cancer: a meta-analysis. Breast Cancer Res Treat. 2012;134(3):957–67.
27. Clark BZ, Onisko A, Assylbekova B, Li X, Bhargava R, Dabbs DJ. Breast cancer global tumor biomarkers: a quality assurance study of intratumoral heterogeneity. Mod Pathol. 2019;32(3):354–66.
28. Lebeau A, Turzynski A, Braun S, Behrhof W, Fleige B, Schmitt WD, et al. Reliability of human epidermal growth factor receptor 2 immunohistochemistry in breast core needle biopsies. J Clin Oncol. 2010;28(20):3264–70.
29. Li S, Yang X, Zhang Y, Fan L, Zhang F, Chen L, et al. Assessment accuracy of core needle biopsy for hormone receptors in breast cancer: a meta-analysis. Breast Cancer Res Treat. 2012;135(2):325–34.
30. Loubeyre P, Bodmer A, Tille JC, Egger JF, Diebold-Berger S, Copercini M, et al. Concordance between core needle biopsy and surgical excision specimens for tumour hormone receptor profiling according to the 2011 St. Gallen classification, in clinical practice. Breast J. 2013;19(6):605–10.
31. Park SY, Kim KS, Lee TG, Park SS, Kim SM, Han W, et al. The accuracy of preoperative core biopsy in determining histologic grade, hormone receptors, and human epidermal growth factor receptor 2 status in invasive breast cancer. Am J Surg. 2009;197(2):266–9.
32. Tamaki K, Sasano H, Ishida T, Miyashita M, Takeda M, Amari M, et al. Comparison of core needle biopsy (CNB) and surgical specimens for accurate preoperative evaluation of ER, PgR and HER2 status of breast cancer patients. Cancer Sci. 2010;101(9):2074–9.
33. Kuerer HM, Rauch GM, Krishnamurthy S, Adrada BE, Caudle AS, DeSnyder SM, et al. A clinical feasibility trial for identification of exceptional responders in whom breast cancer surgery can be eliminated following neoadjuvant systemic therapy. Ann Surg. 2018;267(5):946–51.
34. Symmans WF, Peintinger F, Hatzis C, Rajan R, Kuerer H, Valero V, et al. Measurement of residual breast cancer burden to predict survival after neoadjuvant chemotherapy. J Clin Oncol. 2007;25(28):4414–22.
35. Provenzano E, Bossuyt V, Viale G, Cameron D, Badve S, Denkert C, et al. Standardization of pathologic evaluation and reporting of postneoadjuvant specimens in clinical trials of breast cancer: recommendations from an international working group. Mod Pathol. 2015;28(9):1185–201.
36. Diaz J, Stead L, Shapiro N, Newell R, Loudig O, Lo Y, et al. Mitotic counts in breast cancer after neoadjuvant systemic chemotherapy and development of metastatic disease. Breast Cancer Res Treat. 2013;138(1):91–7.
37. von Minckwitz G, Huang CS, Mano MS, Loibl S, Mamounas EP, Untch M, et al. Trastuzumab Emtansine for residual invasive HER2-positive breast cancer. N Engl J Med. 2019;380(7):617–28.
38. Masuda N, Lee SJ, Ohtani S, Im YH, Lee ES, Yokota I, et al. Adjuvant Capecitabine for breast cancer after preoperative chemotherapy. N Engl J Med. 2017;376(22):2147–59.
39. Cortazar P, Zhang L, Untch M, Mehta K, Costantino JP, Wolmark N, et al. Pathological complete response and long-term clinical benefit in breast cancer: the CTNeoBC pooled analysis. Lancet. 2014;384(9938):164–72.
40. Jones RL, Lakhani SR, Ring AE, Ashley S, Walsh G, Smith IE. Pathological complete response and residual DCIS following neoadjuvant chemotherapy for breast carcinoma. Br J Cancer. 2006;94(3):358–62.

41. Mazouni C, Peintinger F, Wan-Kau S, Andre F, Gonzalez-Angulo AM, Symmans WF, et al. Residual ductal carcinoma in situ in patients with complete eradication of invasive breast cancer after neoadjuvant chemotherapy does not adversely affect patient outcome. J Clin Oncol. 2007;25(19):2650–5.
42. von Minckwitz G, Untch M, Blohmer JU, Costa SD, Eidtmann H, Fasching PA, et al. Definition and impact of pathologic complete response on prognosis after neoadjuvant chemotherapy in various intrinsic breast cancer subtypes. J Clin Oncol. 2012;30(15):1796–804.
43. Fisher B, Brown A, Mamounas E, Wieand S, Robidoux A, Margolese RG, et al. Effect of preoperative chemotherapy on local-regional disease in women with operable breast cancer: findings from National Surgical Adjuvant Breast and Bowel Project B-18. J Clin Oncol. 1997;15(7):2483–93.
44. Rastogi P, Anderson SJ, Bear HD, Geyer CE, Kahlenberg MS, Robidoux A, et al. Preoperative chemotherapy: updates of National Surgical Adjuvant Breast and Bowel Project Protocols B-18 and B-27. J Clin Oncol. 2008;26(5):778–85.
45. Fisher B, Bryant J, Wolmark N, Mamounas E, Brown A, Fisher ER, et al. Effect of preoperative chemotherapy on the outcome of women with operable breast cancer. J Clin Oncol. 1998;16(8):2672–85.
46. Amin MB, Edge S, Greene F, Byrd D, Brookland R, Washington M, et al. AJCC cancer staging manual. 8th ed. Springer International Publishing: American Joint Commission on Cancer; Switzerland. 2017.
47. Carey LA, Metzger R, Dees EC, Collichio F, Sartor CI, Ollila DW, et al. American Joint Committee on Cancer tumor-node-metastasis stage after neoadjuvant chemotherapy and breast cancer outcome. J Natl Cancer Inst. 2005;97(15):1137–42.
48. Cheng E, Ko D, Nguyen M, Moo TA, Andreopoulou E, Hoda SA, et al. Residual pure Intralymphatic breast carcinoma following neoadjuvant chemotherapy is indicative of poor clinical outcome, even in node-negative patients. Am J Surg Pathol. 2017;41(9):1275–82.
49. Symmans WF, Wei C, Gould R, Yu X, Zhang Y, Liu M, et al. Long-term prognostic risk after neoadjuvant chemotherapy associated with residual cancer burden and breast cancer subtype. J Clin Oncol. 2017;35(10):1049–60.
50. Sheri A, Smith IE, Johnston SR, A'Hern R, Nerurkar A, Jones RL, et al. Residual proliferative cancer burden to predict long-term outcome following neoadjuvant chemotherapy. Ann Oncol. 2015;26(1):75–80.
51. Peintinger F, Sinn B, Hatzis C, Albarracin C, Downs-Kelly E, Morkowski J, et al. Reproducibility of residual cancer burden for prognostic assessment of breast cancer after neoadjuvant chemotherapy. Mod Pathol. 2015;28(7):913–20.
52. Ogston KN, Miller ID, Payne S, Hutcheon AW, Sarkar TK, Smith I, et al. A new histological grading system to assess response of breast cancers to primary chemotherapy: prognostic significance and survival. Breast. 2003;12(5):320–7.
53. Chollet P, Abrial C, Durando X, Thivat E, Tacca O, Mouret-Reynier MA, et al. A new prognostic classification after primary chemotherapy for breast cancer: residual disease in breast and nodes (RDBN). Cancer J. 2008;14(2):128–32.
54. Mittendorf EA, Jeruss JS, Tucker SL, Kolli A, Newman LA, Gonzalez-Angulo AM, et al. Validation of a novel staging system for disease-specific survival in patients with breast cancer treated with neoadjuvant chemotherapy. J Clin Oncol. 2011;29(15):1956–62.
55. Boughey JC, Ballman KV, Le-Petross HT, McCall LM, Mittendorf EA, Ahrendt GM, et al. Identification and resection of clipped node decreases the false-negative rate of sentinel lymph node surgery in patients presenting with node-positive breast cancer (T0-T4, N1-N2) who receive neoadjuvant chemotherapy: results from ACOSOG Z1071 (Alliance). Ann Surg. 2016;263(4):802–7.
56. Caudle AS, Yang WT, Krishnamurthy S, Mittendorf EA, Black DM, Gilcrease MZ, et al. Improved axillary evaluation following neoadjuvant therapy for patients with node-positive breast cancer using selective evaluation of clipped nodes: implementation of targeted axillary dissection. J Clin Oncol. 2016;34(10):1072–8.

57. Caudle AS, Yang WT, Mittendorf EA, Black DM, Hwang R, Hobbs B, et al. Selective surgical localization of axillary lymph nodes containing metastases in patients with breast cancer: a prospective feasibility trial. JAMA Surg. 2015;150(2):137–43.
58. Caudle AS, Kuerer HM, Krishnamurthy S, Shin K, Hobbs BP, Ma J, et al. Feasibility of fine-needle aspiration for assessing responses to chemotherapy in metastatic nodes marked with clips in breast cancer: a prospective registry study. Cancer. 2019;125(3):365–73.
59. Newman LA, Pernick NL, Adsay V, Carolin KA, Philip PA, Sipierski S, et al. Histopathologic evidence of tumor regression in the axillary lymph nodes of patients treated with preoperative chemotherapy correlates with breast cancer outcome. Ann Surg Oncol. 2003;10(7):734–9.
60. Fisher ER, Wang J, Bryant J, Fisher B, Mamounas E, Wolmark N. Pathobiology of preoperative chemotherapy: findings from the National Surgical Adjuvant Breast and Bowel (NSABP) protocol B-18. Cancer. 2002;95(4):681–95.
61. Wong SM, Almana N, Choi J, Hu J, Gagnon H, Natsuhara K, et al. Prognostic significance of residual axillary nodal micrometastases and isolated tumor cells after neoadjuvant chemotherapy for breast cancer. Ann Surg Oncol. 2019;26(11):3502–9.
62. Tadros AB, Yang WT, Krishnamurthy S, Rauch GM, Smith BD, Valero V, et al. Identification of patients with documented pathologic complete response in the breast after neoadjuvant chemotherapy for omission of axillary surgery. JAMA Surg. 2017;152(7):665–70.
63. Samiei S, van Nijnatten TJA, de Munck L, Keymeulen K, Simons JM, Kooreman LFS, et al. Correlation between pathologic complete response in the breast and absence of axillary lymph node metastases after neoadjuvant systemic therapy. Ann Surg. 2020;271(3):574–80.
64. Bi Z, Liu J, Chen P, Liu Y, Zhao T, Wang C, et al. Neoadjuvant chemotherapy and timing of sentinel lymph node biopsy in different molecular subtypes of breast cancer with clinically negative axilla. Breast Cancer. 2019;26(3):373–7.
65. Montagna G, Sevilimedu V, Fornier M, Jhaveri K, Morrow M, Pilewskie ML. How effective is Neoadjuvant Endocrine Therapy (NET) in downstaging the axilla and achieving breast-conserving surgery? Ann Surg Oncol. 2020;27(12):4702–10.
66. Rossi L, McCartney A, Risi E, De Santo I, Migliaccio I, Malorni L, et al. Cyclin-dependent kinase 4/6 inhibitors in neoadjuvant endocrine therapy of hormone receptor-positive breast cancer. Clin Breast Cancer. 2019;19(6):392–8.
67. Ellis MJ, Tao Y, Luo J, A'Hern R, Evans DB, Bhatnagar AS, et al. Outcome prediction for estrogen receptor-positive breast cancer based on postneoadjuvant endocrine therapy tumor characteristics. J Natl Cancer Inst. 2008;100(19):1380–8.
68. Ellis MJ, Suman VJ, Hoog J, Goncalves R, Sanati S, Creighton CJ, et al. Ki67 proliferation index as a tool for chemotherapy decisions during and after neoadjuvant aromatase inhibitor treatment of breast cancer: results from the American College of Surgeons Oncology Group Z1031 Trial (Alliance). J Clin Oncol. 2017;35(10):1061–9.
69. Dowsett M, Smith IE, Ebbs SR, Dixon JM, Skene A, A'Hern R, et al. Prognostic value of Ki67 expression after short-term presurgical endocrine therapy for primary breast cancer. J Natl Cancer Inst. 2007;99(2):167–70.
70. Dowsett M, Smith IE, Ebbs SR, Dixon JM, Skene A, Griffith C, et al. Short-term changes in Ki-67 during neoadjuvant treatment of primary breast cancer with anastrozole or tamoxifen alone or combined correlate with recurrence-free survival. Clin Cancer Res. 2005;11(2 Pt 2):951s–8s.
71. Ellis MJ, Rosen E, Dressman H, Marks J. Neoadjuvant comparisons of aromatase inhibitors and tamoxifen: pretreatment determinants of response and on-treatment effect. J Steroid Biochem Mol Biol. 2003;86(3–5):301–7.

Chapter 14
Guidelines for Neoadjuvant Systemic Therapy

Kristie Bobolis

Introduction

Breast cancer has become the most commonly diagnosed cancer among women in the United States and globally. The outcome, however, for contemporary women diagnosed with early stage breast cancer in the United States has significantly improved over the past 40 years compared to patients treated in the 1980s. Although this is true for all subtypes of breast cancer, including hormone-receptor-positive breast cancer, this is particularly true for women with HER2-positive and triple-negative breast cancer [1]. This is due in part due to advancements in each specialty field, including breast imaging, surgery, pathology, radiation and medical oncology, with care typically delivered by a multidisciplinary breast care team. This is also due to widespread use of adjuvant systemic therapy and development of more effective systemic treatments for HER2-positive and triple-negative subtypes [1, 2]. Although current treatments are more effective, late relapses are still seen in patients with hormone-receptor-positive tumors with an early peak of recurrence in patients with hormone-receptor-negative cancers.

With the adoption of widespread population screening for breast cancer in the United States in the 1980s, there has been a reduction in breast cancer mortality in women who undergo regular screening [3–6]. Mammography screening increases the likelihood of detecting small breast cancers that are amenable to breast conservation therapy [7]. Several breast cancer screening guidelines exist for women considered at average and higher than average risk for breast cancer as put forth by the U.S. Preventive Services Task Force [8], the American Cancer Society [9], the American College of Obstetricians and Gynecologists [10], the American College

K. Bobolis (✉)
Department of Medicine, Sutter Roseville Medical Center, Roseville, CA, USA
e-mail: Bobolik@sutterhealth.org

A. Soran, F. Nakhlis (eds.), *Management of the Breast and Axilla in the Neoadjuvant Setting*, https://doi.org/10.1007/978-3-030-88020-0_14

of Radiology [11], and the American College of Physicians [12]. Women at higher than average risk, particularly women at genetically high risk for breast are recommended to start screening at a younger age than average-risk women and with supplemental imaging such as contrast enhanced breast MRI, as mammography alone does not perform as well for this subgroup of individuals [13–17].

Despite benefits of mammographic screening with clear reduction in breast cancer mortality [18], there are limitations to mammography. Biologically more aggressive cancers can become clinically obvious as an "interval cancer" in the time after a normal mammogram and some screen detected cancers are detected when already at a locally advanced stage [19]. Additionally, there are many women who do not participate in breast cancer screening, either by choice, lack of access to care, pregnancy, or because they fall outside of screening guidelines by virtue of age. Many young women at elevated risk for breast cancer based on family history, prior thoracic radiation for Hodgkin's lymphoma or genetic predisposition, are often not identified as high-risk individuals and are not afforded the opportunity to participate in high-risk screening for early cancer detection. This group of women, when diagnosed with breast cancer, present with palpable disease, often more advanced than screen-detected asymptomatic breast cancer, where optimal management requires more intensive systemic management, more extensive local-regional measures with a less favorable long-term outcome.

Surgical resection of breast cancer remains the cornerstone of therapy for patients diagnosed with *early stage breast cancer*. Systemic therapy (chemotherapy, endocrine therapy, or targeted therapy) can reduce the risk of systemic relapse in patients with early stage breast cancer by killing disseminated cancer cells that escape the primary breast or local regional lymph nodes. *Adjuvant* systemic therapy refers to chemotherapy, endocrine therapy and/or targeted therapy delivered after definitive surgery and is the mainstay of treatment for early-stage breast cancer. The goal of adjuvant treatment is to eradicate micro metastatic disease and improve the likelihood of long-term survival. Recommendations for *adjuvant* systemic therapy are developed with knowledge of complete *pathologic* characterization of the tumor, including tumor size, regional nodes, histologic subtype, grade, and biologic prognostic factors (ER, PR, and HER2 expression). Selection of optimal adjuvant chemotherapy and targeted therapy for early breast cancer has been the subject of expert panel review with recent published updates [20, 21] and has evolved in recent decades with advancement in our knowledge of biologic subtypes of breast cancer. In patients with early stage ER positive breast cancer, in addition to clinical-pathologic features, gene expression profile assays have been developed and studied prospectively (Oncotype DX Recurrence Score and MammaPrint) to help with clinical decision-making when determining whether to offer adjuvant systemic chemotherapy in addition to endocrine therapy or if chemotherapy can be safely omitted [22–25].

Neoadjuvant systemic therapy refers to the application of systemic therapy (chemotherapy, endocrine therapy, or targeted therapy) prior to definitive surgical management. It is the treatment of choice for inflammatory breast carcinoma, which is an aggressive subtype of breast cancer with rapid disease progression and propensity for early distant metastases [26, 27]. Before active systemic therapy for breast cancer was available, this subtype of breast cancer was associated with a very poor outcome with poor disease control with surgery alone or combined with radiation therapy [28, 29]. Advances in multimodality therapy for inflammatory breast cancer have resulted in substantial improvements in survival in recent years with biologic subtype and response to neoadjuvant systemic therapy representing important factors in predicting both local control and distant recurrence [27–29].

The initial application of neoadjuvant systemic therapy in the 1970s was for treatment of inoperable or locally advanced breast cancer where the risk of positive surgical margins was considered high or not achievable if surgical intervention were to be attempted first [30, 31]. Neoadjuvant systemic therapy was subsequently studied in the 1980s and 1990s for technically operable breast cancer with the goal of downstaging disease, improving candidacy for breast conservation [32, 33]. The primary goal was met in improving breast conservation rate. There was no difference noted in long-term outcome measures, including disease-free survival and overall survival based when systemic therapy was delivered prior surgery compared to the same regimen given after surgery. There was noted in these early trials, an improvement in pathologic complete response with more active regimens and emergence of subgroups that appeared to benefit from this approach [33, 34]. With advances in knowledge of breast cancer biology, it is now understood that response to contemporary systemic therapy, whether delivered before or after surgical intervention, is driven by breast cancer subtype [35–37].

Because the primary tumor remains intact during therapy, treatment strategies using neoadjuvant therapy allow for monitoring of response to treatment. Disease progression, while infrequent, can occur while receiving neoadjuvant systemic therapy. Patients should be evaluated regularly during treatment. Early identification of progression should prompt discontinuation of systemic therapy and allow the patient to move on to surgical intervention [38]. Outside of a clinical trial, surgical intervention should not be omitted after neoadjuvant systemic therapy, even in the presence of a good clinical response as a significant risk of local-regional disease recurrence has been reported when primary systemic treatment was not accompanied by surgical intervention (i.e., treated with radiation alone) [39].

It was observed from initial trials of neoadjuvant systemic therapy that patients who achieve a pathologic complete response have a significantly better prognosis than those with residual disease [40, 41]. A pooled analysis of 12 neoadjuvant breast cancer clinical trials published in 2014 demonstrated that patients who attained pathologic complete response (pCR) defined as ypT0 ypN0 or ypT0/is ypN0 had improved survival [42]. This pooled analysis also showed the prognostic value of achieving pCR was greatest in aggressive tumor subtypes, particularly patients with triple-negative and HER2-positive disease [42, 43]. A trend toward significance has also been observed for hormone-receptor-positive tumors, likely driven by higher grade tumors. As our understanding of biologic subtypes of breast cancer has advanced in recent decades, more tailored approaches of systemic therapy have been adopted in trials studying neoadjuvant treatments [44–46]. From a research perspective, the neoadjuvant setting has become a model for translational research allowing opportunity to study tumor response in the intact tumor. This remains an active area of study for evaluation of predictive markers, efficacy of novel agents and surrogate endpoints [47–50].

The association between achievement of pathologic complete response and improved long-term outcomes in aggressive subtypes of breast cancer is thought to reflect tumor biology and systemic clearance of micro metastatic disease [42, 43]. This concept has highlighted the potential of optimizing therapy in the *adjuvant* setting based on pathologic response to neoadjuvant therapy. Although the association of pathologic complete response with improved long-term outcomes is recognized for HER2-positive and triple-negative breast cancer, this is less understood for lower grade hormone-receptor-positive breast cancer where PCR is less commonly achieved, and adjuvant endocrine therapy is the mainstay of systemic therapy [42, 43].

Developing an optimal neoadjuvant systemic approach depends on the ability to accurately assess the anatomic stage of disease based on clinical findings. This includes estimated tumor size, typically by imaging, histologic subtype, grade, biomarkers, including ER, PR and HER2 status (based on core needle sampling of the tumor), and clinical assessment of regional nodes by imaging. Clinically suspicious nodes should be assessed with needle biopsy [20, 21]. As with adjuvant systemic therapy, selection of systemic therapy is guided by tumor histology, grade, ER, PR, HER2 analysis, and menopausal status of the patient [21].

As therapeutic decisions regarding neoadjuvant systemic therapy are based on the ability to assess stage up-front, this approach should be reserved for patients where an accurate clinical assessment of stage can be ascertained prior to surgery. In patients with operable breast cancer, where pathologic information from surgical resection such as accurate size of invasive disease, nodal status, or a gene expression profile assay is needed to determine if chemotherapy should be recommended or withheld, the patient should be offered up-front surgery. Otherwise, there is the possibility of over- or underestimating clinical stage, resulting in overtreatment or undertreatment of the patient. Physical examination and results obtained with imaging modalities can be less accurate or uncertain than surgical staging. Accurate nodal staging may affect radiation therapy options [51]. The optimal management of patients appropriate for neoadjuvant systemic therapy requires delivery of care by a multidisciplinary breast care team. Guidelines for the application of neoadjuvant systemic therapy, including goals, patient selection, benefits, and limitations, will be the focus of this chapter.

Goals of Neoadjuvant Systemic Therapy

The term "neoadjuvant systemic therapy" refers to delivery of systemic therapy (chemotherapy, endocrine therapy, and targeted therapy) in the preoperative setting. The goal of systemic therapy, whether administered prior to or after surgery to patients with non-metastatic invasive breast carcinoma, is to reduce the risk of emergence of distant disease and improve the likelihood of long-term disease-free survival.

The additional goals of administering neoadjuvant systemic therapy prior to surgery are several. For locally advanced inoperable disease, the goal is to create surgical opportunities as part of local management of disease. For patients with inflammatory breast cancer, neoadjuvant therapy is considered a standard of care given poor outcome when surgery is attempted first due to local regional extent of disease, involvement of skin lymphatics with tumor emboli, and propensity for disseminated microscopic disease at presentation.

In individuals with operable locally advanced disease, the goal is to downstage disease, reducing the extent of surgery needed to provide local regional control of disease. Downstaging of disease prior to surgery may allow breast conservation rather than mastectomy or less extensive axillary surgery reducing the risk of morbidity from local regional therapy, including pain and lymphedema [35, 37, 51, 68].

Administering systemic therapy prior to surgery in patients with clinically measurable disease allows for monitoring of response and discontinuing of therapy in the uncommon event of progression [38]. Neoadjuvant systemic therapy can also permit evaluation of the effectiveness of systemic therapy as determined by degree of pathologic response. For newly diagnosed breast cancer, where up-front surgery is feasible without the need to downsize disease, the application of neoadjuvant systemic therapy has become recommended for certain subtypes such as high-risk triple-negative and HER2 overexpressing breast cancer, where pathologic response to initial therapy has strong prognostic implications and can be used to tailor adjuvant therapy recommendations [66, 67, 77].

For patients that are candidates for surgery and candidates for adjuvant systemic therapy, but have a need to delay surgery, neoadjuvant systemic therapy can be considered. Examples where patient may need to delay surgery would include, awaiting results of cancer genetic testing to assist with surgical decisions, allowing time to consider options for breast reconstruction or operating room availability as was affected in many centers during the height of the COVID 19 pandemic [69].

Multidisciplinary Management

Patients undergoing neoadjuvant systemic therapy should optimally receive management by a multidisciplinary breast care team to assure optimal patient outcome. Engagement of the multidisciplinary breast care team is recommended early in pretreatment evaluation and management of patients with locally advanced breast carcinoma. Early involvement of plastic surgery can aid in surgical planning. Patients should be assessed for eligibility for clinical trials when available. Early involvement of genetic counseling should be considered, as results of testing may inform surgical decisions. Referral for lymphedema evaluation should be considered early for patient education and baseline arm measurements as patients with locally advanced disease at presentation are at elevated risk for developing lymphedema. Fertility counseling should be offered for premenopausal women. Psychosocial support should be offered to assure the patient is able to fully understand and navigate treatment options. Optimal patient outcomes require coordinated management and input by the entire breast care team. Goals of care should be carefully communicated with patient engagement in decision-making [2].

Patient Selection for Neoadjuvant Systemic Therapy

Locally Advanced Inoperable *Breast Cancer*

Definition

The need to identify locally advanced inoperable breast carcinoma as a separate group of disease arose from recognition of the high associated rate of local regional and systemic failure despite the best efforts of surgeons to remove locoregional spread of the disease in its entirety. The definition of locally advanced, inoperable breast cancer has changed in time with changes in paradigms for breast cancer management. In the early 1900s, when the radical mastectomy was the surgical standard for management of breast cancer, criteria for breast cancer operability were set forth in a publication in 1943 [52]. These criteria were based on an inclusive review of 1040 cases of breast carcinoma seen at the Presbyterian Hospital New York during the period of 1915 to 1934. At the time, there were surgeons who would perform radical mastectomies in very advanced cases of breast cancer, holding to the theory that patients should be given the potential opportunity for cure even when the likelihood was exceeding small. To improve the results achieved with radical mastectomy, early criteria were established describing *"grave signs of locally advanced breast carcinoma"* not considered curable even by radical surgery. Signs of inoperability at the time included ulceration of the skin, edema of the skin, tumor fixation to the chest wall, axillary lymph nodes measuring at least 2.5 cm, fixation of axillary nodes to the skin or deeper structures of the axilla [52, 53].

The American Joint Commission on Cancer (AJCC) published the first edition of the TNM staging system in 1977 to define extent of disease categories for breast cancer. The TNM system refers to primary tumor size (T), regional nodal status (N), and the presence or absence of distant organ metastases (M). There are defined subsets in each category based on clinical pathologic measurements with overall stage assigned based on subset grouping. The TNM staging system has evolved over the past five decades along with the contemporary era of clinical trials and has undergone several revisions since this initial publication [54]. The definition of locally advanced breast cancer has changed in time with the refinements in multimodality treatment as has the outcome in this select group of patients with very advanced local-regional disease.

It is noteworthy that many studies cited on the topic of neoadjuvant systemic therapy used prior editions of the TNM staging system to define patients with locally advanced breast carcinoma and outcomes from clinical trials [37, 39, 55]. The current eighth edition of the AJCC cancer staging manual includes two staging systems, the anatomic and pathologic stages. The anatomic stage focuses on anatomic extent of disease based on tumor size, nodal status, and distant metastasis. The prognostic stage system incorporates tumor grade, hormone-receptor status, HER2 status, and results of gene expression array, if obtained, to more accurately predict a patient's outcome. Where guidelines for patient selection are discussed in this chapter, the staging system as provided in the eighth edition forth in the eighth edition of the AJCC staging manual is used [54].

Presently, locally advanced breast carcinoma breast cancer can be defined as a subset of breast cancers characterized by the most advanced stages of disease in the absence of distant metastases [56, 57]. Approximately 10–15% of breast cancer is diagnosed at a locally advanced stage. Locally advanced breast cancers are further divided into operable or inoperable based on the probability of achieving negative margins on histopathologic examination, with the initial surgical approach performed as part of long-term reduction in local regional recurrence. Locally advanced breast carcinoma encompasses a very heterogeneous group of breast cancer, including patients with large breast masses at least 5 cm in size with positive axillary lymph nodes, chest wall invasion, and/or skin involvement such as satellite nodules or ulceration, and patients with extensive involvement of regional nodes with or with significant disease in the breast. In some cases of locally advanced breast cancer there may be secondary inflammatory changes. These cases are more frequently seen in individuals or communities that lack resources for appropriate screening and treatment [57]. Individuals with locally advanced inoperable disease have a higher risk of local regional relapse and distant relapse with lower rates of long-term survival compared to individuals who receive treatment for early-stage breast carcinoma. The outcome for patients with locally advanced breast cancer has improved, however, with contemporary systemic therapy and multimodality therapy, including the application of neoadjuvant systemic therapy and delivery of postsurgical local regional radiation therapy [57].

Inflammatory breast carcinoma is a rare form of locally advanced breast carcinoma. It is considered inoperable up front due to the aggressive nature of this disease, high risk of systemic spread, and involvement of skin with tumor emboli in dermal lymphatics [58]. True de novo inflammatory breast carcinoma represents a more uniform entity with a distinct biological identity often occurring in younger women. Although a rare entity, representing 2–3% of breast cancers diagnosed annually in the United States, inflammatory breast cancer accounts for 8–10% of breast cancer-related death [58].

Pretreatment Evaluation for Non-inflammatory Locally Advanced Breast Cancer

Initial evaluation should include a history and physical exam, including clinical examination of the breast, skin, and regional nodes. CBC and comprehensive metabolic panel, including liver function tests, should be assessed. Diagnostic breast imaging should include diagnostic mammogram and ultrasound of the affected breast and regional nodes as well as screening images of the unaffected breast if not recently performed per NCCN guidelines [62]. MRI may be considered to assess the extent of breast involvement, assess for chest wall involvement, extent of nodal involvement, and can serve as a baseline for monitoring response to neoadjuvant therapy, particularly when extent of disease is not well defined on diagnostic mammography and ultrasound [59, 60].

Image-guided core-needle biopsy of the breast with placement of an image detectable marker of the breast abnormality is required for confirmation of the diagnosis of invasive carcinoma. Pathology assessment should include tumor histology, estimated grade, biomarkers including estrogen receptor (ER), progesterone receptor (PR), and HER2 status. The use of gene expression assays has not been validated at this time for use in the preoperative setting for clinical decision-making. Palpable or clinically suspicious nodes on imaging should undergo either core- or fine-needle aspiration for a more accurate determination of tumor stage given its prognostic value. The placement of a biopsy clip should be strongly considered when performing a core-needle biopsy, as use of the clip can improve the rate of successful surgical resection of biopsy-proven metastatic axillary lymph nodes [61, 62].

Evaluation for distant disease is appropriate in this subgroup of patients, even in the absence of symptoms as patients with locally advanced disease are at higher risk for having disseminated disease at presentation. Laboratory evaluation should include CBC and complete metabolic panel. Nuclear bone scan and contrast-enhanced CT of the chest, abdomen, and pelvis are usually adequate in assessing for clinical metastases. Additional imaging, including positron emission tomography and MRI, may be required in some situations. Areas suspicious for distant metastases should undergo biopsy, if feasible, to confirm presence of metastatic disease. Brain MRI is recommended for patients with CNS symptoms.

Pretreatment Evaluation for Inflammatory Breast Cancer

The diagnosis of inflammatory breast carcinoma is based on the clinical presentation and presence of invasive carcinoma on breast core-needle biopsy. Patients typically present with rapidly progressive inflammation of the breast, skin changes, including increased warmth, skin color changes (pink flushed, red, or purplish hue), and a thickening of the skin. The nipple may appear flattened or retracted. An associated palpable mass may be noted as well as adenopathy on clinical exam.

Breast imaging should include diagnostic mammogram and ultrasound of the affected breast and regional nodes as well as screening on the contralateral side. Breast MRI can be considered to assess extent of breast involvement, find a target for core-needle biopsy, assess for chest wall abnormalities, assess the contralateral breast, and provide a baseline for monitoring response to neoadjuvant therapy [59, 60].

Core-needle biopsy of the area of concern in the breast is necessary for the initial diagnosis of invasive carcinoma. Full-thickness skin punch biopsy may be obtained to assess for dermal lymphatic invasion by tumor cells which is a clinical feature observed in most cases, but is not necessary to make the diagnosis of inflammatory breast carcinoma. Estrogen receptor, progestin receptor, and HER2 testing is required to guide neoadjuvant systemic therapy. Palpable or clinically suspicious nodes on imaging should also undergo either core- or fine-needle aspiration for a more accurate determination of tumor stage given its prognostic value, with clip placement for identification at the time of surgery if core biopsy is performed [61, 62].

Staging and pretreatment evaluation include complete blood count, liver function tests, serum alkaline phosphatase. Contrast enhanced CT scans of the chest, abdomen, and a bone scan are recommended to rule out metastatic disease at presentation. An FDG PET-CT can be performed at the same time as diagnostic CT and may be helpful in situations where standard imaging studies are equivocal or suspicious. FDG PET-CT may also be helpful in identifying unsuspected regional nodal disease and or distant metastases in locally advanced breast cancer, when used in addition to standard staging studies [62]. Brain imaging should be obtained if there are clinical concerns for CNS metastasis.

Inflammatory breast carcinoma is designated as T4d in the American Joint Commission on Cancer (AJCC) Tumor, Node, Metastasis (TNM) staging system [54]. The following diagnostic criteria must be met: Rapid onset of breast erythema, edema, peau d'orange and/or breast warmth with or without an underlying palpable mass; duration of history no more than 6 months; erythema occupying at least one third of the breast; and pathologic confirmation of invasive breast carcinoma [58].

Clinical Stage Assignment

Once the above information is assessed, patients should be assigned a clinical stage according to the AJCC Cancer Staging System [54]. Table 14.1 summarizes definitions for tumor size (T), Table 14.2 summarizes the definitions for regional lymph node (N), and Table 14.3 summarizes definitions for distant metastases (M), as put forth in this edition. The designation "c" prior to each category refers to clinical stage. The designation "p" refers to pathologic stage. Clinical prognostic stage is provided in this chapter when discussing clinical scenarios. The current AJCC Cancer Staging Manual should be referenced for full staging information. This may also be found in the current NCCN Guidelines for breast cancer [54, 62].

Table 14.1 America Joint committee on Cancer (AJCC) staging. Clinical and pathologic primary tumor (T) category

T category[a]	T criteria
T0	No evidence of primary tumor
Tis (DCIS)	Ductal carcinoma in situ
T1	Tumor ≤20 mm in greatest dimension
T1mi	Tumor ≤1 mm in greatest dimension
T1a	Tumor >1 mm but ≤5 mm
T1b	Tumor >5 mm but ≤10 mm
T1c	Tumor >10 mm but ≤20 mm
T2	Tumor >20 but ≤50 mm in greatest dimension
T3	Tumor >50 mm in greatest dimension
T4	Tumor of any size with direct extension to the chest wall and or to the skin (ulceration or skin nodules); invasion of the dermis alone does not qualify as T4
T4a	Extension to the chest wall; invasion or adherences to pectoralis muscle in the absence of invasion of chest wall structures does not qualify as T4
T4b	Ulceration and/or ipsilateral macroscopic satellite nodules and or edema (including peau d'orange) of the skin that does not meet the criteria for inflammatory carcinoma
T4c	Both T4 a and T4b are present
T4d	inflammatory carcinoma

After neoadjuvant therapy, prefix yp is used

[a]Based on the largest contiguous focus of residual invasive cancer, if present. When multiple foci of tumor are present, the (m) modifier is used

Table 14.2 America Joint committee on Cancer (AJCC) staging. Clinical regional lymph nodes (cN) category

cN category[a]	cN criteria
cN0	No regional lymph node metastasis
cN1	Metastases to movable ipsilateral level I, II axillary lymph node(s)
cN1mi[b]	Micrometastases (200 cells, larger than 0.2 mm, but none larger than 2.0 mm)
cN2	Metastasis in ipsilateral level 1, 2 axillary lymph nodes that are clinically fixed or matted (cN2a) *or* in ipsilateral internal mammary nodes in the absence of axillary lymph node metastases (cN2b)
cN3	Metastases to ipsilateral infraclavicular (level 3) axillary lymph nodes (cN3a) Metastasis to the ipsilateral internal mammary nodes detected by imaging studies (including CT scan and ultrasound) or by clinical examination in conjunction with level I, II, lymph node metastases (cN3b) Metastases to ipsilateral supraclavicular (level III) axillary lymph nodes regardless of presence or absence of axillary or internal mammary nodal involvement (cN3c)

Note: (sn) and (f) specifics should be added to the end category to denote confirmation of metastasis by sentinel node biopsy or fine-needle aspiration/core-needle biopsy, respectively

[a]Includes lymph nodes detected by clinical examination or imaging

[b]cN1mi is rarely used but may be appropriate in cases where sentinel node biopsy is performed before tumor resection

Table 14.3 America Joint committee on Cancer (AJCC) staging. Distant metastases (M)

M0	No clinical or radiographic evidence of distant metastases
cM0 (+)	No clinical or radiographic evidence of distant metastases in the presence of tumor cells or deposits larger than 0.2 mm detected microscopically or by molecular techniques and circulating blood, bone marrow, or other non -regional nodal tissue in patient without symptoms or signs of metastases
cM1	Distant metastases detected by clinical and radiographic means
pM1	Any histologically proven metastases and distant organs; or if in non-regional nodes, metastases greater than 0.2 mm.

Clinical Scenario 1: Inflammatory Breast Cancer

Clinical Prognostic Stage IIIC, cT4d, cN2b, cM0, ER, PR, and HER2 Negative

A patient in her early 30s presents with left breast pain, swelling, skin changes, including erythema, increased warmth, and heaviness of the breast of a few weeks' duration. The patient also notes a palpable mass in the superior aspect of the left breast. There is a paternal family history of breast cancer in two aunts diagnosed before the age of 40. Exam is remarkable for swelling, erythema, edema involving the entire left breast with a palpable mass involving the superior left breast spanning 5–6 cm.

Diagnostic breast imaging is obtained with diagnostic mammograms (Fig. 14.1a) and ultrasound demonstrating a suspicious irregular mass upper outer left breast, possible regional distortion and diffuse left breast skin thickening. Multiple enlarged nodes are noted on ultrasound. Breast MRI more accurately demonstrates extent of disease in this patient (Fig. 14.1b).

Core biopsy, ultrasound-guided left breast demonstrates invasive, poorly differentiated carcinoma. Estimated grade 3, ER negative, PR negative, HER2 negative. Core biopsy of a left axillary node demonstrates metastatic carcinoma, poorly differentiated. Labs are normal. Staging PET-CT (Fig. 14.2) confirms locally advanced, non-metastatic breast carcinoma.

The patient meets NCCN criteria for genetic testing based on her age of presentation and family history [72]. A pathogenic mutation in *BRCA1* is identified on cancer genetic testing.

Clinical Prognostic Stage: IIIC, cT4d, cN3b, cM0, high grade, ER, PR, and HER2 negative

Neoadjuvant chemotherapy is the standard initial approach for inflammatory breast carcinoma. The optimal chemotherapy regimen and schedule for inflammatory breast carcinoma is not defined. Based on expert consensus recommendations, an anthracycline and taxane-based neoadjuvant regimen is typically recommended for patients with inflammatory breast carcinoma, such as dose dense doxorubicin and cyclophosphamide followed by paclitaxel [26, 27]. For tumors that overexpress HER2, inclusion of HER2-directed agents are indicated with polychemotherapy.

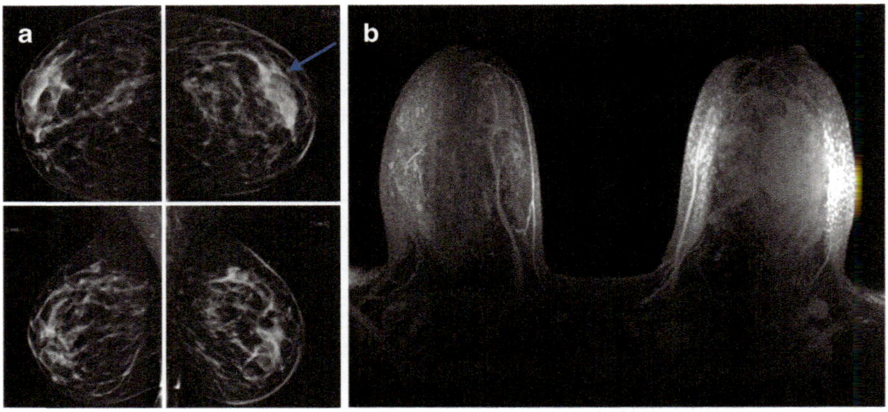

Fig. 14.1 Diagnostic mammograms (**a**) left breast with suspicious irregular mass upper outer left breast and possible regional distortion left cc view with diffuse left breast skin thickening as pointed out by arrow. Limited left breast ultrasound (not pictured) with multiple enlarged left axillary lymph nodes. MRI breast images (**b**) more accurately demonstrates extent of disease in this patient with combination of mass and non-mass regional enhancement throughout the superior aspect left breast extending up to 10 cm with additional scattered areas of mass and non-mass enhancement seen inferiorly in the breast suspicious for multicentric disease. Left axillary adenopathy, including level 3, in addition to left internal mammary lymphadenopathy is noted on MRI

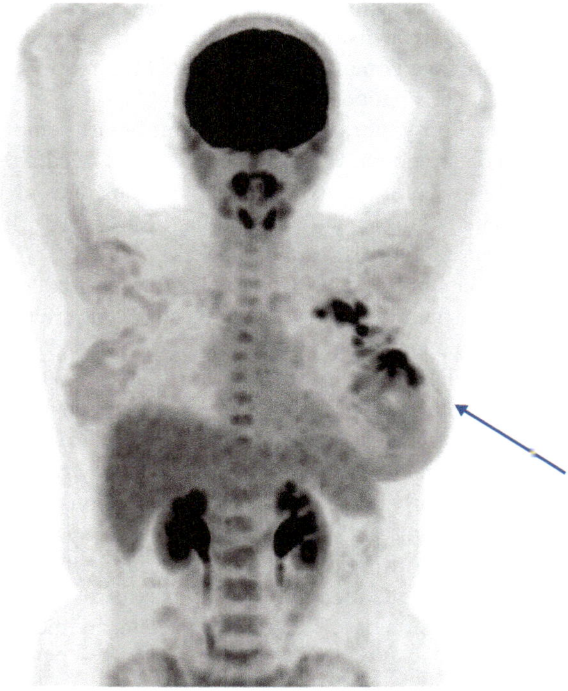

Fig. 14.2 PET-CT with hypermetabolic mass within the left superior lateral breast compatible with primary breast carcinoma. Large areas of increased radiotracer throughout the left breast fibro-glandular tissue concerning for multicentric tumor involvement. Multiple FDG-avid left axillary and internal mammary lymph nodes are noted. Presence of skin thickening is designated by arrow

Patients with inflammatory breast carcinoma who have operable disease following neoadjuvant therapy should proceed with mastectomy and axillary dissection. Skin sparing mastectomy is contraindicated in inflammatory breast carcinoma given the high risk for local failure. Immediate reconstruction following surgery should be avoided given the high risk for local recurrence. Radiation therapy is recommended following mastectomy [26–29]. Patients with high-risk residual disease following neoadjuvant chemotherapy may be considered for additional systemic therapy—as offered for non-inflammatory locally advanced breast carcinoma with residual disease.

Care by a multidisciplinary breast team is key to help the patient with decision-making regarding the role contralateral prophylactic mastectomy versus high-risk screening for the remaining breast in the setting of a BRCA 1 mutation. Fertility preservation options should be addressed prior to starting neoadjuvant therapy, but should be provided in a timely manner given urgency of initiating systemic therapy for individuals with inflammatory breast carcinoma. Gynecology oncology should be engaged for discussion of risk reducing salpingo-oophorectomy, including appropriate timing of this procedure and whether to consider hysterectomy with salpingo-oophorectomy in the setting of a BRCA1 pathogenic variant.

Clinical Scenario 2: Locally Advanced, Inoperable Breast Cancer, ER Positive, Premenopausal

Clinical Prognostic Stage IIIB, cT4b, cN2, cM0, Grade 2 Invasive Ductal Carcinoma

A female in her mid-30s presents with a palpable mass right breast of several months' duration. Exam is remarkable for a very large mass spanning more than 10 cm with edema and erythema although not meeting clinical criteria for inflammatory breast cancer. Several enlarged axillary nodes are palpated on clinical exam.

Diagnostic mammograms demonstrate heterogeneously dense breast tissue with suggestion of architectural distortion craniocaudal view right breast (Fig. 14.3a) and asymmetrically enlarged right axillary nodes (Fig. 14.3b). Ultrasound right axilla demonstrates several enlarged axillary nodes with abnormal morphology, thickened cortex. Breast MRI (Fig. 14.4) demonstrates extensive enhancement throughout the anterior two thirds of the right breast measuring $9 \times 9 \times 8$ cm. Multiple enlarged right axillary lymph nodes are also noted. An area of non-mass enhancement left breast was also noted designating an area of suspected DCIS (Fig. 14.4).

Image-guided core biopsy right breast: Invasive ductal carcinoma, estimated grade 2, ER positive, PR positive, and HER2 negative. Core biopsy right axillary node: Metastatic carcinoma.

Contrast-enhanced CT chest, abdomen, and pelvis demonstrate a large right breast mass with axillary adenopathy. Nuclear medicine bone scan demonstrates no evidence of osseous metastases.

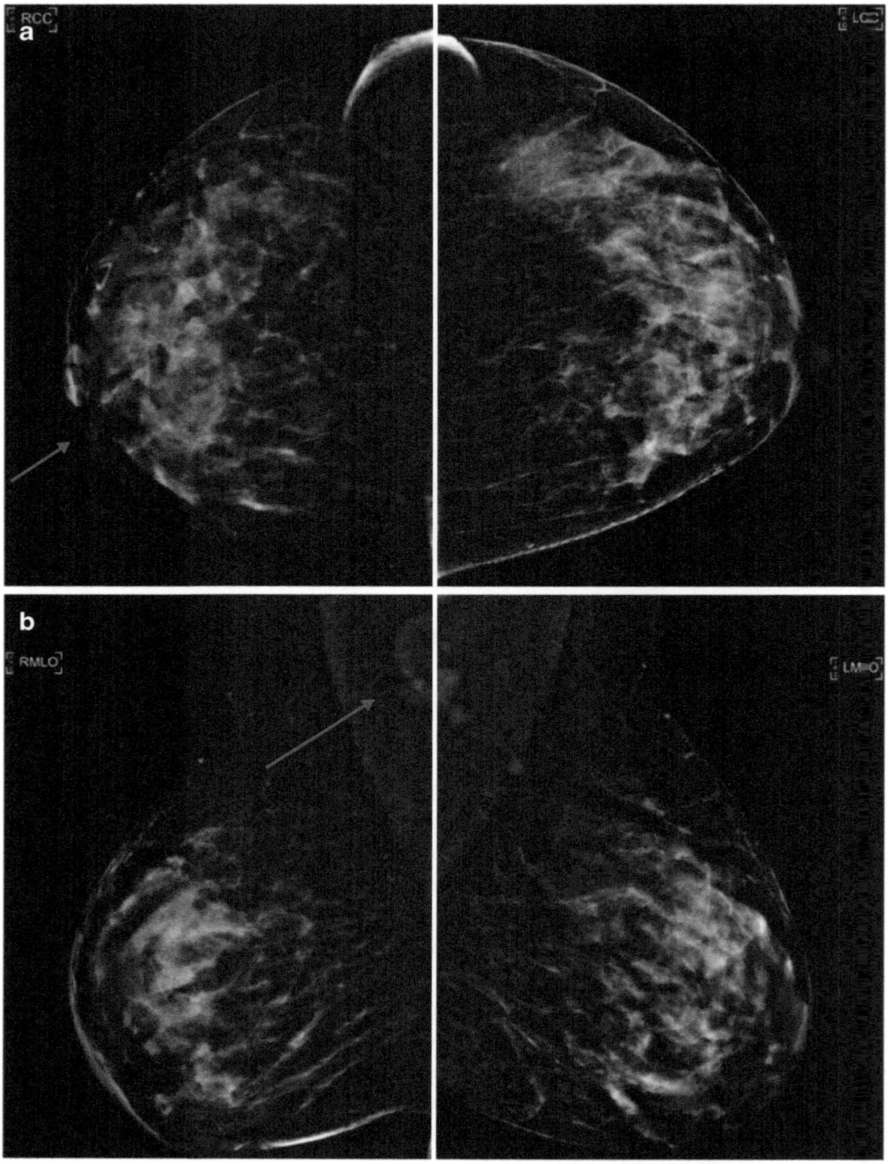

Fig. 14.3 Diagnostic mammograms with demonstrated heterogeneously dense breast tissue with suggestion of architectural distortion (arrow) right breast CC view (**a**) and asymmetrically enlarged right axillary nodes (arrow) right MLO view (**b**)

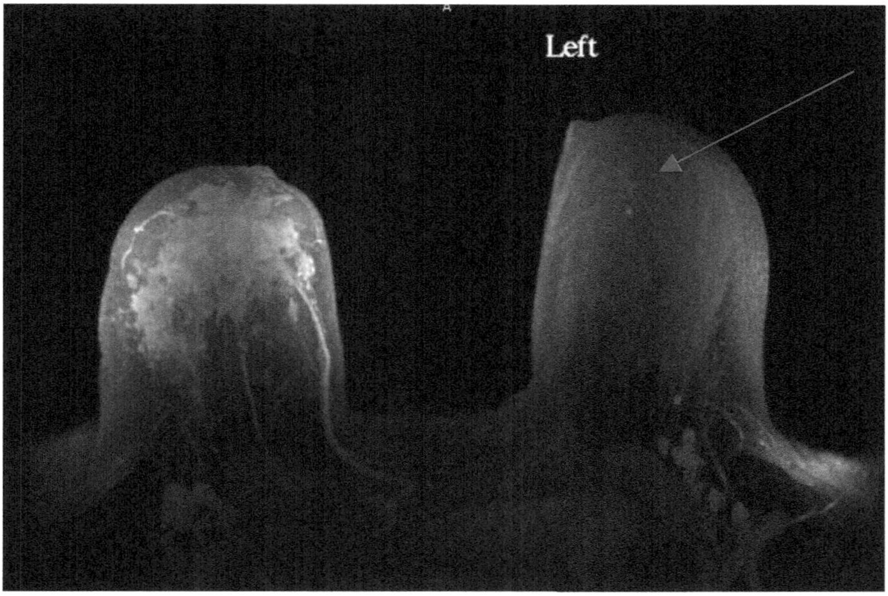

Fig. 14.4 Breast MRI: extensive enhancement throughout the anterior two-thirds of the right breast measuring 9 × 9 × 8 cm. Multiple enlarged right axillary lymph nodes. Extent of disease is much better appreciated on MRI compared to mammography in this young woman with dense breast tissue. An area of non-mass enhancement left breast denotes an area of suspected DCIS, confirmed on biopsy (arrow)

Genetic testing is offered with results negative for pathogenic variant in an 11 gene breast caner panel. Fertility counseling is also offered. Patient is G2P2 and opted not to pursue fertility counseling.

The patient is considered locally advanced, nonoperable by virtue of the very large right breast cancer measuring close to 10 cm with overlying skin changes.

Clinical prognostic stage is IIIB (cT4b, cN2, cM0) grade 2, invasive ductal carcinoma, ER positive, PR positive, and HER2 negative.

Neoadjuvant systemic chemotherapy is prescribed with dose-dense Adriamycin Cytoxan followed by weekly Taxol with a favorable, although incomplete, clinical response to therapy. The large central right breast mass becomes significantly smaller on exam (5–6 cm) after neoadjuvant chemotherapy with marked reduction in palpable adenopathy and complete resolution of skin erythema and edema overlying central lateral inferior breast. A restaging MRI prior to surgery (Fig. 14.5) confirms a favorable response to therapy by imaging.

The patient undergoes right mastectomy with right axillary node dissection for local regional management after neoadjuvant chemotherapy. Right breast pathology demonstrates invasive mammary/ductal carcinoma with lobular features, poorly

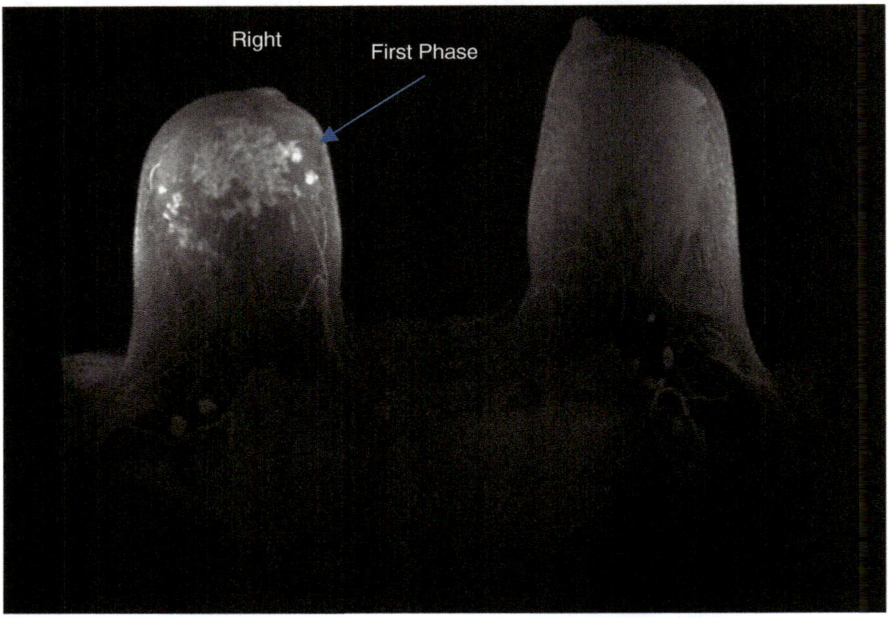

Fig. 14.5 Breast MRI post-neoadjuvant chemotherapy. Findings are consistent with moderate imaging response to neoadjuvant chemotherapy with patchy areas of residual enhancement right breast (arrow). Less enhancement of left breast DCIS also noted

differentiated, grade 3. Tumor size measures at least 9 cm, central site with involvement of all four quadrants. Margins are uninvolved by 6 mm. Treatment effect is present. Metastatic carcinoma is noted in 13 of 30 lymph nodes.

Pathologic Stage: ypT3, ypN3a, M0 ER positive, PR negative, and HER2 negative.

She opts for simple left mastectomy. Left breast pathology: Ductal carcinoma in situ, intermediate nuclear grade. Architectural patterns: Solid, cribriform, and comedo patterns with microcalcifications and lobular extension. Estimated extent 2.6 cm. Tumor site: Retroareolar. Margins are widely uninvolved.

Pathologic Stage 0: ypTis, cN0

Adjuvant radiotherapy post-mastectomy is recommended to the right chest wall and comprehensive nodal basin. Adjuvant endocrine therapy is also recommended with consideration for ovarian suppression along with an endocrine agent.

Referral to plastics is recommended early during the course of treatment to discuss the option of delayed reconstruction. Early referral for lymphedema assessment is also recommended given the high risk for developing lymphedema in this clinical scenario due to extent of axillary node involvement and need for both axillary dissection and radiation for local regional management.

Clinical Scenario 3: Locally Advanced, Inoperable Breast Cancer, HER2 Positive

Clinical Prognostic Stage IIIC, cT1mi, cN3, cM0, ER *Negative*, PR *Negative*, and HER2 *Positive*

A female in her early 60s presents with left axillary discomfort and a sizable mass palpable left axilla. She last participated in screening 3 years ago. She reports a family history of breast cancer in a paternal aunt in her 60s. Diagnostic mammogram and ultrasound (not shown) reveal confluent multiple pathologic-appearing left axillary nodes with subtle asymmetric distortion and microcalcifications left upper outer breast. Biopsy of left breast calcifications: high grade DCIS with microinvasive high-grade ductal carcinoma, ER 0, PR 0, HER2 3+, 100% by immunohistochemistry. Biopsy of axillary node reveals metastatic carcinoma.

Breast MRI (Fig. 14.6) demonstrates multiple abnormally enlarged lymph nodes spanning left axillary levels 1 through 3, including bulky adenopathy level 1 as well as supraclavicular versus low cervical adenopathy.

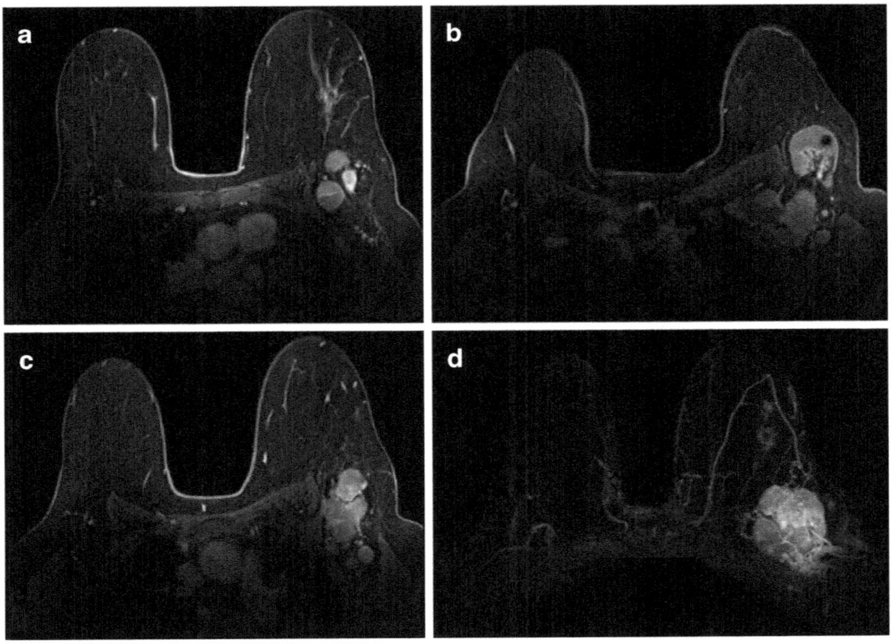

Fig. 14.6 MRI breast: non-mass enhancement in the upper outer quadrant left breast spanning several cm with signal void related to biopsy clip (**a**). There are multiple abnormally enlarged lymph nodes spanning left axillary levels 1 through 3 with a 3.6 cm node level 1 region containing a biopsy marker clip (**b**). The largest level 1 axillary node measures 5 cm (**c**). There is a supraclavicular node measuring 1.8 cm (not pictured). No internal mammary adenopathy noted. MIP image (**d**) demonstrates marked axillary involvement

Systemic staging with PET-CT demonstrates multiple abnormal nodes, involving the left supraclavicular, left axillary, and left subpectoral regions (Fig. 14.7).

Clinical Prognostic Stage is IIIB, cTmi, cN3c, cM0, grade 3, invasive microinvasive ductal carcinoma left breast, ER negative, PR negative, HER2 positive.

Given presence of bulky, fixed left axillary adenopathy, the patient is not a candidate for up-front surgical resection. There is also a high likelihood disseminated microscopic disease in this aggressive subtype of breast cancer which is HER2 positive. Neoadjuvant systemic polychemotherapy incorporating HER2-targeted monoclonal antibodies is indicated to reduce risk of emergence of systemic disease and downstage disease prior to surgery.

Despite presenting with advanced inoperable breast carcinoma, this subtype of breast cancer can be highly responsive to neoadjuvant systemic polychemotherapy combined with dual anti-HER2 antibodies. Pathologic response to upfront polychemotherapy and HER2-targeted monoclonal antibodies is highly prognostic in this setting and will influence recommendations for adjuvant anti-HER2 therapy. Adjuvant radiotherapy, including comprehensive nodal basin irradiation, would be appropriate after surgery. The goal of therapy is cure. The extent of adenopathy as well as the extent of local regional therapy needed to achieve local regional control of disease places this patient at high risk for therapy-related lymphedema. It would be appropriate to refer for lymphedema evaluation early in the course of care as well as plastic surgery to discuss the option of delayed reconstruction.

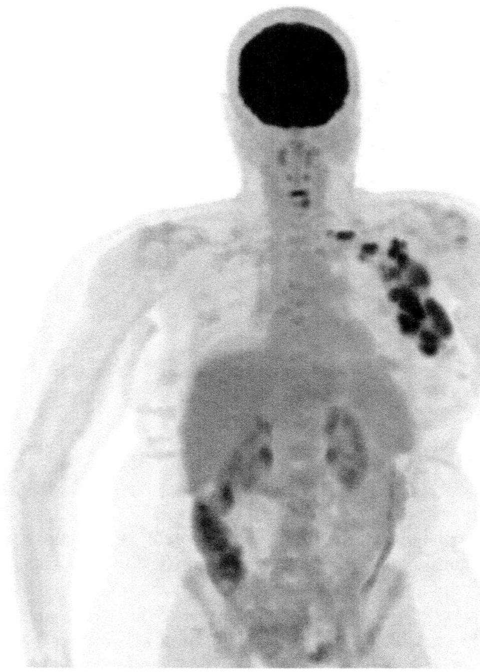

Fig. 14.7 PET-CT image above demonstrates multiple abnormal nodes, including supraclavicular, left axillary, and left subpectoral regions. Subtle findings of architectural distortion noted with mild left FDG activity noted along the left lateral aspect of the left breast at the site of biopsy proven DCIS with microinvasion

Clinical Scenario 4: Locally Advanced, Inoperable Breast Cancer, Triple-Negative Breast Cancer

A female in her late 50s presents with painless swelling in her left axilla. She last participated in screening 18 months ago. Diagnostic mammograms (Fig. 14.8a) and targeted ultrasound of the left breast reveal two masses, each less than 2 cm (Fig. 14.9a, b). Extensive suspicious left axillary adenopathy is noted on mammography (Fig. 14.10a). Ultrasound of the left axilla demonstrates multiple abnormal prominent lymph nodes accounting for patient's clinical presentation (Fig. 14.10c).

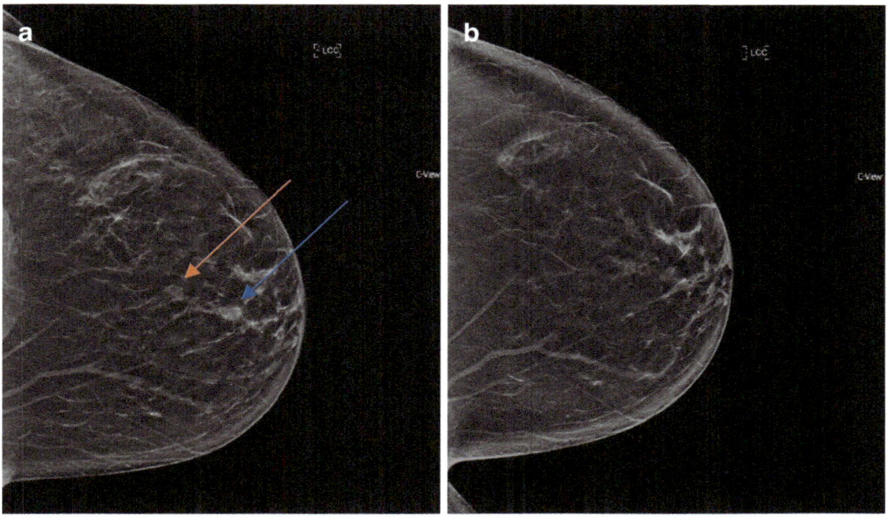

Fig. 14.8 Diagnostic mammogram CC view (**a**) demonstrates two new masses, central left breast. More anterior mass measures 1.3 cm (blue arrow). The mass at middle depth measures 1.2 cm (red arrow). These masses were not present on screening study 18 months prior (**b**)

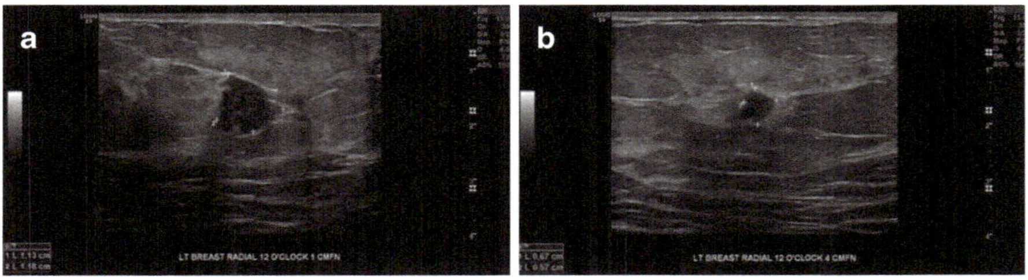

Fig. 14.9 Ultrasound of left breast 12:00 position, 1 cm from the nipple demonstrated an irregular hypoechoic mass measuring 1.2 × 1.1 × 1.0 cm (**a**). Ultrasound of the left breast 12 o'clock position, 4 cm from the nipple demonstrated a similar but smaller mass measuring 0.7 × 0.6 × 0.6 cm (**b**)

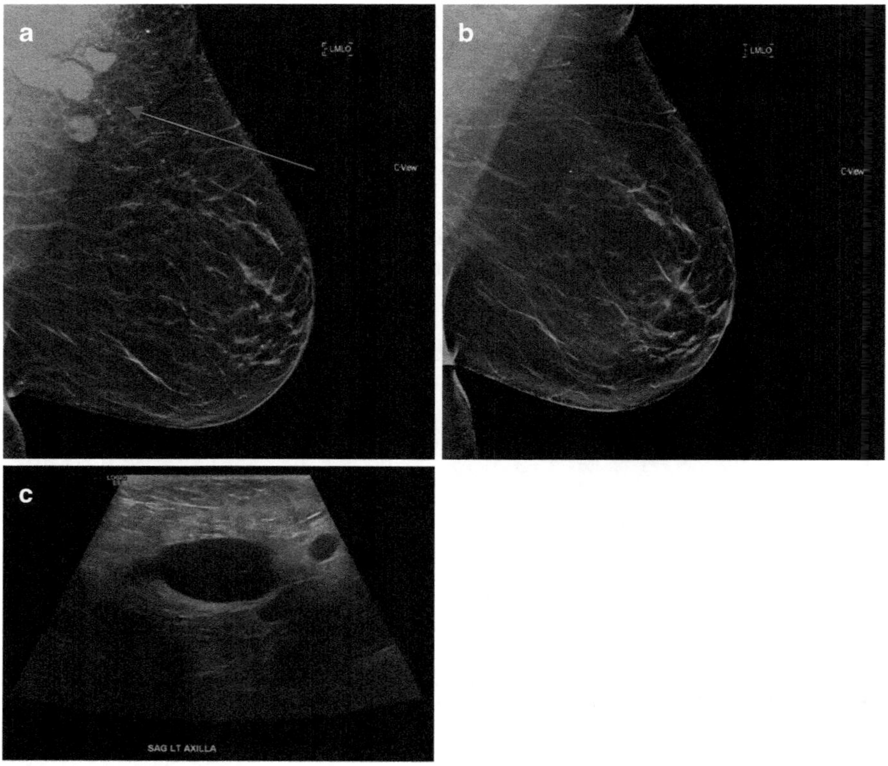

Fig. 14.10 Mammogram LMLO view demonstrated multiple asymmetrically prominent abnormal lymph nodes (**a**). These nodes were not noted on screening mammogram 18 months prior (**b**). Ultrasound of the left axilla demonstrates multiple abnormal prominent lymph nodes corresponding to the patient's palpable concern (**c**)

Core-needle biopsy of both breast lesions demonstrate invasive ductal carcinoma, grade 3, ER negative, PR negative, and HER2 negative. Left axillary needle biopsy demonstrates metastatic carcinoma.

Breast MRI (Fig. 14.11) confirms two masses in the left breast with very extensive adenopathy left axilla involving levels 1–3. FDG PET-CT (Fig. 14.12) demonstrated extensive hypermetabolic left axillary nodal metastases but no evidence of distant metastases.

Clinical prognostic stage is IIIC, cT1c (m), cN3a, cM0, grade 3 invasive ductal carcinoma left breast, ER negative, PR negative, and HER2 negative.

This patient meets criteria for locally advanced inoperable breast carcinoma based on the massive extent of axillary disease. There is also a high likelihood of disseminated microscopic disease in this aggressive subtype of breast cancer. The

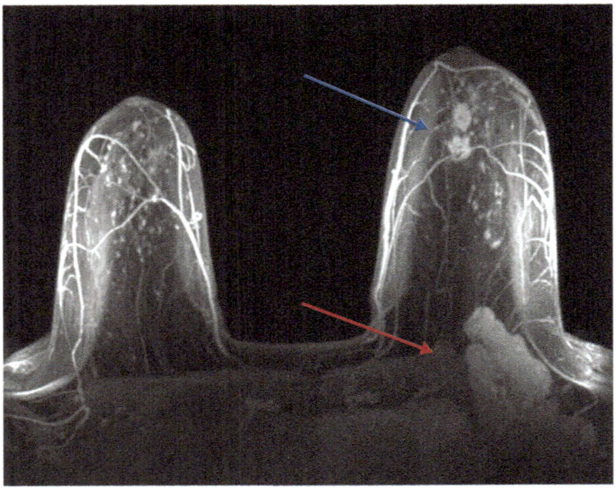

Fig. 14.11 MRI demonstrates two masses in the left breast representing biopsy-proven malignancy (blue arrow). There is extensive left axillary adenopathy involving levels 1 through 3 (red arrow). No evidence of malignancy in the right breast

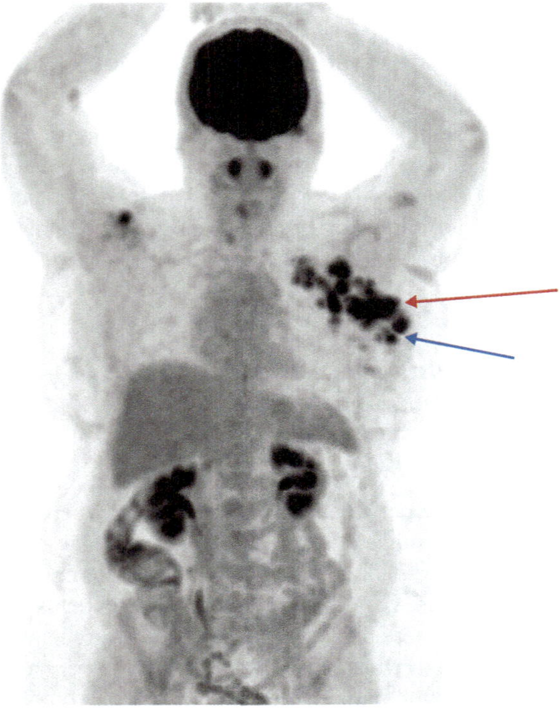

Fig. 14.12 PET-CT shows two mildly hypermetabolic left breast masses compatible with biopsy-proven invasive mammary carcinoma (blue arrow). Extensive hypermetabolic left axillary lymph node metastases (red arrow)

patient is appropriate for neoadjuvant systemic chemotherapy with an anthracycline and a taxane containing regimen with the goal of reducing local-regional disease and addressing micro metastatic disease. Carboplatin can be considered in the neoadjuvant setting in patients with triple-negative breast cancer to increase the likelihood of pathologic complete response.

Pathologic response to neoadjuvant systemic chemotherapy is highly prognostic in patients with high grade triple-negative breast carcinoma. If less than a complete pathologic response is achieved, the patient should be considered for adjuvant therapy with capecitabine or considered for a clinical trial.

Patients with triple-negative breast cancer diagnosed before age 60 meet NCCN criteria for genetic testing [72]. Given the extent of lymph node involvement, adjuvant radiation after surgery, including comprehensive nodal fields is recommended. Lymphedema evaluation is also recommended early in the management of patients with extensive nodal disease given the high risk for lymphedema related to the volume of disease at presentation and extent of local regional measures needed for management of disease.

Neoadjuvant Systemic Therapy for Operable Breast Cancer

Beyond established use for inflammatory, unresectable, and potentially resectable disease, selected patients with operable breast cancer warrant consideration of neoadjuvant systemic therapy. In appropriately selected patients, neoadjuvant systemic therapy can allow for improved surgical outcomes, prognostic information, and optimization of adjuvant therapy.

Downstaging Disease (Stage IIB–IIIA)—Tailoring Surgical Options

Neoadjuvant systemic therapy has been used for more than two decades in patients with operable but locally advanced disease where downstaging is desired to reduce the extent of surgery required for local regional management.

This would include patients with large but operable tumors (**T3**, select T4) with or without disease in the axilla (N0, N1). Patients with **large T2** lesions relative to breast size where breast conservation is desired can also be considered in this subgroup where downstaging of disease in the breast is the goal of neoadjuvant systemic therapy to improve cosmetic outcome from surgery.

For patients who present with **N1** nodal involvement, effective neoadjuvant systemic therapy may allow downstaging to pN0 by sentinel lymph node biopsy with avoidance of axillary dissection, reducing morbidity and reducing risk of lymphedema.

The choice between breast conservation and mastectomy after neoadjuvant treatment is dependent on treatment response. In general, patients who experience local regional progression, but not distant spread while on neoadjuvant systemic therapy, should proceed with surgery rather than switching systemic therapy.

The choice of chemotherapy, endocrine therapy, or targeted therapy is guided by the same principles used to determine systemic treatment in the adjuvant setting, including tumor histology, grade, stage and estrogen, progesterone, and HER2 expression.

Prognostic Information

Several studies have highlighted the prognostic significance of pathologic complete response after neoadjuvant chemotherapy. Achievement of a pathologic complete response after neoadjuvant chemotherapy is associated with significantly improved event-free survival and overall survival, particularly for aggressive biologic subtype such as triple-negative and HER2-positive breast cancer. The achievement of pathologic complete response as defined as ypT0 ypN0 or ypT0/is ypN0 is highly prognostic in this subgroup of patients and is thought to reflect tumor biology and systemic clearance of micro metastatic disease.

Patients with hormone-receptor-positive disease who achieve a pathologic complete response to neoadjuvant systemic therapy also have an improved outcome relative to those who do not. However, pathologic complete response to neoadjuvant therapy is less common in patients with hormone-receptor-positive breast cancer and does not hold the same prognostic value in this subset of patients where prolonged exposure to an endocrine agent (5–10 years) plays a significant role in impacting micro metastatic disease [41].

Impact on Adjuvant Systemic Recommendations—Tailoring Medical Therapy

There are select patients with operable breast cancer where downstaging per se is not necessary to accomplish surgical goals, but assessing the degree of response to therapy is useful in tailoring adjuvant therapy recommendations. Neoadjuvant systemic therapy can be considered in **high-risk HER2-positive (Stage IIA, cT2 N0 or T0-1 N1), and triple-negative breast cancer (Stage IA if cT1c N0—IIA, cT0-1 N1 or cT2 N0)**, as presence or absence of residual disease in this subgroup of patients is highly prognostic and would guide recommendations for adjuvant therapy. Achieving complete pathologic response identifies patients who are highly sensitive to up-front chemotherapy. Patients in this subgroup with residual disease are at higher risk for distant relapse and benefit from tailoring adjuvant therapy strategies to improve long-term outcome.

Delay in Surgery Is Needed

Patients with operable breast cancer who are candidates for surgery and candidates for adjuvant systemic therapy but have a need to delay surgery, can be considered for neoadjuvant systemic therapy. Examples where patient may need to delay surgery would include awaiting results of cancer genetic testing to assist with surgical decisions. Allowing time to consider options for breast reconstruction can represent another scenario where neoadjuvant systemic therapy can be considered. Intercurrent illness or operating room availability, as was affected in many centers during the height of the COVID 19 pandemic [53], may also represent a situation where neoadjuvant systemic therapy can be considered.

Pretreatment Evaluation

Workup prior to preoperative systemic therapy should include a history and physical exam. Diagnostic bilateral mammogram with ultrasound as indicated. Breast MRI is a consideration, particularly for mammographically occult tumors and where extent of disease is not well defined on mammography or ultrasound.

Image-guided core biopsy of the breast abnormality with placement of an image detectable marker is necessary to confirm the histologic diagnosis of invasive breast carcinoma and to provide tissue to assess ER, PR, and HER2 status.

Axillary assessment should be performed with physical exam and dedicated axillary ultrasound with image-guided biopsy of suspicious nodes. An image-detectable clip should be placed at the time of image-guided biopsy to permit verification that the biopsy-positive lymph node is removed at the time of definitive surgery.

Pathology review of the core specimens are performed to establish the histopathologic type of invasive breast cancer with estimated grade when possible. ER, PR, and HER2 status should be determined.

Genetic counseling should be considered if patient is at risk for hereditary breast cancer. Counseling for fertility options should be addressed if the patient is premenopausal.

Laboratory testing should include CBC, comprehensive metabolic panel, including liver function tests and alkaline phosphatase.

Evaluation of distant disease: Routine systemic staging is not indicated for early breast cancer in the absence of symptoms (stage I and II). Diagnostic contrast-enhanced CT scan of the chest and abdomen and bone scan should be performed if clinical concern for metastatic disease, unless there is a contraindication because of contrast allergy. It is not unreasonable to consider systemic staging imaging for patients with Stage III disease, even in the absence of symptoms, as there is a higher risk for systemic disease in this subgroup. FDG PET-CT can be considered if contrast enhanced CT cannot be performed or if standard staging studies are equivocal or suspicious. FDG PET-CT may also be helpful in identifying unsuspected regional nodal disease in cases of locally advanced breast cancer when used in addition to standard staging studies [58].

Multidisciplinary Management

Management of patients recommended neoadjuvant systemic therapy optimally involves a multidisciplinary team that should include surgery, medical oncology, radiation oncology, pathology, radiology and, in certain cases, plastic surgery, genetics provider, and research staff. As optimization of systemic and local therapies continues to evolve, participation in clinical trial should be considered for eligible patients.

Communication between the patient and clinician is very important when recommending neoadjuvant systemic therapy for breast cancer. Clear communication regarding goals of delivering systemic treatment prior to surgery must be aligned with the patient's goals of care whether for downstaging to reduce extent of surgery, allowing time for genetic results or plastics referral, or individualizing adjuvant therapy. Clinicians recommending neoadjuvant systemic therapy must also have a clear understanding of the goals of therapy and work closely with the multidisciplinary breast care team to assure that the team is also aligned regarding goals of care for an individual patient.

As there are differences in goals and indications for neoadjuvant systemic therapy in patients with operable breast carcinoma depending on breast cancer subtype, the next sections will provide guidelines for selection of patients who are hormone-receptor positive, HER2 positive, and triple negative.

Hormone-Receptor-Positive Breast Carcinoma

Hormone-receptor-positive breast cancer is the most common subtype of breast cancer, comprising 70–80% of all breast cancers. For women participating in routine screening, most of these cancers are screen detected at an early stage (T1-T2-N0) where up-front surgery can be performed without the need to downstage for optimal surgical results. When possible, patients diagnosed with early-stage hormone-receptor-positive breast (Stage IB-IIA) cancer should be offered surgery first to allow for assignment of clinical risk based on complete pathologic assessment (tumor size, nodal status, grade, degree of ER/PR expression). Where results of a gene expression assay would be useful in considering the use of systemic chemotherapy versus endocrine therapy alone for operable lower stage hormone-receptor-positive breast cancer, surgery should, in most situations, be performed first. Results from the long-term analysis of the phase III MINDACT trial and TAILORx trial have provided high quality data to help inform treatment decisions for many women with early stage breast cancer [20–23].

The main indication for neoadjuvant systemic therapy in hormone-receptor-positive breast cancer is to downstage disease in more locally advanced patients allowing for less extensive surgery needed to achieve local regional management. Patients with locally advanced breast cancer, stage IIIA (T3, N1) as well as a subset of stage IIB cancers with T2, N1 or T3, N0 disease would fall in this category [55, 63, 70].

For patients with stage IIA disease, either primary surgery or neoadjuvant therapy may be used in patients who desire breast-conserving surgery and are not candidates up-front due to a high tumor size (large T2) relative to breast size.

Hormone-receptor-positive, HER2-negative cancers are less likely to respond to neoadjuvant chemotherapy than other biologic subtypes, such as HER2-positive or triple-negative breast cancer. Lower grade hormone-receptor-positive cancers are less likely to respond to neoadjuvant chemotherapy than higher grade tumors. This observation does not necessarily negate a benefit of systemic chemotherapy in locally advanced disease if downstaging is desired, but should serve to set expectations when selecting patients for this approach.

Pathologic complete response is not common in hormone-receptor breast cancer compared to other biologic subtypes, such as HER2-positive or triple-negative breast cancer where the greatest benefit of pCR is observed. Among hormone-receptor-positive tumors, pCR rates with neoadjuvant systemic chemotherapy are higher and the relationship with long-term outcomes is stronger among grade 3 tumors compared to lower grade tumors. Although response to therapy has some prognostic value in this subgroup as a whole, it is less tied to long-term outcome than in HER2-positive or triple-negative breast cancer given the important role of subsequent adjuvant endocrine therapy in long-term disease control. While traditionally neoadjuvant *chemotherapy* has been used to downstage locally advanced and unresectable breast carcinomas, several studies have highlighted the role of neoadjuvant endocrine therapy as an alternative option to chemotherapy and hormone-receptor-positive, postmenopausal women [63, 70].

Case scenarios are provided to highlight selection of hormone-receptor-positive patients appropriate to consider for neoadjuvant systemic therapy.

Clinical Scenario 1: Hormone-Receptor-Positive, Postmenopausal Patient. Clinical Stage IIIA cT2, cN2b, cM0

Goal: Downstaging—Tailoring Surgical Options

A postmenopausal female in her late 60s presents with a palpable mass inferior medial aspect left breast. Last participated in screening 6 years ago. Diagnostic bilateral mammograms (Fig. 14.13a, b) with targeted ultrasound (Fig. 14.14a) demonstrate a 2.6 cm mass lower inner quadrant posterior depth with benign appearing axillary nodes. Ultrasound-guided core biopsy right breast demonstrates invasive ductal carcinoma, high grade with tumor infiltrating lymphocytes. ER strongly positive, PR negative, Ki-67 positive; percentage of positive nuclei 70%. HER2 negative. There is a maternal family history of breast cancer, lymphoma, and pancreatic cancer and a paternal family history of breast cancer. Genetic testing with a broad cancer gene panel is negative. Breast MRIs (Figs. 14.14b and 14.15a) demonstrate a multilobulated enhancing mass in the inferomedial left breast at posterior depth, 8:00 position which at least abuts the chest wall with question of possible pectoralis muscle invasion. No axillary lymphadenopathy is noted. A 6 mm left internal mammary lymph node is noted (Fig. 14.15b).

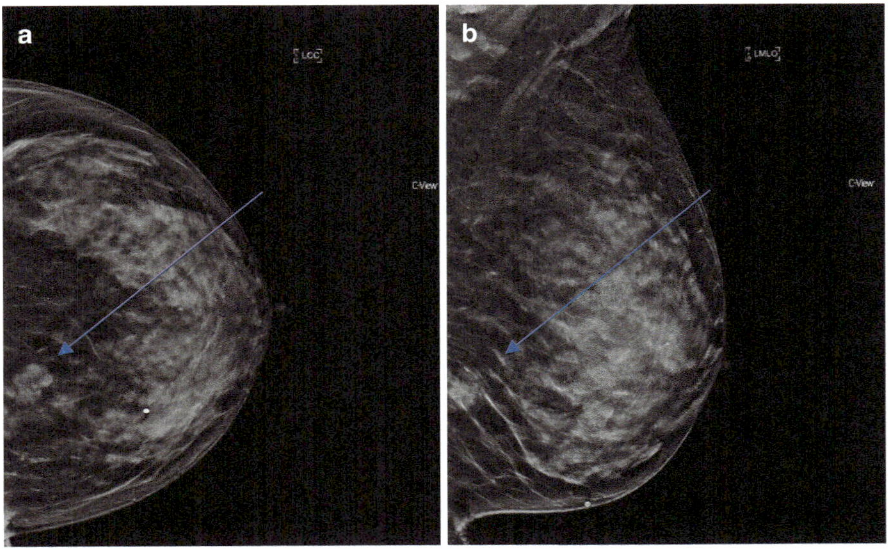

Fig. 14.13 Diagnostic mammograms CC view (**a**) and MLO view (**b**) demonstrate a partially visualized 3 cm irregular mass left lower inner quadrant posterior depth (arrow)

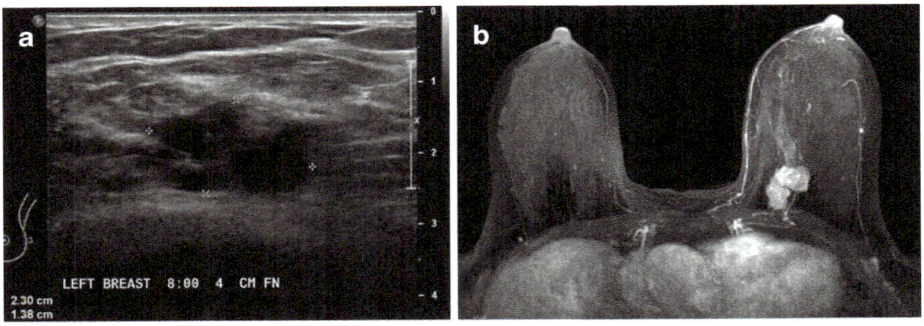

Fig. 14.14 Targeted ultrasound (**a**) demonstrates a 2.3 cm irregular mass 8:00 position with benign appearing lymph nodes left axilla. MRI (**b**) demonstrated a multilobulated enhancing mass in the inferomedial left breast posterior depth at 8:00 measuring 2.4 × 2.6 × 2.6 cm. The mass at least abuts the chest wall—concern raised for possible pectoralis muscle involvement

PET CT—demonstrates a multilobulated enhancing mass posterior left breast 8:00 abutting the chest wall (Fig. 14.16a). Mild FDG uptake on PET-CT (Fig. 14.16c) correlates with the 6 mm internal mammary lymph node.

Clinical prognostic stage IIIA, cT1, cN2b, cM0, grade 3 invasive ductal carcinoma, ER positive, PR negative HER2 negative.

This patient presents with a high-grade hormone-receptor-positive T2 primary breast cancer with a highly suspicious internal mammary node. Neoadjuvant systemic chemotherapy is recommended in this scenario with the goal of improving the extent of surgery needed for breast conservation given the size of the tumor in the

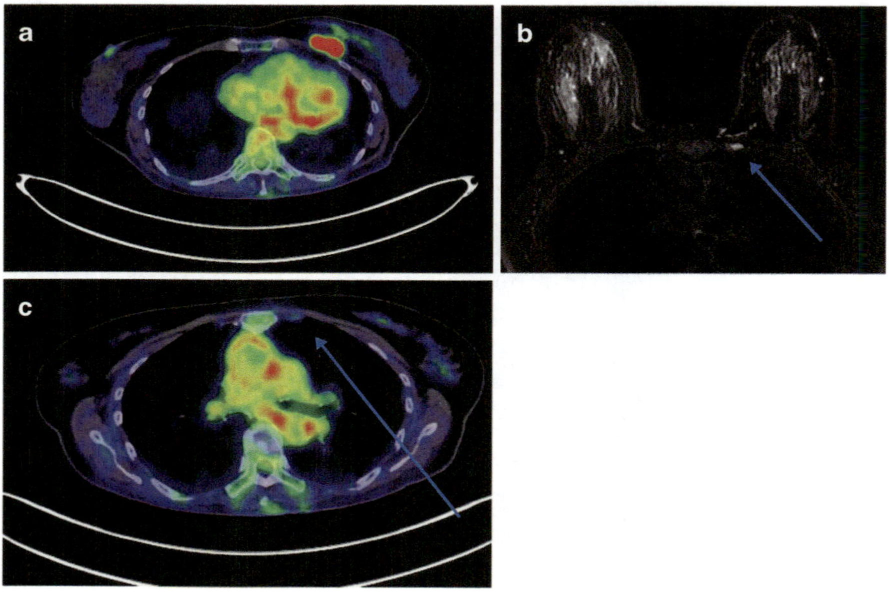

Fig. 14.15 MRI demonstrates a 6 mm left internal mammary node (**b**). PET CT demonstrates an FDG-avid mass abutting the chest wall (**a**). Mild FDG on PET-CT correlates with the 6 mm internal mammary lymph node noted on breast MRI (**c**)

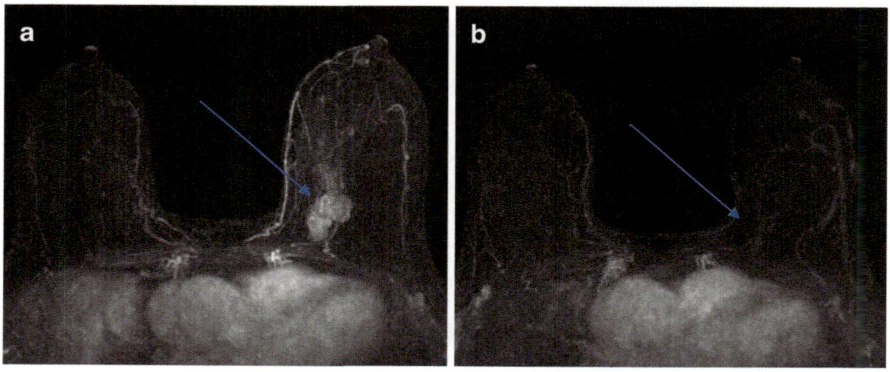

Fig. 14.16 Restaging breast MRI demonstrates a good response to therapy with decrease in size of left breast mass from 2.6 cm prior to therapy (**a**) to 2.2 × 1.0 × 1.8 cm post-therapy (**b**) and decrease in size of left internal mammary lymph node now measuring 3 mm in short axis. There is continued extension of tumor posteriorly to the pectoralis without invasion

inferior breast which abuts and possibly invades the chest wall. The goal of therapy is to reduce the size of the primary and improve the likelihood of clear margins with breast conservation. One can comfortably offer systemic chemotherapy prior to surgery, as this patient would be offered systemic chemotherapy in addition to a hormone blocker were surgery to be performed first, given the size, grade, and stage of disease with internal mammary node involvement by imaging.

MRI after therapy (Fig. 14.16b) demonstrates a good response to therapy with decreased size left 8:00 breast mass and decreased size left internal mammary lymph node compared to preoperative imaging (Fig. 14.16a).

The patient undergoes left axillary sentinel lymph node excision and left breast lumpectomy, revealing breast tissue with treatment-related changes and biopsy-related changes with no residual malignancy identified (pCR). Sentinel lymph nodes are negative for malignancy.

When pathologic complete response occurs in patients with hormone-receptor-positive breast cancer, it is associated with improved long-term outcome as with other aggressive subtypes of breast cancer. Adjuvant radiation and adjuvant endocrine therapy are both recommended post-lumpectomy. Given pretreatment knowledge of a positive internal mammary node noted on MRI and PET-CT, the internal mammary region is included in treatment planning for adjuvant radiotherapy.

Clinical Scenario 2: Hormone-Receptor-Positive, Premenopausal Patient. Clinical Stage IIB, cT2, cN1, cM0

Goal: Downstaging—Tailoring Surgical Options

A patient in her mid-40s presents with a palpable mass right breast. She reports having a normal screening study 3 years ago. There is no family history of breast carcinoma, although family history is limited. She meets NCCN guidelines for genetic counseling [72]. Cancer genetic testing is negative for a pathogenic variant in 36 cancer genes analyzed.

Diagnostic mammogram and ultrasound demonstrate a highly suspicious mass upper outer right breast with a suspicious level I right axillary lymph node. Ultrasound-guided needle biopsy demonstrates grade 3, invasive mammary/ductal carcinoma. ER positive, PR positive, and HER2 negative. Right axillary lymph node core biopsy is also positive for metastatic carcinoma.

Breast MRI (Fig. 14.17) is requested to better assess extent of disease and demonstrates a heterogeneously enhancing mass 12:00 measuring 3.4 × 2.7 × 2.8 cm. A

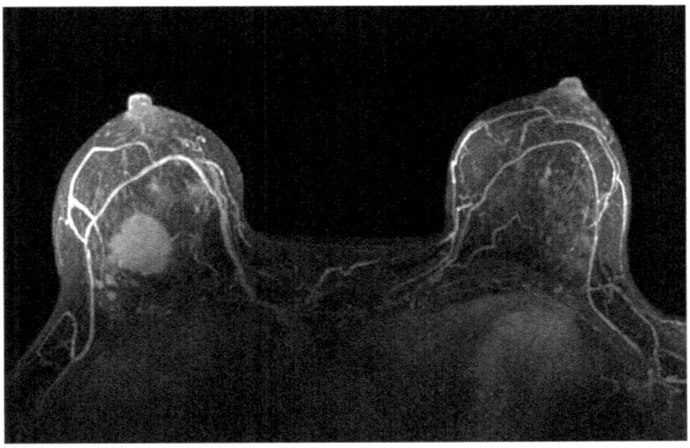

Fig. 14.17 Breast MRI with a 3.4 × 2.7 × 2.8 cm irregular heterogeneously enhancing mass 12:00 p.m. right breast with an associated tissue marker clip

right axillary node is noted with tissue marker clip. Patient desires consideration for breast conservation.

Clinical prognostic stage is IIB, cT2, cN1, grade 3 invasive ductal carcinoma, ER positive, PR positive, HER2 negative.

Given the size of the tumor relative to breast size, downsizing the tumor prior to surgery may allow for breast conservation. Neoadjuvant systemic chemotherapy would be a reasonable consideration in this scenario as this is a premenopausal patient with high grade, T2, node positive breast cancer who would be a candidate for systemic chemotherapy if surgery were to be performed first. One would not need to order a gene expression assay to assist with this recommendation.

As the primary tumor is high grade, it is reasonable to expect a clinical response from therapy. Among hormone-receptor-positive tumors, response rates to neoadjuvant systemic chemotherapy rates are higher among grade 3 tumors compared to lower grade tumors. Although pathologic response can provide prognostic information in high-grade, ER positive breast cancers, complete pathologic response is less commonly seen in this subgroup of patients compared to patients with triple-negative or HER2-positive breast cancer and is not requisite for long-term disease control, where endocrine therapy remains the mainstay of adjuvant treatment.

The main goal of neoadjuvant systemic therapy in this scenario is to downstage disease, allowing for breast-conserving surgery followed by adjuvant radiation. Although pCR is rare, it can sometimes be seen in this subgroup of patients. Regardless of degree of response to up-front systemic chemotherapy, all patients with hormone-receptor-positive cancers should be offered adjuvant endocrine therapy for a prolonged period (5–10 years) to improve long-term disease control.

Clinical Scenario 3: Low Grade ER Positive, Postmenopausal Patient. Clinical Stage IIB, cT2, cN1, cM0

Goal: Downstaging—Tailoring Surgical Options

A female in her late 60s presents with a palpable left breast mass and nipple inversion. Diagnostic mammogram (Fig. 14.18a, b) and ultrasound demonstrate a highly suspicious 4.5 cm mass 1:00 left breast (Fig. 14.18c). Two small axillary nodes are noted in the lower outer aspect of the axillary tail on ultrasound (Fig. 14.18d).

Ultrasound-guided core needle biopsy demonstrates invasive lobular carcinoma, estimated low grade. ER strongly positive, PR strongly positive, HER2 negative. Core biopsy of one of the axillary nodes demonstrates metastatic carcinoma.

Clinical prognostic stage is Stage IIA, cT2, cN1, cM0, grade 1, invasive lobular carcinoma, ER positive, PR positive, and HER2 negative.

The patient desires attempt at breast conservation. Neoadjuvant endocrine therapy with an aromatase inhibitor is prescribed. Significant clinical benefit is noted with 6 months of neoadjuvant endocrine therapy with resolution of the palpable mass on exam and resolution of nipple areolar inversion.

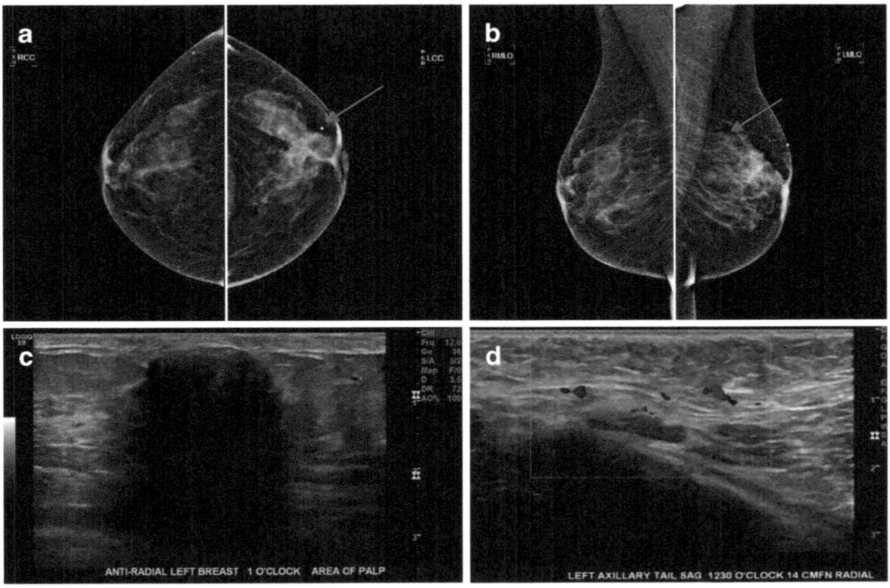

Fig. 14.18 Mammograms CC (**a**) and MLO views (**b**) show heterogeneously dense breast tissue with a focal asymmetry in the left upper outer breast (arrow). Ultrasound left breast (**c**) demonstrates a solid hypoechoic mass 1:00 a.m. peri-areolar position corresponding to the palpable mass measuring 4.5 × 2.3 × 1.8 cm. Two closely adjacent left axillary lymph nodes noted lower outer aspect of the axillary tail (**d**), larger measuring 7 mm with near complete effacement of the fatty hilum and cortical thickness of 3.4 mm

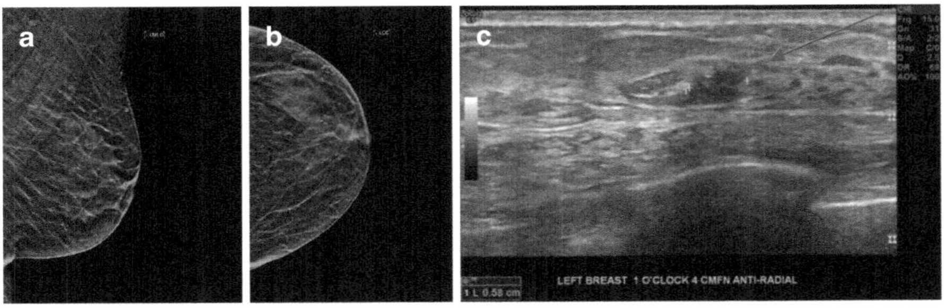

Fig. 14.19 Mammogram findings MLO (**a**) and CC views (**b**) demonstrate marked improvement in the asymmetric density previously noted in the retro-areolar and upper outer middle to anterior one third of left breast. Ultrasound shows marked improvement as well with residual 4 × 6 mm irregular hypoechoic lesion 1 o'clock position 4 cm from the nipple (**c**)

Repeat diagnostic mammogram (Fig. 14.19a, b) and US (Fig. 14.19c) demonstrate marked improvement in the mass. Breast MRI shows no suspicious enhancement in either breast, specifically no suspicious enhancement seen around the biopsy marker at the site of the known biopsy-proven invasive lobular carcinoma.

Pathology findings at the time of breast-conserving surgery demonstrate evidence of treatment effect, but residual invasive lobular carcinoma, essentially spanning the specimen, estimated at least 4.5 cm with multiple positive margins and metastatic carcinoma in 5 of 12 axillary nodes, largest measuring 0.7 cm with no extra-nodal extension. Although clinical response is impressive, this case illustrates the challenges in treating diffuse invasive lobular carcinoma as imaging findings often underestimate the extent of disease [63, 70]. Despite efforts at breast conservation completion, mastectomy is necessary in this patient for local control as well as post-mastectomy radiotherapy with continued adjuvant endocrine therapy.

Clinical Scenario 4: Hormone-Receptor-Positive (Premenopausal Patient) with Clinical Stage IIA, Multifocal cT2, cN1a, cM0 Grade 2 Invasive Ductal Carcinoma, ER Positive, PR Positive, and HER2 Negative

Goal: Reducing Delay in Initiating Systemic Therapy While Surgery and Reconstruction Are Being Planned

A patient in her mid-30s presents with a palpable mass left breast and axilla. She is 16 months post-partum and breastfeeding at the time. Diagnostic mammogram and ultrasound demonstrate multiple solid masses within the left breast and axilla, the largest measuring 3.5 cm. Ultrasound-guided breast biopsy demonstrates invasive mammary carcinoma, estimated grade 3, with focal mucinous features. ER positive, PR positive, and HER2 negative. Biopsy of a left axillary node measuring 2.5 cm demonstrates metastatic carcinoma with mucinous features. MRI breast demonstrates the biopsy-proven left breast carcinoma 12:00 position and metastatic left axillary lymph node with multiple additional enhancing masses involving all four quadrants, especially in the anterior one third of the left breast (Fig. 14.14a). There is a family history of colon cancer and lymphoma. Cancer genetic testing is negative. Staging CT scans and bone scan are negative for systemic disease.

Clinical prognostic stage IIA, cT2, cN1, cM0, grade 2 invasive ductal carcinoma, ER positive, PR positive, HER2 negative.

The patient is not a candidate for breast conservation given multifocal extent of disease in the breast. Pathology demonstrates a grade 2 invasive ductal carcinoma where neoadjuvant systemic chemotherapy is expected to be less effective at reducing local-regional disease than higher grade ER positive tumors and would not result in a change in surgery needed for local regional management. Delay in surgery is desired, however, while exploring surgical options, including reconstruction. Given the young age and stage of disease, this patient would be offered systemic chemotherapy in addition to adjuvant endocrine therapy if surgery were performed first. It is thus reasonable to offer neoadjuvant systemic chemotherapy with the goal of therapy of initiating systemic therapy while awaiting surgical planning. It is important to set the expectation that pathologic complete response is not expected and not tied to long-term outcome as adjuvant endocrine therapy will play an important part of adjuvant systemic therapy.

The patient is treated with neoadjuvant chemotherapy while awaiting surgical planning. Overall imaging supports a favorable response to chemotherapy

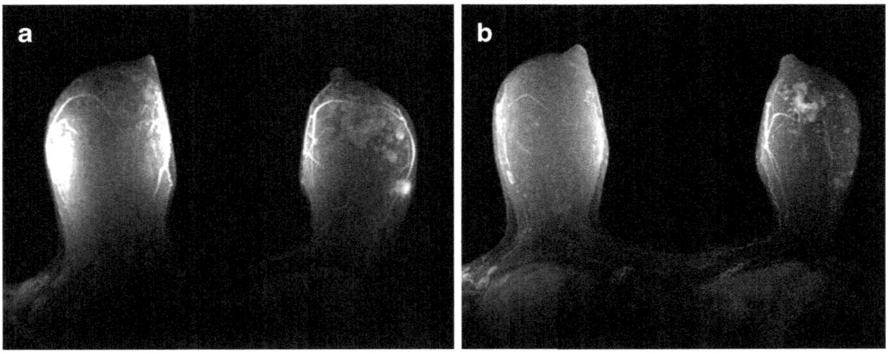

Fig. 14.20 MRI breast demonstrates the biopsy-proven left breast carcinoma 12:00 position and metastatic left axillary lymph node with multiple additional enhancing masses involving all four quadrants, especially in the anterior one third of the left breast. No areolar, pectoral, or skin involvement seen (**a**). Post-neoadjuvant chemotherapy MRI (**b**) with favorable response at all sites of measurable disease although residual multicentric disease is noted (**b**) as well as left axillary adenopathy (not pictured)

(Fig. 14.20b) with improvement at all sites of measurable disease, but with residual multicentric disease as well as left axillary adenopathy.

Mastectomy with left axillary dissection and first stage reconstruction is accomplished with placement of a tissue expander. Pathology demonstrates invasive carcinoma with focal mucinous features, grade 2, multifocal with at least 8 foci present. The largest tumor size is 2.4 cm in greatest dimension with metastatic carcinoma in 2 of 15 lymph nodes. There is evidence of treatment effect. Pathologic stage classification: ympT2, pN1a, cM0.

Referral for post-mastectomy radiotherapy is appropriate in this patient given positive axillary nodes at time of axillary dissection. Referral for lymphedema evaluation is also appropriate given the risk of developing lymphedema related to local-regional disease. Extended adjuvant endocrine therapy will be the mainstay of adjuvant therapy.

HER2-Positive Breast Cancer

Locally Advanced, Node Positive or High-Risk Node Negative

HER2-positive breast cancer is a particularly aggressive subtype which accounts for 20–25% of breast cancer cases diagnosed yearly. This is also a heterogeneous subtype of breast cancer defined by HER2 oncoprotein overexpression as detected by IHC staining or amplification of the HER2 oncogene by in situ hybridization and includes both ER positive and ER negative cancers.

HER2-positive breast cancer used to carry the worst outcome before effective therapy was developed for this subtype of disease. HER2-overexpression tumors display increased sensitivity to cytotoxic chemotherapy. A higher percentage of HER2-positive patients achieve a complete pathologic response to neoadjuvant chemotherapy, particularly when combined with HER2-directed therapy when compared to other subtypes of breast cancer.

Neoadjuvant chemotherapy is the favored approach for patients with operable locally advanced HER2-positive breast cancer. This would be defined by patients with stage IIIA cancer (cT3, N1) as well as the subset of IIB cancers with (T3, N0 and T2, N1) disease.

Patients with Stage IIA (T2, N0) disease may also be candidates for neoadjuvant systemic therapy, particularly if the patient is not an optimal candidate for breast-conserving surgery up-front due to tumor location or size relative to the size of the patient's breast (T2).

Patients with limited axillary nodal involvement (N1) may be also be considered for neoadjuvant systemic therapy with the goal of downstaging to pN0 by sentinel lymph node biopsy with avoidance of axillary node dissection [68].

Patients with stage II–IIIA operable HER2-positive breast cancer should be offered polychemotherapy with anti-HER2-directed antibodies, including trastuzumab and pertuzumab if node positive. Given the high sensitivity of this sub-group of breast cancer to cytotoxic chemotherapy, particularly combined with HER2-targeted antibodies, patients are likely to respond and can expect an improvement in surgical options. This can translate to less extensive surgery, fewer mastectomies, and potentially less extensive axillary surgery.

Approximately 50–60% of patients with HER2-positive tumors achieve a pathologic complete response after neoadjuvant therapy with higher response rates if ER negative and HER2 positive. Given the highly prognostic significance of achieving a complete pathologic response in the HER2-positive breast cancer subgroup, response to neoadjuvant systemic therapy is useful in guiding recommendations for adjuvant therapy. Patients with highly sensitive disease who achieve a complete pathologic response are expected to do well with continued adjuvant anti-HER2-directed antibody therapy. For patients with residual disease, the long-term prognosis is less favorable [71]. Based on improved outcomes reported in patients with residual disease in the KATHERINE trial, patients can be offered a switching strategy to adjuvant TDM1 [65]. Additional adjuvant strategies depend on ER status and nodal status at presentation and will be discussed in a subsequent chapter. There are ongoing trials looking at minimizing therapy for highly sensitive patients [72], as well as trials looking to improve the outcome in high-risk individuals with residual disease [73].

Patients with clinical stage I disease should be offered surgery first. This is because chemotherapy and HER2-directed therapy can be withheld in patients with T1a disease. Patients with pT1b-T1c, N0 can be offered more minimal systemic therapy with paclitaxel and Herceptin for 12 weeks followed by Herceptin for a year with excellent reported outcomes [74].

In circumstances where surgery will be postponed while awaiting plastics consultation or results of genetic testing, neoadjuvant systemic therapy can be considered in this subgroup of patients if they meet criteria for which adjuvant therapy would be recommended.

Clinical Scenario 1: HER2-Positive Breast Carcinoma. Clinical Stage IIIA, cT2, cN2a, cM0, ER Negative, PR Negative, HER2 Positive

Goal: Downstage Disease to Improve Surgical Options and to Tailor Adjuvant Therapy Recommendations Based on Pathologic Response to Therapy

A patient in her late 60s is diagnosed with Clinical Stage IIIA (cT2, cN2) high-grade invasive ductal carcinoma left breast, ER negative, PR negative, and HER2 positive, 3+, 100% by IHC. Presents with a palpable mass lower outer left breast. Last participated in screening 5 years ago. Diagnostic breast imaging including MRI demonstrate a 3 cm mass in the lower outer left breast (Fig. 14.21a, b) with enlarged axillary nodes level 1 and 2. Systemic staging, including PET-CT, confirms an intensely hypermetabolic mass in the left lateral breast with numerous hypermetabolic lymph nodes in the left axilla and left lateral subpectoral regions (Fig. 14.22).

This patient is not an optimal candidate for up-front surgery due to stage of disease with extensive axillary adenopathy involving levels 1 and 2. Neoadjuvant poly chemotherapy is recommended combined with dual anti-HER-2 antibodies.

The patient derives an excellent clinical response to neoadjuvant systemic chemotherapy with HER2-targeted dual antibody although therapy was abbreviated because of side effects and challenges getting through the entire course of treatment. Restaging MRI demonstrates interval resolution of the biopsy-proven mass (Fig. 14.23b) and axillary adenopathy.

Lumpectomy using a non-wire localization technique is performed with sentinel node and limited axillary dissection, including the node where a marker was placed at the time of biopsy. There is evidence of treatment effect and complete pathologic response in the breast and nodes. Adjuvant radiotherapy to the left breast and regional lymphatics is recommended post-lumpectomy as part of local regional

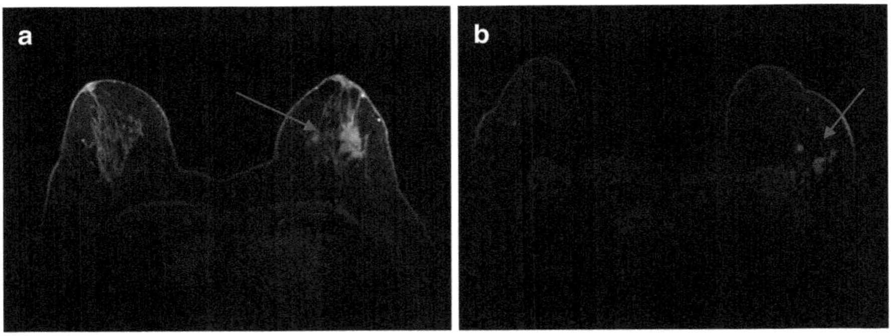

Fig. 14.21 Breast MRI demonstrates a mass at 4–5 o'clock, 3 cm from the nipple, measuring 2.9 × 1.7 × 2.6 cm (**a**) with heterogeneous enhancement including washout kinetics (arrow). Left axillary adenopathy is noted. A biopsy marker is noted in the 1.3 cm biopsy-proven axillary node metastases (**b**) with closely adjacent enlarged lymph nodes at both level 1 and 2 (arrow)

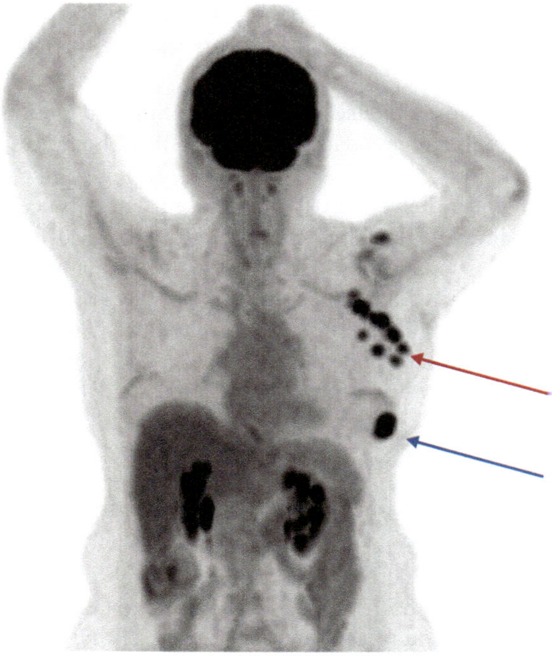

Fig. 14.22 PET-CT with intensely hypermetabolic 2.2 cm density left lateral breast consistent with the patient's known left breast carcinoma (blue arrow). Numerous, approximately 12–15 hypermetabolic lymph nodes in the left axillary and left lateral subpectoral regions (red arrow), consistent with relatively extensive local regional and nodal disease

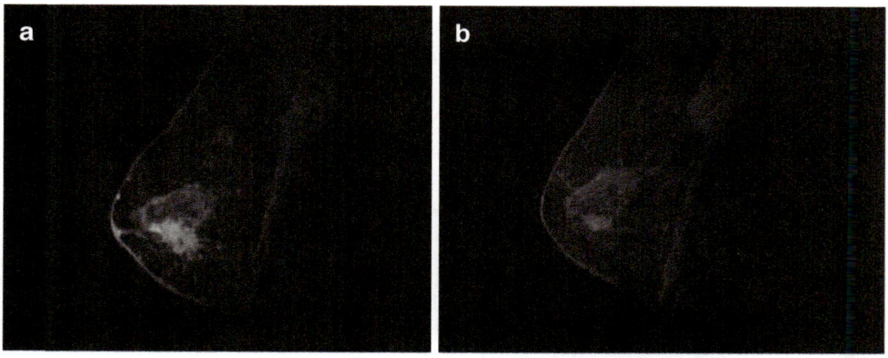

Fig. 14.23 MRI shows the 3 cm left breast mass prior to systemic therapy (**a**) with interval resolution of biopsy-proven left 4:00 carcinoma (**b**) and abnormal left lymph nodes (not pictured) following neoadjuvant chemotherapy. No discrete suspicious residual enhancement, mass, or adenopathy is noted

management. Given high sensitivity demonstrated to neoadjuvant therapy with pCR achieved, continued adjuvant dual anti-HER2 antibody therapy is recommended for 1 year. Referral for lymphedema evaluation is warranted as the risk of lymphedema is high in this individual given extent of nodal involvement at presentation, extent of axillary surgery, and radiation therapy.

Clinical Scenario 2: Clinical Stage IIB HER2-Positive Breast, ER Positive Breast Cancer

Goal: Downstage Disease to Improve Surgical Options and to Tailor Adjuvant Therapy Based on Pathologic Response to Therapy

A patient in her mid-40s is diagnosed with Clinical Stage IIB, cT3, cN2a, cM0, high-grade invasive ductal carcinoma of the left breast, ER moderately positive, PR moderately positive, and HER2 3+ 100% positive, by immunohistochemistry. She presents with several small palpable masses left breast and left axillary adenopathy. Diagnostic breast imaging including breast MRI (Fig. 14.24a) demonstrates extensive non-mass enhancement occupying the lower outer and upper outer quadrants of the left breast spanning more than 8 cm with left axillary adenopathy at levels 1 and 2.

Systemic polychemotherapy with dual anti-HER2 antibody therapy is initiated in this scenario with the goal of improving surgical options and to tailor adjuvant systemic therapy based on response to neoadjuvant therapy. The patient is not a candidate for breast conservation or nipple sparing mastectomy given the proximity of this process to the nipple areolar region, but the patient is more likely to achieve clear margins and may require less extensive axillary surgery with up-front systemic therapy.

Restaging breast MRI after completing 6 cycles of neoadjuvant systemic therapy demonstrates near complete resolution of carcinoma in the upper outer and lower outer quadrants of the breast with scattered residual non mass enhancement and near complete resolution of left axillary adenopathy (Fig. 14.24b).

At the time of mastectomy, there is residual invasive ductal carcinoma and DCIS spanning more than 6 cm with treatment effect and involvement of 2 of 3 sentinel

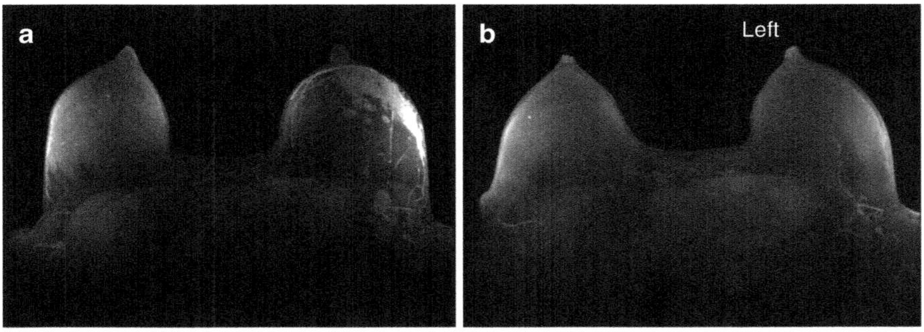

Fig. 14.24 Breast MRI demonstrates extensive non-mass enhancement occupying the lower outer and upper outer quadrants of the left breast spanning more than 8 cm with left axillary adenopathy at levels 1 and 2 (**a**). Restaging breast MRI after completing 6 cycles of neoadjuvant systemic therapy revealed near complete resolution of carcinoma in the upper outer and lower outer quadrants of the breast with scattered residual non mass enhancement and near complete resolution of left axillary adenopathy (**b**)

and 2 of 10 axillary nodes. Adequate surgical margins are achieved. Adjuvant radiotherapy is recommended as well as a switch to adjuvant TDM1 for 14 cycles given lack of pCR to up-front systemic therapy. Adjuvant endocrine therapy is recommended as well. Long-term prognosis is less favorable in this scenario given extent of residual disease after neoadjuvant therapy.

Clinical Scenario 3: Clinical Stage IIA HER2 ER Negative, HER2 Positive Breast Cancer

Goal: Downstage Disease to Improve Surgical Options and to Tailor Adjuvant Therapy Based on Pathologic Response to Therapy

A female in her early 40s is diagnosed with Clinical Prognostic Stage IIA, right breast carcinoma, cT1, cN1, cM0 grade 3 invasive ductal carcinoma, ER negative, PR negative, HER2 3+ positive, 100% by IHC. She presents with a palpable mass in the lower outer right breast. Screening mammograms 18 months prior were negative. Diagnostic breast imaging including MRI (Fig. 14.25) demonstrates a 1.9 cm mass right breast lower outer quadrant with a 4.3 cm right axillary mass consistent with known axillary metastases. Staging PET-CT (Fig. 14.26) demonstrates findings consistent with biopsy-proven lower outer quadrant right breast carcinoma with right axillary lymph node metastases.

The patient has a history of thyroiditis and a paternal family history of breast cancer in several relatives. Genetic testing with a 35 gene cancer panel is negative.

Clinical pathologic stage is IIA cT1c, cN1, cM0, grade 3 invasive ductal carcinoma, ER negative, PR negative, and HER2 negative.

Neoadjuvant systemic polychemotherapy with dual HER-2-directed antibody therapy is recommended with several goals in mind. The likelihood of response to

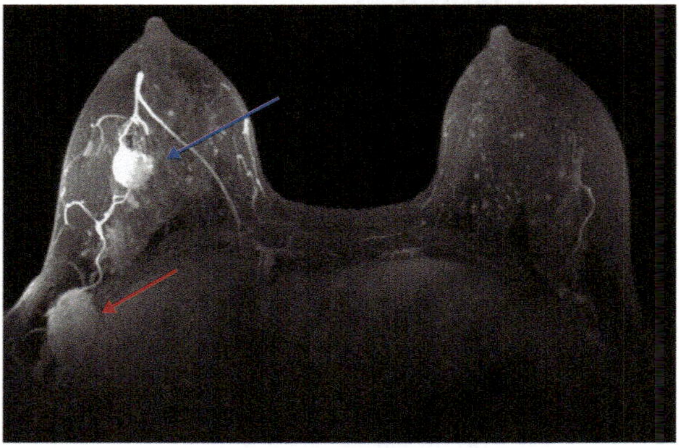

Fig. 14.25 Breast MRI demonstrates a 1.9 cm mass lower outer quadrant right breast (blue arrow) with 4.3 cm right axillary mass (arrow) consistent with known axillary metastasis. Additional nodes noted measuring up to 1.3 cm

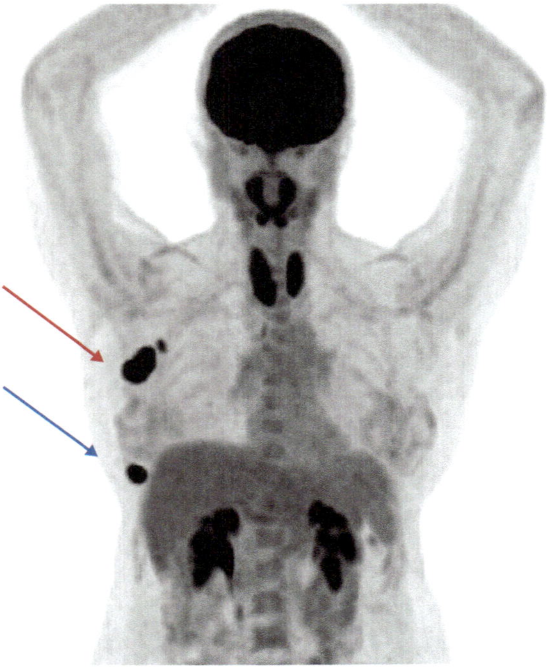

Fig. 14.26 Findings consistent with biopsy-proven lower outer quadrant right breast carcinoma (blue arrow) with right axillary lymph node metastasis (red arrow). Diffuse uptake noted in both lobes of thyroid consistent with patient's history of thyroiditis

therapy is high in individuals with high grade ER negative, HER2-positive breast cancer. Less extensive surgery would be required in the breast and axilla by downstaging with systemic therapy prior surgery. The effectiveness of systemic therapy would also provide prognostic information and inform options for adjuvant systemic therapy recommendations based on extent of residual disease after neoadjuvant chemotherapy. The patient is also afforded more time to complete genetic testing and explore surgical opinions while deciding whether to pursue breast-conserving surgery or mastectomy for local regional management as she was initially leaning toward.

Restaging MRI after neoadjuvant systemic therapy revealed marked diminution of the right breast mass and axillary adenopathy. The patient underwent a lumpectomy and axillary node surgery with targeted axillary node dissection. A complete pathologic response to neoadjuvant therapy is achieved. Pathologic stage ypT0, ypN0, cM0. Post-lumpectomy radiotherapy is recommended with continued systemic therapy with dual anti-HER2 antibody therapy for 1 year.

Clinical Scenario 4: Clinical Stage IA, cT1c, cN0 Breast Carcinoma, ER Negative, HER2 Positive

Upfront Surgery Is Preferred for Accurate Staging with Adjuvant Systemic Therapy Based on Pathologic Staging

A patient in her mid-40s is diagnosed with clinical stage IA, cT1c(m), cN0, high-grade invasive ductal carcinoma of the left breast, ER negative, PR negative, and HER2 positive associated with extensive high-grade ductal carcinoma in situ. She presents with a small palpable mass in the upper outer left breast.

Diagnostic mammograms (Fig. 14.27a, b) reveal linear branching calcifications within the left upper inner quadrant extending to the nipple. An irregularly shaped mass is identified in the posterior 3rd of the left breast at the 2 o'clock position (Fig. 14.27c) corresponding to the palpable mass with an additional 1.2 cm mass noted on ultrasound at 12 o'clock. Biopsy of the mass at 2:00 demonstrates high-grade infiltrating ductal carcinoma (Fig. 14.27e) ER negative, PR negative, and HER2 positive, 3+, 100% by IHC. Core biopsy of calcifications demonstrates ductal

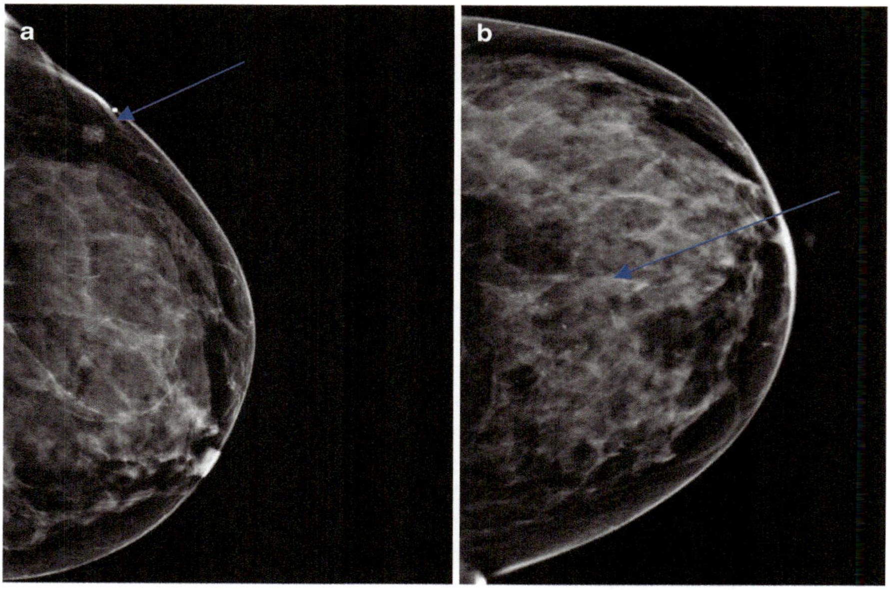

Fig. 14.27 Exaggerated Left CC mammogram highlighting palpable mass (**a**) with LCC mammogram demonstrating linear branching calcifications (**b**). An irregularly shaped mass measuring 0.9 cm was identified 2:00 on US corresponding to the palpable mass (**c**). MRI demonstrates multifocal invasive breast carcinoma with extensive non-mass enhancement (**d**). Biopsy of the mass noted on US demonstrates high-grade infiltrating ductal carcinoma, ER, 0, PR 0, HER2 positive (**e**). Stereotactic core biopsy of calcifications demonstrated ductal carcinoma, high nuclear grade with necrosis (**f**)

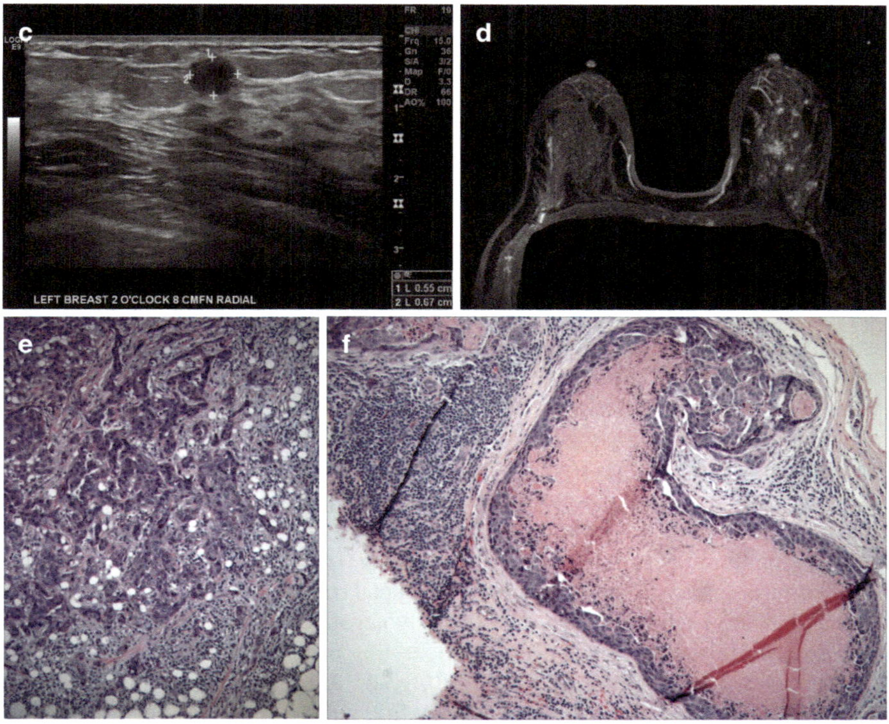

Fig. 14.27 (continued)

carcinoma in situ, high nuclear grade (Fig. 14.27f). An MRI supports the findings of multifocal invasive carcinoma with extensive non-mass-like enhancement within the left breast (Fig. 14.27d).

There is a maternal family history of breast cancer and ovarian cancer. Genetic testing with a 35-gene panel is negative.

The patient is not a candidate for breast conservation given the extent of high-grade DCIS. Neoadjuvant systemic therapy is not clearly indicated in this patient who presents with clinical stage IA disease. Even with downstaging of disease, mastectomy would be indicated, regardless of response to therapy. It is challenging to precisely stage this patient with extensive DCIS and multifocal invasive carcinoma. Pathologic staging would be most helpful in defining precise stage of disease with adjuvant therapy recommendations based on firm clinical data.

The patient undergoes mastectomy with final pathology revealing multifocal invasive ductal carcinoma with extensive high-grade ductal carcinoma in situ spanning an area of 11 cm (Fig. 14.27f) corresponding to the microcalcifications seen in the upper inner quadrant. The invasive carcinoma is described as grade 3 measuring 1.2 cm and 0.9 cm, respectively (Fig. 14.27e). Five sentinel nodes are negative. First stage implant-based reconstruction is accomplished at the time of mastectomy.

Adjuvant systemic therapy is recommended with 12 weeks of single-agent paclitaxel and trastuzumab followed by trastuzumab to 1 year [76]. Radiation is not indicated post-mastectomy given node negative status and clear surgical margins.

Clinical Scenario 5. Clinical Stage IA, cT1c, cN0, HER2-Positive, ER Positive Breast Carcinoma

Planned Surgery Is Expected to Be Delayed

A patient in her mid-30s presents with a palpable mass upper outer left breast. She is 10 months postpartum with her 5th child and is breastfeeding at the time she notes this mass. Diagnostic workup including mammograms and targeted ultrasound which demonstrate a 15 × 14 × 12 mm mass 2 o'clock position left breast corresponding to the area of palpable concern. Core biopsy demonstrates invasive ductal carcinoma, grade 2, ER positive, PR positive, and HER2 positive. She discontinues breastfeeding with this diagnosis. Breast MRI (Fig. 14.28) confirms an irregular shaped mass at the 2:00 position measuring 1.4 × 1.3 × 1.7 cm in maximal dimension. A smaller mass is noted at 10:00 measuring 0.6 × 0.5 × 0.4 cm. Biopsy of the smaller mass demonstrates grade 2 invasive ductal carcinoma, ER positive, PR positive, and HER2 negative. Nodes are clinically negative by imaging. There is a family history of breast cancer. Cancer genetic testing is negative.

Clinical Stage IA, cT1c(m), cN0, cM0, grade 2 invasive ductal carcinoma ER positive, PR positive, and HER2 positive at 2:00 left breast. A smaller T1b grade 2 invasive ductal carcinoma is identified at the 10 o'clock position is ER positive, PR positive, and HER2 negative.

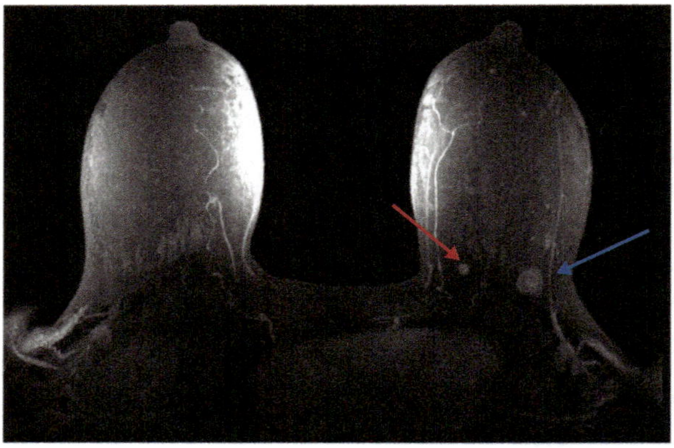

Fig. 14.28 MRI demonstrates a 1.4 × 1.3 × 1.7 cm enhancing mass left breast at 2:00, 11 cm from the nipple (blue arrow) with biopsy of this lesion under US demonstrating grade 2 invasive ductal carcinoma, ER, PR, and HER2 positive. There is also a smaller enhancing mass at 10:00, 12 cm from the nipple measuring 0.7 × 0.5 × 0.4 cm (red arrow) with US-guided biopsy demonstrating infiltrating ductal carcinoma, grade 2, ER, PR positive, and HER2 negative

The patient is seeking multiple opinions regarding surgery and is contemplating bilateral mastectomies with reconstruction. She is not comfortable waiting to initiate systemic therapy until this decision is made. She is not an appropriate candidate for a standard neoadjuvant systemic regimen, which is polychemotherapy with trastuzumab. This would represent overtreatment in this individual. One could extrapolate from adjuvant data for patients with favorable node negative HER2-positive breast cancer with primaries less than 2 cm and consider providing weekly paclitaxel with trastuzumab prior to surgery with continued trastuzumab and an endocrine agent postoperatively.

Triple-Negative Breast Cancer

Locally Advanced, Node Positive or High-Risk Node Negative

Triple-negative breast cancer is defined as a type of breast cancer that lacks expression of the estrogen receptor, progesterone receptor, and HER2 oncoprotein. Breast carcinomas that do not express ER, PR, and HER2 represent a heterogeneous group of breast carcinoma with respect to histology, genomics, prognosis, and response to treatment. Triple-negative breast carcinoma in general is considered an aggressive subtype of breast carcinoma and account for approximately 15% of breast cancers diagnosed yearly. Triple-negative breast carcinoma is more commonly diagnosed in women under 40 years of age compared to women over 50 and appears to be relatively more common among Black women compared to white women. Risk factors associated with the diagnosis of triple-negative breast carcinoma include presence of a germline pathogenic variant in BRCA, particularly in BRCA1. Up to 20% of patients with triple-negative breast carcinoma are found to harbor a pathogenic variant in a cancer risk allele vs. less than 6% of other breast cancer subtypes. For this reason, patients with triple-negative breast carcinoma, including patients age 60 and younger, should be offered cancer genetic counseling and testing for identification of a BRCA germline mutation in BRCA.

Triple-negative breast cancer presents with rapid growth and are more likely to be diagnosed clinically rather than mammographically than ER-positive breast cancers or as interval cancers. Triple-negative breast cancer is usually high grade with infiltrating ductal carcinoma representing the most common histology. Rare histologic subtypes such as medullary carcinoma and metaplastic and adenoid cystic carcinomas are typically triple-negative. Triple-negative breast cancers can exhibit geographic necrosis, a pushing border of invasion and presence of stromal lymphocytic infiltration. Unlike other subtypes of breast cancer (Hormone-receptor-positive, HER2 positive) there are no approved targeted treatments for non-metastatic triple-negative breast carcinoma. However, this subtype is associated with a relatively high PCR rate following chemotherapy [77].

Preferred regimens for triple-negative breast cancer are listened in the NCCN guidelines and commonly consist of anthracycline-, alkylator-, and taxane-based regimens—typically administered in a dose-dense fashion. Non-anthracycline-based regimens are appropriate alternatives for patients with lower-risk triple-negative breast cancer, such as node-negative or less than 1 cm, or those with a contraindication to anthracyclines. As PCR is highly prognostic in this subgroup, platinum agents such as carboplatin can be offered to select higher risk/stage patients with triple-negative breast cancer in the neoadjuvant setting to increase the likelihood of complete pathologic response. There can be increased nausea and myelosuppression when platinum agents are incorporated into neoadjuvant regimens and the effect on long-term outcome is less clear. Immune checkpoint inhibitors have also been studied in this setting, although there is currently not sufficient evidence to support incorporation into standard neoadjuvant therapy regimens.

Patients with residual disease at the end of treatment are at increased risk of recurrence. This relationship is particularly true of patients with triple-negative breast carcinoma as well as HER2-positive disease. If there is residual disease after preoperative therapy with taxane-, alkylator-, and anthracycline-based chemotherapy, adjuvant capecitabine can be offered versus participation on a clinical trial. As additional information from ongoing clinical trials assessing the role of immunotherapy mature, these treatment recommendations are expected to evolve.

Administration of neoadjuvant systemic therapy is the favored approach in patients with locally advanced breast cancer, Stage IIB–III to downstage disease, improve surgical options, and to monitor effectiveness of systemic treatment. Prognostic information is also gained by assessing the extent of residual disease after neoadjuvant chemotherapy and can guide recommendations for adjuvant therapy. For patients with highly sensitive disease to neoadjuvant chemotherapy, achieving a pathologic complete response is associated with improvement in disease-free survival [74, 75]. Additionally, patients with less advanced but high-risk disease, such as T1c or N1 disease, may be offered neoadjuvant therapy, particularly if a candidate for additional treatment in the adjuvant setting should residual disease be identified. Patients with small node-negative triple-negative breast carcinoma, T1a, or T1b should not routinely be offered neoadjuvant therapy.

Scenario 1. Premenopausal Patient with Clinical Stage IIIC Triple-Negative Breast Cancer. BRCA2 Carrier

Goals: Downstage Disease to Improve Surgical Options and to Tailor Adjuvant Therapy Based on Pathologic Response to Therapy

A patient age 50 is diagnosed with Clinical Stage IIIC, cT2, cN1, cM0, grade 3, triple-negative infiltrating ductal carcinoma of the right breast. Presents with an asymptomatic screening abnormality demonstrating an ill-defined nodular density deep in the lateral aspect of the right breast. Screening 1 year prior demonstrated heterogeneously dense breast tissue, but no other findings concerning for

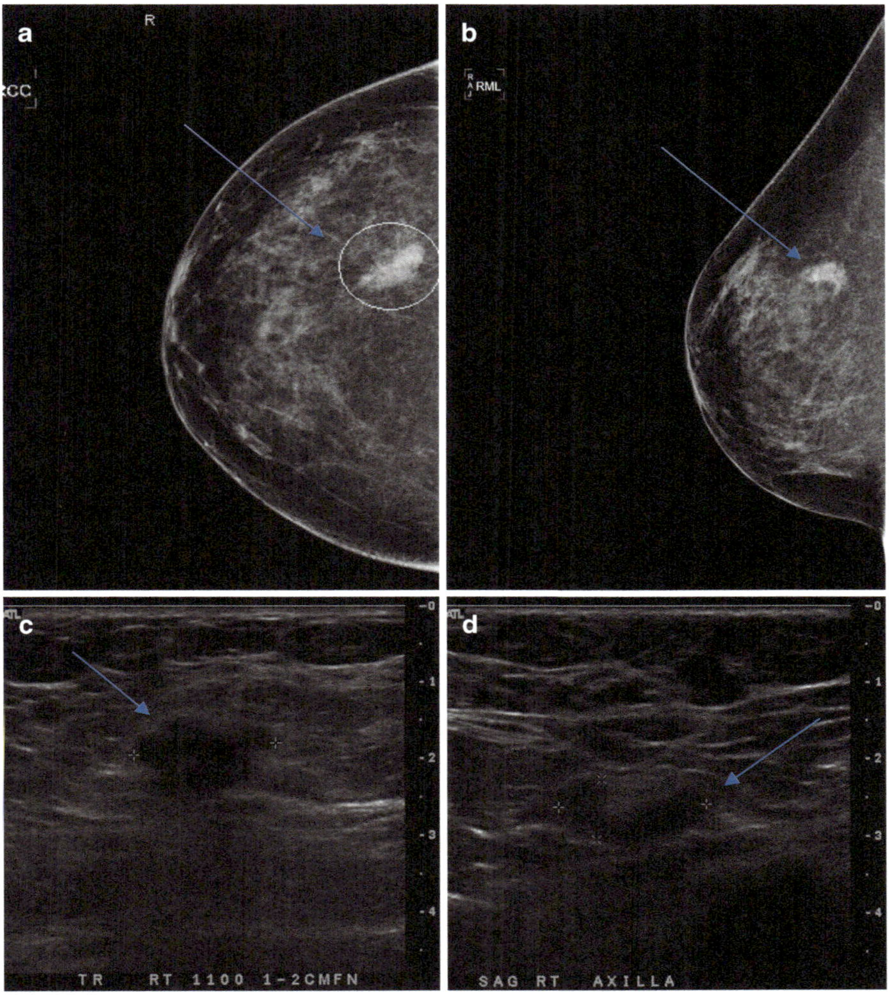

Fig. 14.29 Mammograms RCC (**a**) and RML views (**b**) right breast demonstrate an ill-defined nodular density lateral aspect right breast (arrow). There is a 1.8 × 1.0 × 0.7 cm irregularly marinated lobulated hypoechoic mass right breast 11:00, 12 cm from the nipple (**c**). A 1.9 × 0.8 × 1.7 cm lymph node is noted right axilla with lobulated margins (**d**)

malignancy. Diagnostic mammogram (Fig. 14.29a, b) and targeted ultrasound (Fig. 14.29c) demonstrate an irregular lobulated hypoechoic mass on ultrasound highly suspicious for malignancy. A 1.9 cm lymph node is noted right axilla with lobulated cortical margins (Fig. 14.29d).

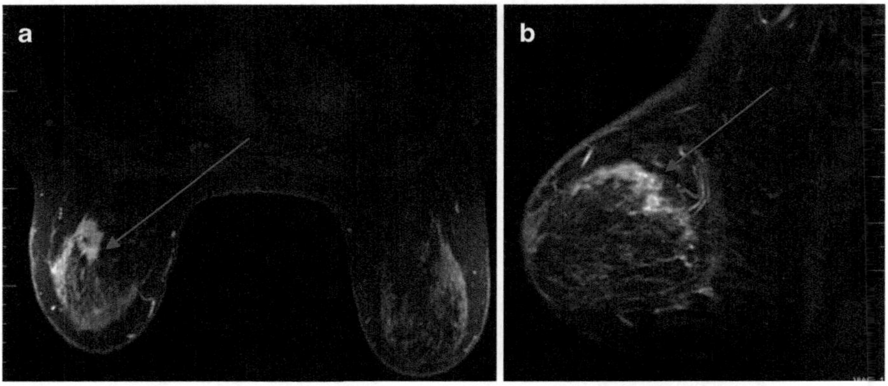

Fig. 14.30 MRI breast axial (**a**) and sagittal images (**b**) demonstrates a 3.2 cm mass upper outer right breast (arrow) with additional areas of aggressive enhancement extending 4 cm anterior an inferior to the main mass and 2 cm anterior and superior to the main mass, in total spanning over 7 cm. All areas of enhancement were within the upper outer quadrant

Ultrasound-guided biopsy of the right breast mass demonstrates poorly differentiated infiltrating ductal carcinoma, ER, PR, and HER2 negative. Biopsy of the right axillary node demonstrates metastatic poorly differentiated carcinoma.

Breast MRI (Fig. 14.30a, b) demonstrates a 3 × 2 cm mass upper outer right breast with additional areas of aggressive enhancement extending an additional 4 cm anterior and inferior to the main mass and an area of enhancement extending 2 cm anterior and inferior to the main tumor mass. All areas of abnormal enhancement are in the upper outer quadrant. CT chest, abdomen, and pelvis, contrast enhanced, and bone scan are negative for systemic disease.

Clinical prognostic Stage IIIC, cT3, cN1, cM0, grade 3 invasive ductal carcinoma right breast, ER negative, PR negative, and HER2 negative.

The patient is recommended neoadjuvant systemic chemotherapy with a regimen containing an anthracycline—with an alkylator, followed by a taxane delivered in a dose-dense fashion. Goals of therapy are to reduce local-regional disease prior to surgery, address management of micro metastatic disease and to monitor response to therapy.

Restaging breast MRI demonstrates no residual abnormal enhancement in the upper outer quadrant. Given initial extent of disease, right mastectomy sentinel node excision and limited axillary surgery, including removal of the clipped axillary node, is performed. There is evidence of treatment effect with no residual carcinoma within the breast or axilla—ypT0, ypN0.

She is referred for post-mastectomy radiotherapy given initial stage of disease. The patient meets criteria for cancer genetic counseling given histologic subtype of cancer [72]. Genetic testing identifies a pathogenic variant in BRCA2. Patient is referred for risk-reducing bilateral salpingo-oophorectomy and is followed with high-risk screening protocol for the remaining breast as she contemplates the option of prophylactic contralateral mastectomy with bilateral reconstruction.

Clinical Scenario 2. Anatomic Stage IIB (cT2, cN1) Triple-Negative Breast Carcinoma

Goals: Downstage Disease to Improve Surgical Options and to Tailor Adjuvant Therapy Based on Pathologic Response to Therapy

A female in her late 40s presents with a palpable mass right breast upper outer quadrant. She last participated in screening 5 years prior. Diagnostic mammograms and targeted ultrasound (Fig. 14.31) demonstrate a 3.5 cm oval mass in the posterior third right breast upper outer quadrant corresponding to the palpable mass with at least two enlarged right axillary nodes, each measuring close to 3 cm. Ultrasound-guided core biopsy right breast (with clip placement at the time of biopsy) demonstrates invasive ductal carcinoma associated with a component of high-grade ductal carcinoma in situ. Estimated grade 3. ER negative, PR negative, and HER2 negative. Biopsy of the right axillary node (with clip placement) demonstrates metastatic carcinoma.

MRI breast (Fig. 14.32a) demonstrates a 3.4 cm necrotic mass right breast 10:30 position and at least 6 abnormal right axillary level 1 lymph nodes. Mild right lateral breast subcutaneous edema is noted post-biopsy.

Staging with PET-CT demonstrates right breast carcinoma with multiple metastasis to right axillary level 1 lymph nodes. Clinical prognostic stage is IIIB, cT2, cN1, cM0, grade 3, invasive ductal carcinoma, ER, PR, and HER2 negative. The patient reports no family history of cancer and cancer genetic testing is negative.

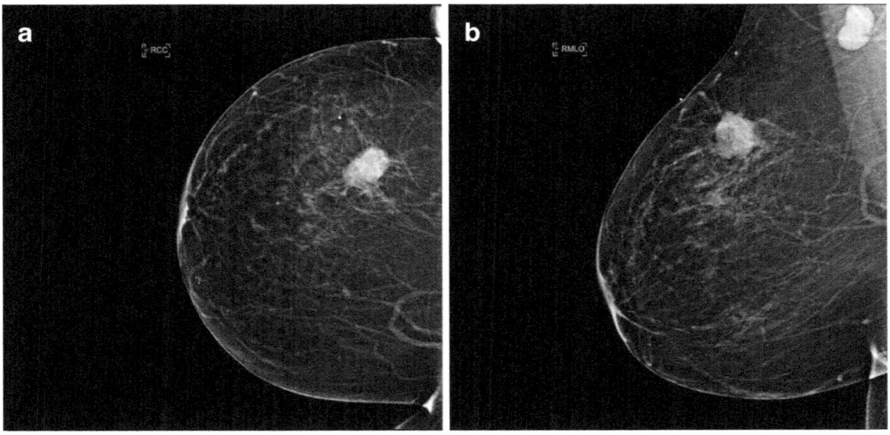

Fig. 14.31 Diagnostic Mammogram confirms a highly suspicious mass in the right upper outer quadrant on CC view (**a**) and suspected right axillary metastatic lymphadenopathy on MLO view (**b**)

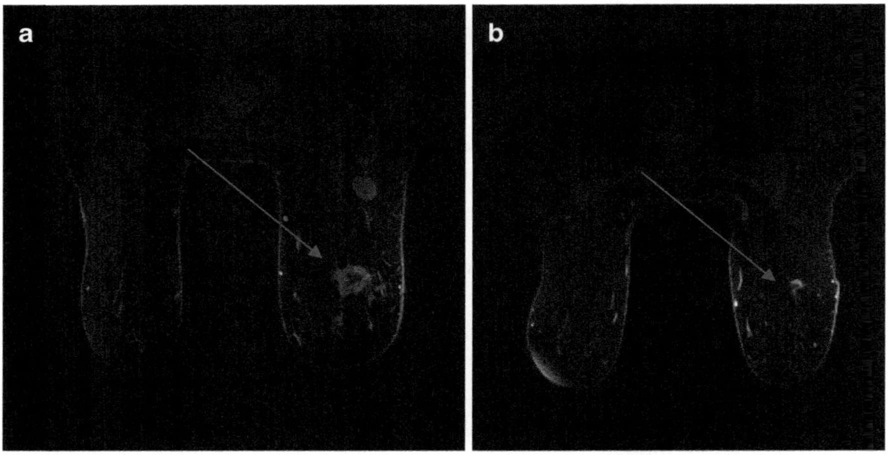

Fig. 14.32 Breast MRI demonstrates a 3.5 cm necrotic mass at the right 10:30 position corresponds to the biopsy-proven index carcinoma (arrow). Approximate 3 cm non mass enhancement extends anterolaterally from the mass. At least 6 abnormal right axillary level I lymph nodes (a). MRI post-neoadjuvant chemotherapy (**b**) demonstrates marked interval response to therapy with decrease in index lesion to 1.4 cm (arrow) and resolution of the anterolateral non mass enhancement. Marked interval decrease in right axillary adenopathy

Neoadjuvant systemic chemotherapy is recommended with a regimen containing an anthracycline—with an alkylator followed by a taxane delivered in a dose-dense fashion. Goals of therapy are to reduce local-regional disease to reduce the extent of surgery and to monitor response to therapy.

Response to neoadjuvant systemic chemotherapy is excellent on clinical exam but incomplete on reimaging (Fig. 14.32b). The patient opts for right mastectomy axillary dissection with the findings of residual invasive ductal carcinoma, 1.7 cm grade 3 with LVI, associated ductal carcinoma in situ comprising less than 5% of the carcinoma and metastatic carcinoma in 6 of 13 axillary nodes with the largest focus measuring 0.7 cm. Treatment effect is noted. Pathologic Stage classification (ypT1c, ypN2a, cM0).

As pathologic response to therapy is highly prognostic in this subgroup of patients, adjuvant systemic therapy is recommended with capecitabine versus participation in a clinical trial. The patient is a candidate for post-mastectomy radiotherapy and is at high risk for lymphedema given extent of axillary involvement, extent of axillary surgery and need for post-mastectomy radiotherapy as part of local regional management.

Clinical Scenario 3. Clinical Stage IIB, cT2, cN1 Triple-Negative Breast Carcinoma

Goal: Downstage Disease to Improve Surgical Options and to Tailor Adjuvant Therapy Based on Pathologic Response to Therapy

A female in her early 40s presents with a palpable mass left breast. Diagnostic mammograms and targeted ultrasound demonstrate heterogeneously dense breast tissue with a new asymmetry in the retro areolar region of the left breast. Ultrasound demonstrates a mass at 12:00, 3 cm from the nipple measuring 3.4 × 2.7 × 3.5 cm with a single left axillary node with asymmetric lobular cortex. Ultrasound-guided core biopsy of the left breast mass demonstrates invasive, poorly differentiated ductal carcinoma, estimated grade 3. ER 0, PR 0, and HER2 negative. Image-guided biopsy of the left axillary node with clip placement demonstrates metastatic carcinoma. Breast MRI (Fig. 14.33a) demonstrates an intensely hypermetabolic 3.3 cm mass left breast with a left axillary node measuring 3 × 1.5 × 1.9 cm.

Clinical prognostic stage is IIIA, cT2, cN1, high-grade invasive ductal carcinoma, ER/PR and HER2 negative.

The patient is of African Ancestry. She meets criteria for cancer genetic testing [72] with reported results negative for a pathogenic mutation in 47 genes analyzed. The patient receives neoadjuvant systemic chemotherapy with dose dense Adriamycin and Cytoxan followed by weekly Taxol with the **goals of downstaging**

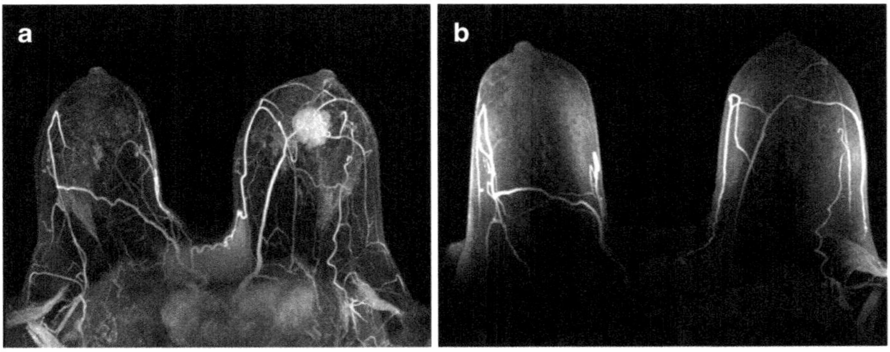

Fig. 14.33 MRI prior to neoadjuvant systemic therapy (**a**) demonstrates an intensely hypermetabolic 3.3 cm mass—left superior breast with a left axillary node measuring 3.0 × 1.5 × 1.9 cm. Following neoadjuvant systemic therapy, breast MRI (**b**) demonstrates 1 cm residual transverse enhancement in the area of the biopsy marker corresponding to known breast cancer. Corresponding to biopsy-proven metastatic left axillary level 1 node, residual lymph node measures up to 1 cm cranial caudal

disease and assessing degree of pathologic response. She appears to have a near complete response on restaging MRI (Fig. 14.33b).

Breast-conserving surgery is performed. Pathology reveals residual invasive ductal carcinoma, poorly differentiated, grade 3 measuring 1.3 cm in greatest dimension. Treatment effect is noted in the breast. Three axillary sentinel nodes, including the node with the biopsy marker, are all negative for carcinoma. Pathologic stage classification is ypT1c, ypN0, cM0. Repeat tumor profile testing demonstrates ER 0, PR 0, and negative HER2 status. Adjuvant radiotherapy is administered. As pathologic complete response is prognostic in this subtype of breast cancer, the patient should be offered adjuvant systemic therapy with capecitabine or participation on a clinical trial.

Clinical Scenario 4: Clinical Stage IIB, cT2, cN0, Triple-Negative Breast Carcinoma

Goals: To Downstage Local-Regional Disease and Assess Pathologic Response to Therapy

A patient in her early 60s is diagnosed with clinical stage IIA, cT2, cN0, grade 2 invasive ductal carcinoma left breast, ER negative, PR negative, and HER2 negative. Patient presents with a palpable mass left breast. Diagnostic breast imaging, including mammograms (Fig. 14.34), demonstrate heterogeneously dense breast tissue with mass close to 3 cm in the superior left breast. Most recent screening mammograms 18 months prior demonstrated were negative.

Targeted left breast ultrasound demonstrates a mass close to 3 cm in upper outer left breast (Fig. 14.35a). Additional diagnostic breast imaging with Breast MRI confirms a mass 3.5 × 2.6 × 3 cm in size left breast (Fig. 14.35b).

There is a family history of prostate cancer. Patient is referred for cancer genetic testing with negative results.

Clinical prognostic stage is IIB, cT2, cN0, grade 2, infiltrating ductal carcinoma left breast, ER, PR, and HER2 negative.

Although patient is a candidate for breast-conserving therapy up-front, neoadjuvant systemic chemotherapy is the preferred approach with the **goal of reducing the surgery needed for breast conservation and to assess response to therapy.**

A left breast lumpectomy with sentinel node biopsy is performed with findings of a complete pathologic response to therapy. Adjuvant radiotherapy is recommended post-lumpectomy. As the patient achieved a pathologic complete response to neoadjuvant therapy, there is no role for adjuvant systemic therapy.

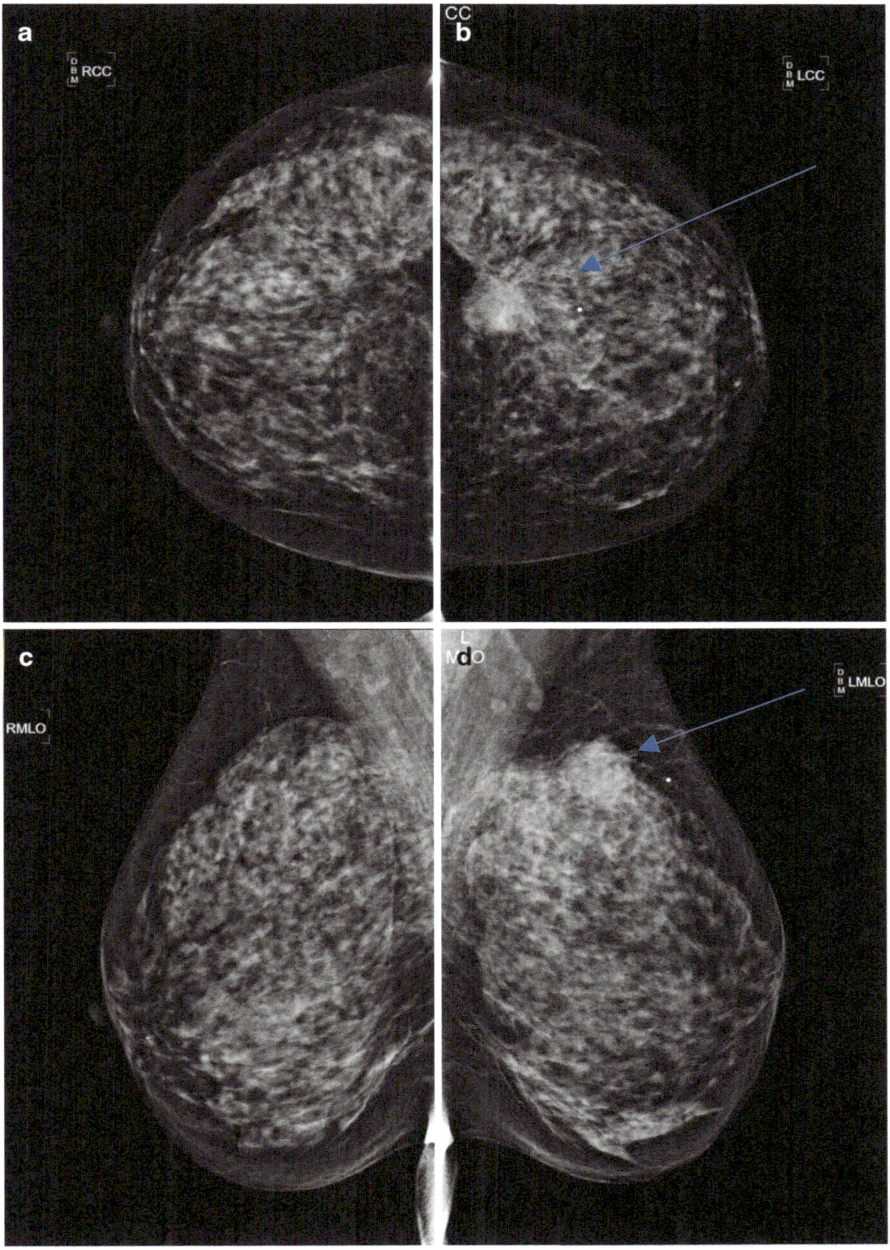

Fig. 14.34 Diagnostic mammograms (**a**–**d**) demonstrate heterogeneously dense breast tissue with a 2.7 cm mass in the 12:00 position posterior third of the left breast (**b**, **d**) (arrow)

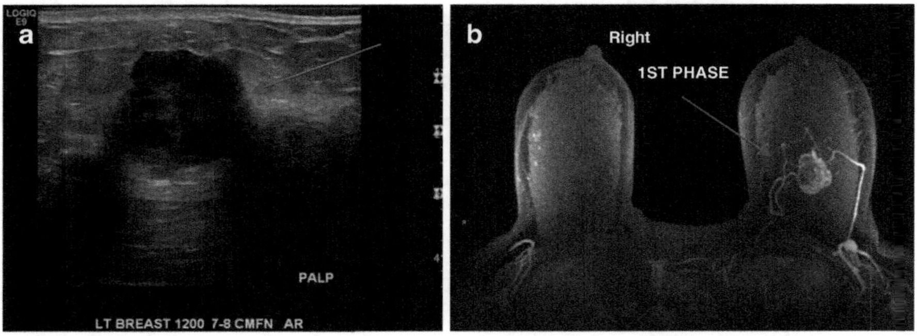

Fig. 14.35 Targeted US right breast palpable mass confirms a 2.4 × 2.7 × 1.9 cm hypoechoic ma s at 12:00 (**a**). MRI breast demonstrates a 3.5 × 2.6 × 3 cm nodular ring enhancement surrounding an area of low signal within the 12:00 position consistent with patients known malignancy with a component of central necrosis (**b**). A mildly prominent node is noted left axilla measuring 1.3 × 0.8 cm with second look US and biopsy showing benign findings

Clinical Scenario 5: Clinical Stage IB, cT1c, cN0, cM0 Triple-Negative Breast Carcinoma

Goals: To Assess Response to Therapy and Inform Options for Adjuvant Therapy

A patient in her mid-40s is diagnosed with clinical pathologic stage IB, triple-negative breast carcinoma. She presents with a palpable mass left breast 6 months after normal screening mammograms.

Diagnostic mammograms (Fig. 14.36a–d) demonstrate heterogeneously dense breast tissue with a new hyperdense mass with lobulated margins in the area of the palpable lump. Targeted left breast ultrasound (Fig. 14.36e) demonstrates a hypoechoic heterogeneous lesion with irregular margins measuring 14 × 20 × 13 mm in diameter. Axillary nodes appear normal by ultrasound. Breast MRI demonstrates an enhancing mass with central necrosis corresponding to the biopsy-proven carcinoma at the 11 to 12 o'clock position left breast. The mass measures 2.0 × 1.5 × 2.0 cm. There is no evidence of adenopathy or chest wall involvement (Figs. 14.37 and 14.38).

The patient has no family history of cancer but meets criteria for cancer genetic testing [72] with results reported as negative.

Clinical prognostic stage is IB, cT1c, cN0, cM0 grade 3 invasive ductal carcinoma, ER, PR, and HER2 negative.

Although the patient is a candidate for breast-conserving therapy up-front, neoadjuvant systemic chemotherapy is the preferred approach with the **goal of assessing response to therapy for prognostic purposes and guiding recommendations for adjuvant therapy if indicated.** The patient receives neoadjuvant systemic therapy with Adriamycin Cytoxan followed by a taxane. There is a partial clinical response to Adriamycin and Cytoxan therapy, but the patient develops clinical

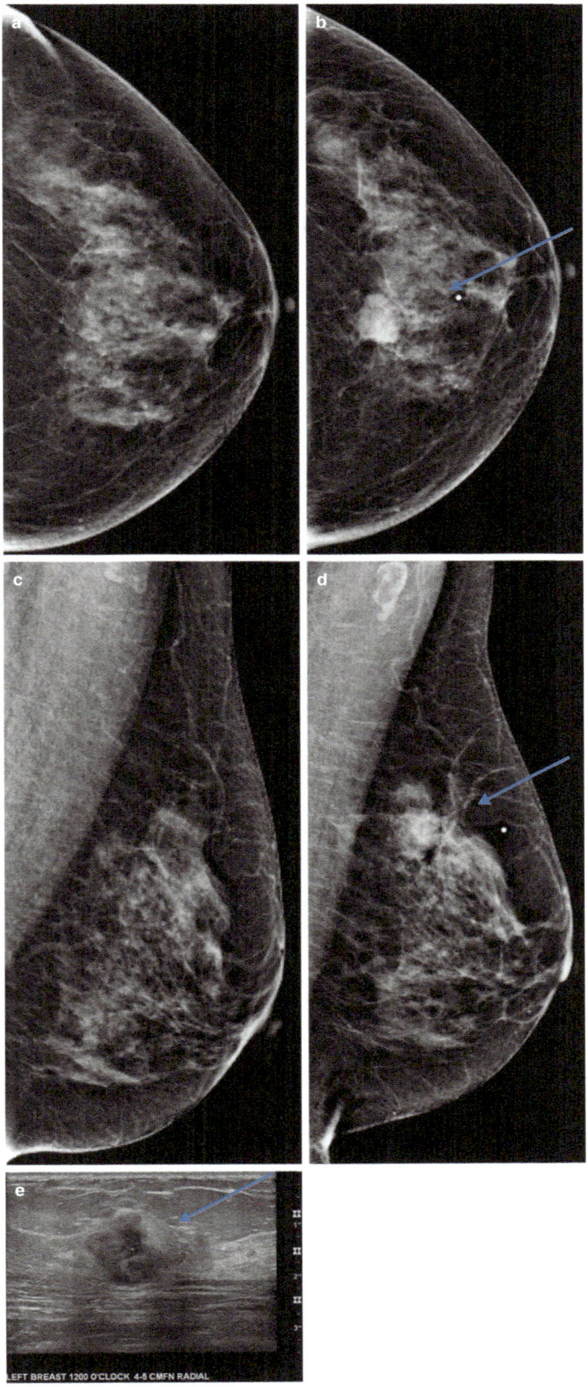

Fig. 14.36 Patient presents with a new hyperdense mass left breast (arrows) on diagnostic mammograms (**b**, **d**) representing an interval finding compared to screening study 6 months prior (**a**, **c**). Sonographic evaluation demonstrated a hypoechoic heterogeneous lesion with irregular margins measuring 14 × 20 × 13 mm in diameter 12:00 position, 4–5 cm from nipple (**e**)

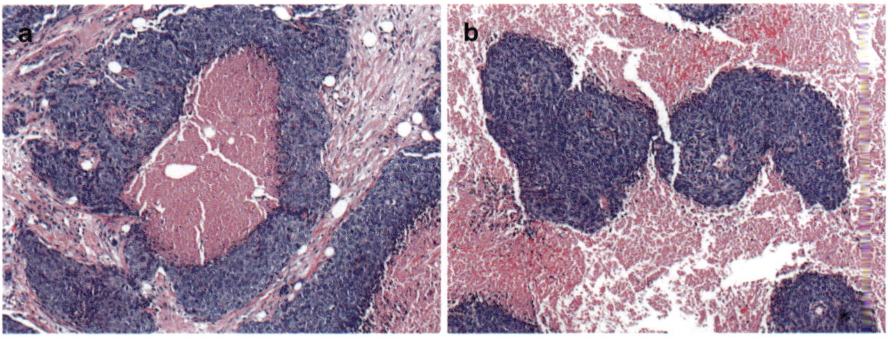

Fig. 14.37 Ultrasound-guided needle biopsy of the left breast mass demonstrates infiltrating ductal carcinoma with extensive necrosis (**a**, **b**). Estimated grade 3, ER negative, PR negative, and HER2 negative

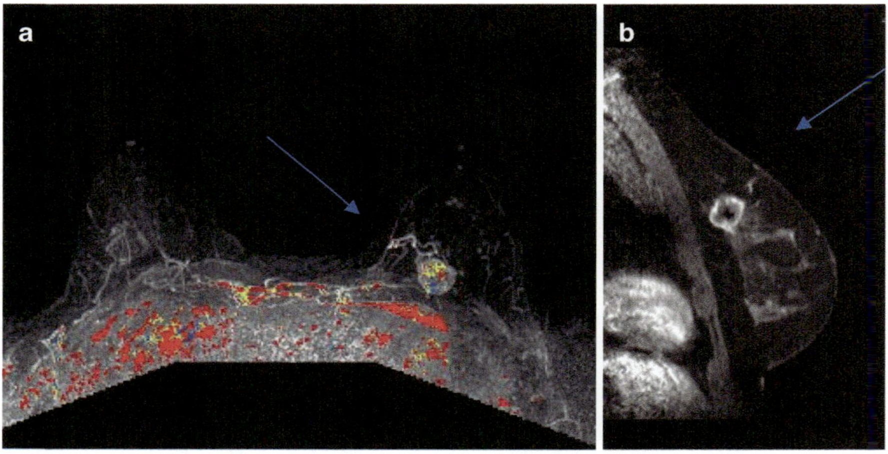

Fig. 14.38 MRI breast demonstrates an enhancing mass axial view (**a**) and sagittal view (**b**) with central necrosis (arrow) corresponding to the biopsy-proven carcinoma at the 11 to 12 o'clock position left breast. The mass measures 2.0 × 1.5 × 2.0 cm. There is no evidence of adenopathy or chest wall involvement

progression while receiving a taxane. Carboplatin is added without substantial response. Further neoadjuvant systemic therapy is abandoned and the patient undergoes left breast lumpectomy and axillary surgery. Pathology findings demonstrate a 3.8 cm triple-negative breast carcinoma with metastatic carcinoma in 1 of 7 axillary nodes. Pathologic stage classification ypT2, ypN1, cM0. She receives postoperative radiation therapy. It is important to remember that some patients are resistent to upfront therapy. If progression occurs, it is best to move to surgery for local regional management before the patient becomes inoperable [38]. Progression on neoadjuvant systmeic therapy carries a poor prognosis. Adjuvant systemic therapy, preferably as part of a clinical trial is indicated.

Clinical Scenario 6: Clinical Stage IA, cT1a, cN0 Triple-Negative Breast Carcinoma

Upfront Surgical Management Is Indicated for Accurate Staging with Adjuvant Systemic Therapy If Indicated Based on Pathologic Staging

A patient in her early 50s presents for cancer risk assessment. She has a history of DCIS right breast, intermediate grade, ER, PR positive presenting 5 years prior with clustered microcalcifications on screening mammograms. DCIS spanned 1 cm. Patient was managed with breast-conserving therapy and received 5 years of tamoxifen. She reports a family history of breast cancer in several maternal relatives. She is referred for cancer genetic counseling and genetic testing reveals a pathogenic mutation in BRCA 1.

Breast MRI is ordered for screening in this high-risk patient and demonstrates a new nodular focus of enhancement in the left breast. This is not visible sonographically and was not seen on screening mammograms 6 months prior (Fig. 14.39).

Patient undergoes MRI-guided biopsy demonstrating infiltrating ductal carcinoma, estimated grade 3, ER negative, PR negative, and HER2 negative. Clinical stage IA, cT1a, cN0, cM0. This patient should not receive neoadjuvant systemic therapy, but should be undergo surgery first to assess pathologic stage of disease.

Given BRCA 1 mutation status, the patient opts for bilateral mastectomies with sentinel node procedure on the left. Final pathology reveals a focus of residual infiltrating ductal carcinoma, grade 3, measuring 1.2 mm. There is no lympho-vascular invasion and the left axillary sentinel lymph nodes are negative. Patient's prognosis is excellent, given early detection of her cancer. There is no indication for adjuvant systemic therapy. She is referred for prophylactic salpingo-oophorectomy and cascade testing is offered to her family.

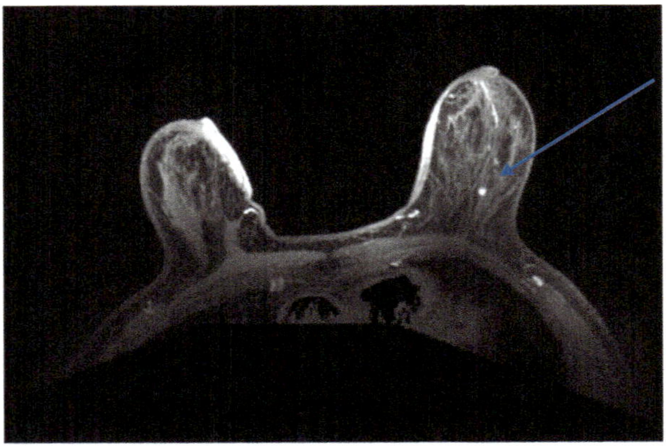

Fig. 14.39 In the central posterior aspect of the breast there is a new enhancing nodule measuring approximately 5 mm in greatest dimension (arrow)

Summary

Guidelines for use of neoadjuvant systemic therapy have evolved over the past 50 years. The goal of systemic therapy, whether administered prior to or after surgery to patients with non-metastatic invasive breast carcinoma, is to reduce the risk of emergence of distant disease and improve the likelihood of long-term disease-free survival. The additional goals of administering neoadjuvant systemic therapy prior to surgery are several. For locally advanced inoperable disease, the goal is to convert patients to operable candidates as part of local regional management of disease. Neoadjuvant therapy is considered standard of care for patients with inflammatory breast cancer, given the poor outcomes noted when surgery is attempted first, due to local regional extent of disease, involvement of skin lymphatics with tumor emboli, and propensity for disseminated microscopic disease at presentation.

In individuals with operable locally advanced disease, neoadjuvant systemic allows the tailoring of surgical options to reduce the extent of surgery needed to provide local regional control of disease. This may allow for breast conservation rather than mastectomy, less extensive axillary surgery, or improvement in cosmetic outcomes by reducing the size of lumpectomy for larger tumors. Administering systemic therapy prior to surgery allows for monitoring of response, including discontinuing therapy in the uncommon event of progression. Neoadjuvant delivery of systemic therapy also allows for evaluation of effectiveness of systemic therapy as determined by pathologic response. This information can be used to tailor adjuvant therapy recommendations, particularly in HER2-positive and triple-negative breast carcinoma, where pathologic response to initial therapy has strong prognostic implications. Ongoing guidelines will continue to change as information from ongoing clinical trials become available [49, 74, 75].

For patients that are candidates for surgery and candidates for adjuvant systemic therapy, but have a need to delay surgery, neoadjuvant systemic therapy can be considered. Examples where patient may need to delay surgery would include, awaiting results of cancer genetic testing to assist with surgical decisions, allowing time to consider options for breast reconstruction or operating room availability as was affected in many centers during the height of the COVID 19 pandemic [69].

The use of chemotherapy, endocrine therapy, or targeted therapy is guided by the same principles used to determine systemic treatment in the adjuvant setting, including tumor histology, grade, stage, and estrogen, progesterone, and HER2 expression. Although there is interest in use of gene expression assays (such as Onco*type* Dx Recurrence Score and MammaPrint) in guiding clinical decisions [64], there have not been prospective trials assessing the clinical utility of using a gene expression assay in the setting of locally advanced breast cancer. Future guidelines and recommendations how best to utilize this clinical approach will continue to evolve as results from ongoing clinical trials mature.

References

1. Cossetti RJD, Tyldesley SK, Speers CH, Zheng Y, Gelmon KA. Comparison of breast cancer recurrence and outcome patterns between patients treated from 1986 to 1992 and from 2004 to 2008. J Clin Oncol. 2015;33:65–73.
2. Saini KS, Taylor C, Ramirez AJ, et al. Role of the multidisciplinary team in breast cancer management: results from a large international survey involving 39 countries. Ann Oncol. 2012;23:853–9.
3. Tabar L, Vitak B, Chen TH, et al. Swedish 2 county trial: impact of mammographic screening on breast cancer mortality during 3 decades. Radiology. 2011;260:65 8–663.
4. Coldman A, Phillips N, Wilson C, et al. Pan-Canadian study of mammography screening and mortality from breast cancer. J Natl Cancer Inst. 2014;106:dju261.
5. Duffy SW, Tabar L, Chen HH, et al. The impact of organized mammography service screening on breast carcinoma mortality in 7 Swedish counties. Cancer. 2002;95:458–69.
6. Tabar L, Dean PB, Chen TH, Yen AM, et al. The incidence of fatal breast cancer measures the increased effectiveness of therapy in women participating in mammography screening. Cancer. 2019;125:515–23.
7. James TA, Wade JE, Sprague BL. The impact of mammographic screening on the surgical management of breast cancer. J Surg Oncol. 2016;113(5):496–500.
8. Sui AL. U.S. Preventive Services Task Force. Screening for breast cancer: U.S. preventive Services Task Force recommendation statement. Ann Intern Med. 2016;164(4):279–96.
9. Oeffinger KC, Fontham ET, Etzioni R, Herzig A, Michaelson JS, Shih YC, Walter LC, Church TR, Flowers CR, et al. Breast cancer screening for women at average risk colon 2015 guideline update from the American Cancer Society. J Am Med Assoc. 2015;314(15):1599–614.
10. Committee on Gynecologic Practice. Committee opinion no. 625. Management of women with dense breasts diagnosed by mammography. Obstet Gynecol. 2015;125(3):750–1.
11. Committee on Practice Bulletins–Gynecology. Practice bulletin number 179: breast cancer risk assessment and screening in average-risk women. Obstet Gynecol. 2017;130(1):e1–e16.
12. Monticciolo DL, Newell MS, Hendrick RE, Helvie MA, Moy L, Monsees B, Kopans DB, Eby PR, Sickles EA. Breast cancer screening for average-risk women: recommendations from the ACR commission on breast imaging. J Am Coll Radiol. 2017;14(9):1137–43.
13. Qaseem A, Lin JS, Reem AM, Horwitch CA, Wilt TJ. Screening for breast cancer in average-risk women: statement from the American College of Physicians. Ann Intern Med. 2019;170(8):547–60.
14. Lehman CD. Role of MRI in screening women at high risk for breast cancer. J Magn Reson Imaging. 2006;24(5):964–70.
15. Committee on Practice Bulletins–Gynecology, Committee on Genetics, Society of Gynecologic Oncology. Practice bulletin No. 182: Hereditary breast and ovarian cancer syndrome. Obstet Gynecol. 2017;t 130(3):e110–e126.
16. Monticciolo DL, Newell MS, Moy L, Niell B, Monsees B, Sickles EA. Breast cancer screening in women at higher-than-average risk: recommendations from the ACR. J Am Coll Radiol. 2018;15(3 Pt A):408–414.
17. Berg WA, Zheng Z, Lehrer D, et al. Detection of breast cancer with addition of annual screening ultrasound or a single screen MRI to mammography in women with elevated breast cancer risk. JAMA. 2020;303(2):168–9.
18. Duffy SW, Tabar L, Yen A, Dean PB, Smith RA, et al. Mammography screening reduces rates of advanced and fatal breast cancers: result in 549, 091 women. Cancer. 2020;126(13):2971–9.
19. Irvin VA, Zhang A, Simon MS, Chlebowski RT, et al. Comparison of mortality among participants of women's health initiative trials with screening detected breast cancers versus interval breast cancers. JAMA Netw Open. 2020;3(6):e207227.

20. Denduluri N, Somerfield MR, Eisen A, et al. Selection of optimal adjuvant chemotherapy regimens for HER-2 negative and HER-2 positive breast cancers: an ASCO guideline adaptation of the Cancer Care Ontario clinical practice guideline. J Clin Oncol. 2016;34:2416–27.
21. Dendaluri N, Chavez-MacGregor M, Telli ML, et al. Selection of optimal adjuvant chemotherapy and targeted therapy for early breast cancer: ASCO clinical practice guideline focused update. J Clin Oncol. 2018;36:2433–43.
22. Sparano AJ, Gray RJ, Ravdin PM, Makower DF, et al. Adjuvant chemotherapy guided by a 21 gene expression assay in breast cancer. N Engl J Med. 2018;379:111–21.
23. Sparano AJ, Gray RJ, Ravdin PM, Makower DF, Pritchard KI, Albain KS, et al. Clinical and genomic risk to guide the use of adjuvant therapy for breast cancer. N Engl J Med. 2019;380:2395–405.
24. Cardoso F, van'tVeer LJ, Bogaerts J, Slaets L, Viale G, et al. 70 gene signature as an aid to treatment decisions and early stage breast cancer. N Engl J Med. 2016;375:71 7–729.
25. Rutgers E, van't Veer LJ, Poncet C, et al. MINDACT: Long-term results of the large prospective trial testing the 70 gene signature MammaPrint as guide for adjuvant chemotherapy in breast cancer patients. 12th European Breast Cancer Conference. Abstract 21. Presented October 3, 2020.
26. Chia S, Swain S, Byrd D, Mankoff D. Locally advanced and inflammatory breast cancer. J Clin Oncol. 2008;26:786–90.
27. Baker JL, Hedge J, Thompson CK, Lee MK, DiNome ML. Local regional management of inflammatory breast cancer. Curr Breast Cancer Rep. 2020;12:326–35.
28. Hance KW, Anderson WF, Devesa SS, Young HA, Levine PH. Trends in inflammatory breast cancer incidence and survival: the surveillance, epidemiology and results program at the National Cancer Institute. J Natl Cancer Inst. 2005;97(13):966–75.
29. Robertson FM, Bondy M, Yang W, Yamauchi H, Wiggins S, et al. Inflammatory breast cancer: the disease, the biology, the treatment. CA Cancer J Clin. 2010;60(6):351.
30. Zucali R, Uslenghi C, Kenda R, Bonadonna G. Natural history a survival of inoperable breast cancer treated with radiotherapy and of radiotherapy followed by radical mastectomy. Cancer. 1976;37(3):1422–31.
31. Rubens RD, Sexton S, Tong D, Winter PJ, et al. Combined chemotherapy and radiotherapy for locally advanced breast cancer. Eur J Cancer Period. 1980;4:351–6.
32. Fisher B, Brown A, Mamounas EP, et al. Effect of preoperative chemotherapy on local regional disease in women with operable breast cancer: findings from the National Surgical Adjuvant Breast and Bowel Project B-18. J Clin Oncol. 1997;15:2483–93.
33. Rastogi P, Anderson SJ, Bear HD, et al. Preoperative chemotherapy: updates of National Surgical Adjuvant Breast and Bowel Project B-18 and B-27. J Clin Oncol. 2008;26:778–85.
34. Bear HD, Anderson S, Smith RE, Geyer CE, Mamounas EP, Fisher B, et al. Sequential preoperative or postoperative docetaxel added to preoperative doxorubicin plus cyclophosphamide for operable breast cancer: National Surgical adjuvant breast and bowel project protocol B-27. J Clin Oncol. 2006;24:2020–7.
35. Chen AM, Meric-Bernstam F, Hunt KK, et al. Breast conservation after neoadjuvant chemotherapy: the MD Anderson Cancer Center experience. J Clin Oncol. 2004;23:2303–12.
36. Mauri D, Pavlidis N, Ionnidis JPA. Neoadjuvant versus adjuvant systemic treatment and breast cancer: a meta-analysis. J Natl Cancer Inst. 2005;97:187–94.
37. Kaufmann M, Hortobagyi GN, Goldhirsch A, Scholl S, Makris A et al: Recommendations from an international expert panel on the use of neoadjuvant (primary) systemic treatment of operable breast cancer: an update. 2006;24:1940–47.
38. Caudle AS, Gonzalez-Angulo AM, Hunt KK, et al. Impact of progression during neoadjuvant chemotherapy on surgical management of breast cancer. Ann Surg Oncol. 2011;18:932–8.
39. Early Breast Cancer Trialists' Collaborative Group (EBCTCG). Long-term outcomes for neoadjuvant versus adjuvant chemotherapy in early breast cancer: meta-analysis of individual patient data from 10 randomized trials. Lancet Oncol. 2018;19:27.

40. Von Minckwitz G, Untch M, Blohmer JU, et al. Definition and impact of pathologic complete response on prognosis after neoadjuvant chemotherapy in various intrinsic breast cancer subtypes. J Clin Oncol. 2012;30:1796.
41. Bonnefoi H, Litere S, Piccart M, et al. Pathological complete response after neoadjuvant chemotherapy is an independent predictive factor irrespective of simplified breast cancer intrinsic subtypes: a landmark and two-step approach analyses from the ERORTC 10994/BIG 1-00 phase III Trial. Ann Oncol. 2014;25:1128–36.
42. Cortazar P, Zhang L, Untch M, et al. Pathologic complete response and long-term clinical benefit in breast cancer: the CTNeoBC pooled analysis. Lancet. 2014;384:16 4–172.
43. Spring LM, Fell G, Arfe A, et al. Pathologic complete response after neoadjuvant chemotherapy and impact on breast cancer recurrence and survival: a comprehensive meta-analysis. Clin Cancer Res. 2020;26:2838–48.
44. von Minckwitz G, Schneeweiss A, Loibl S, et al. Neoadjuvant carboplatin in patients with triple negative and HER2 positive early breast cancer (GeparSexto GBG 66). Lancet Oncol. 2014;15:74 7-756.
45. Sikov WM, Berry DA, Perou CM, et al. Impact of the addition of carboplatin and or bevacizumab to neoadjuvant once per week paclitaxel followed by dose dense doxorubicin and cyclophosphamide on pathologic complete response rates in stage II-III triple negative breast cancer: CALGB 40603 (Alliance). J Clin Oncol. 2015;33:13–21.
46. Giani L, Pinkowski T, Im Y-H, Tseng L-M, Liu M-C, Lluch A, et al. 5-year analysis of neoadjuvant pertuzumab and trastuzumab in patients with locally advanced, inflammatory, or early-stage HER2-positive breast cancer (NeoSphere): a multicentre, open-label, phase 2 randomised trial. Lancet Oncol. 2016;17:791–800.
47. Barker AD, Sigman DD, Kelloff GJ, Hylton, Berry DA, Esserman LJ, et al. I-SPY 2: adaptive breast cancer trial design in the setting of neoadjuvant chemotherapy. Clin Pharmacol Ther. 2009;86:97–100.
48. Bardia A, Baselga J. Neoadjuvant therapy as a platform for drug development and approval in breast cancer. Clin Cancer Res. 2013;19(23):6360–70.
49. Nanda R, Liu MC, Yau C, et al. Effect of Pembrolizumab plus neoadjuvant chemotherapy on pathologic complete response in women with early-stage breast cancer. JAMA Oncol. 2020;6(5):676–84.
50. Wang H, Yee D. I-SPY 2: a neoadjuvant adaptive clinical trial designed to improve outcomes in high-risk breast cancer. Curr Breast Cancer Rep. 2019;11(4):303–10.
51. Pilewski M, Morrow M. Axillary nodal management following neoadjuvant chemotherapy. JAMA Oncol. 2017;3(4):549–55.
52. Haagensen C, Stout A. Carcinoma of the breast II. Criteria of operability. Ann Surg. 1943;118:859.
53. Lawrence W, Fletcher GH. Criteria of operability in advanced breast cancer. In: Fletcher GH, Levitt SH, editors. Non-disseminated breast cancer. Berlin: Springer; 1993. p. 5–9.
54. Hortobagyi GN, Connolly JL, D'Orsi CJ, et al. Breast. In: Amin MB, Edge S, Greene F, et al., editors. American Joint Committee on cancer. AJCC cancer staging manual. 8th ed. New York: Springer; 2017. p. 589–636.
55. Gralow FR, Burnstein HJ, Wood W, et al. Preoperative therapy in invasive breast cancer: pathologic assessment and systemic therapy issues in operable breast disease. J Clin Oncol. 2008;26:814.
56. Garg PJ. Current definition of locally advanced breast cancer. Curr Oncol. 2015;22(5):e409–10.
57. Newman SA. Epidemiology of locally advanced breast cancer. Semin Radiat Oncol. 2009;19(4):195–203.
58. Dawood S, Merajver SD, Viens P, et al. International expert panel on inflammatory breast cancer: consensus statement for standardized diagnosis and treatment. Ann Oncol. 2011;22:515.
59. Dianali V, Chadashvill T, Slanetz PJ. Role of imaging in neoadjuvant therapy for breast cancer. Ann Surg Oncol. 2015;22:1416–24.

60. Rieg B, Heacock L, Lewin A, Cho N, Moy L. Role of MRI to assess response to neoadjuvant therapy for breast cancer. J Magn Reson Imaging. 2020;52:1587–606.
61. Feng Y, Huang R, He Y, et al. Efficacy of physical examination, ultrasound, and ultrasound combined with fine needle aspiration for axillary staging a primary breast cancer. Breast Cancer Res Treat. 2015;149:761–5.
62. National Comprehensive Cancer Network. NCCN clinical guidelines in oncology. Breast cancer. Version 5.2020. NCCN.org.
63. Smith IE, Dowsett M, Ebbs SR, et al. Neoadjuvant treatment of postmenopausal breast cancer with anastrozole, tamoxifen or both in combination. The immediate preoperative anastrozole, tamoxifen or combined with tamoxifen (IMPACT) or multicenter double-blind randomized trial. J Clin Oncol. 2005;23:5 108-5116.
64. Pease AM, Riba LA, Gruner RA, et al. OncotypeDx recurrence score as a predictor of response to neoadjuvant chemotherapy. Ann Surg Oncol. 2019;26:366–71.
65. Le-Petross HT, Christofanilli M, Carkaci S, Krishnamurthy S, et al. MRI features of inflammatory breast cancer. Am J Roentgenol. 2011;197:W769–76.
66. Masuda N, Lee SJ, Ohtani S, et al. Adjuvant capecitabine for breast cancer after preoperative chemotherapy. N Engl J Med. 2017;376:214 7-2159.
67. von Minckwitz G, Huang CS, Mano MS, et al. Trastuzumab emtansine for residual invasive her 2 positive breast cancer. N Engl J Med. 2019;380:617–28.
68. Mamtani A, Barrio AV, King TA, et al. How often does neoadjuvant chemotherapy avoid axillary dissection and patients with histologically confirm nodal metastases question results of a prospective study. Ann Surg Oncol. 2016;23:3467.
69. Soran A, Brufsky A, Gimbel M, Diego E. Breast cancer diagnosis, treatment and follow-up during COVID-19 pandemic. Eur J Breast Health. 2020;16(2):86–8.
70. Lips EH, Mukhtar RA, Yau C, et al. Lobular histology and response to neoadjuvant chemotherapy in invasive breast cancer. Breast Cancer Res Treat. 2012;136:35–43.
71. Bonadonna G, Veronisi U, Brambilli C, et al. Primary chemotherapy to avoid mastectomy in tumors with diameters of three cm or more. J Natl Cancer Inst. 1990;82:1539–45.
72. NCCN Clinical practice guidelines in oncology. Genetic/familial guidelines for genetic/familial high-risk assessment: breast and ovarian. Version 5.2020. NCCN.org.
73. Fernandez-Martinez A, Krop IE, Hillman DW, et al. Survival, pathologic response and genomics in CALGB 00601 (Alliance), a neoadjuvant phase III trial of paclitaxel-trastuzumab with or without lapatinib in HER2 positive breast cancer. J Clin Oncol. 2020;38:4184–93.
74. CompassHER2-pCR: decreasing chemotherapy for breast cancer patients after pre-surgery chemo and targeted therapy. ClinicalTrials.gov Identifier: NCT04266249.
75. CompassHER2 RD trial: T-DM1 and Tucatinib compared with T-DM1 alone in preventing relapses in people with high risk HER2-positive breast cancer. ClinicalTrials.gov Identifier: NCT04457596.
76. Tolaney SM, Barry WT, Dang CT, Yardley DA, Moy D, et al. Adjuvant paclitaxel and trastuzumab for node negative HER2 positive breast cancer. N Engl J Med. 2015;372(2):134–41
77. Liedtke C, Mazouni C, Hess KR, et al. Response to neoadjuvant therapy and long-term survival in patients with triple negative breast cancer. J Clin Oncol. 2008;26:1275.

Chapter 15
Ongoing Clinical Studies and Future Directions

Azadeh Nasrazadani, Juan Luis Gomez Marti, Tara Hyder, Vikram Gorantla, and Adam M. Brufsky

Introduction

The philosophy of the neoadjuvant approach can be traced back to NSABP B-18 [1] and 27 [2], which demonstrated that neoadjuvant therapy reduces the size of breast tumors and decreases incidence of positive nodes at time of surgery. Logical application of the neoadjuvant approach was to downsize the primary and axilla to improve surgical outcomes and reduce morbidity, especially in cancers that were deemed chemosensitive. As understanding and practice of neoadjuvant approach and outcomes grew, so did our realization of the implications of the in vivo response to neoadjuvant treatment vis-à-vis pathologic complete response as a marker of prognosis and surrogate marker for overall survival. Trials evaluating adjuvant therapies for non-responders showed benefit which led to the approval of adjuvant therapy to improve outcomes. These reasons have made the neoadjuvant paradigm an attractive option, allowing for a personalized approach to escalation and de-escalation of care.

Juan Luis Gomez Marti and Tara Hyder contributed equally with all other contributors.

A. Nasrazadani · A. M. Brufsky (✉)
University of Pittsburgh Physicians, Pittsburgh, PA, USA

UPMC Hillman Cancer Center, Magee Women's Hospital, Pittsburgh, PA, USA
e-mail: nasrazadania2@upmc.edu; brufskyam@upmc.edu

J. L. G. Marti · V. Gorantla
Department of Pathology, University of Pittsburgh School of Medicine, Pittsburgh, PA, USA
e-mail: jug59@pitt.edu; gorantlavc2@upmc.edu

T. Hyder
University of Pittsburgh Physicians, Pittsburgh, PA, USA
e-mail: hydert@upmc.edu

A. Soran, F. Nakhlis (eds.), *Management of the Breast and Axilla in the Neoadjuvant Setting*, https://doi.org/10.1007/978-3-030-88020-0_15

Key ongoing trials in this arena are summarized in the following sections and provide insight into the direction toward which the field is moving. Table 15.1 lists details central to study design for all described studies herein.

Hormone-Receptor-Positive Breast Cancer

While neoadjuvant chemotherapy (NAC) is commonly utilized for purposes of tumor shrinkage and downstaging, the role of neoadjuvant endocrine therapy (NET) is less clear. Strongly, estrogen receptor (ER) positive tumors are thought to be prime examples with potential for response to NET in an overall attempt to avoid or reduce need for more toxic therapies. Identification of appropriate cases, however, is key, and in the setting of NET, has led to the development of the preoperative endocrine prognostic index (PEPI). PEPI incorporates recurrence-free survival (RFS) associated factors, including pathological tumor size, pathological node status, clinical response (complete plus partial clinical response vs. stable disease plus progressive disease), surgical specimen ER status (Allred score ≥3 vs. 0 or 2), histological grade (grade 1 vs. grade 2/3), and the Ki-67 level. Validated by the

Table 15.1 Summary of ongoing breast cancer trials in the neoadjuvant setting

ClinicalTrials.gov Number identifier	Number of patients	Phase	Treatment arms	Primary endpoint
Hormone-receptor-positive				
NCT01953588 (alternate)	$N = 1473$	3	Arm 1: Anastrazole Arm 2: Fulvestrant Arm 3: Anastrazole +fulvestrant	1. Rate of endocrine-resistant disease 2. pCR 3. RFS
NCT02206984	$N = 170$	2	Arm 1: Tamoxifen Arm 2: Anastrazole Arm 3: Fulvestrant	Ki-67 level changes from baseline to post-treatment in ILC patients
NCT03969121	$N = 200$	3	Arm 1: Placebo+tamoxifen+leuprorelin or goserelin (postmenopausal also receive letrozole) Arm 2: Palbociclib+tamoxifen+leuprorelin or goserelin (postmenopausal also receive letrozole)	1. PEPI score 2. EndoPredict EPclin score
NCT03447132 (SAFIA)	$N = 400$	3	Arm 1: Placebo+fulvestrant+goserelin Arm 2: Palbociclib+fulvestrant+goserelin	pCR

Table 15.1 (continued)

ClinicalTrials.gov Number identifier	Number of patients	Phase	Treatment arms	Primary endpoint
NCT03628066 (NSABP FB-13)	*N* = 24	2	Premenopausal women divided into 2 cohorts based on baseline breast recurrence score (RS) (cohort 1: RS < 11 or cohort 2: RS 11–26) Both cohorts receive letrozole+palbociclib+goserelin for 6 weeks If core-cut biopsy at 6 weeks has a Ki67 <10% then continue study therapy. If Ki67 ≥10%, then begin neoadjuvant chemotherapy or surgery	Percentage of patients with Ki67 < 2.7%
NCT02764541 (PELOPS)	*N* = 195	2	Premenopausal women with IDC or ILC. Arm 1: Tamoxifen +endocrine therapy Arm 2: Letrozole + endocrine therapy Arm 3: Tamoxifen + endocrine therapy + palbociclib Arm 4: Letrozole + endocrine therapy + palbociclib	1. Ki67 changes from baseline to day 15 2. Residual cancer burden
NCT04109066 (Checkmate 7FL)	*N* = 1200	3	Arm 1: Placebo + neoadjuvant chemotherapy → surgery → placebo + adjuvant endocrine therapy Arm 2: Nivolumab + neoadjuvant chemotherapy → surgery → nivolumab + adjuvant endocrine therapy	1. pCR 2. EFS
NCT03725059 (KEYNOTE-756)	*N* = 1140	3	Arm 1: Placebo + neoadjuvant chemotherapy → surgery → placebo + adjuvant endocrine therapy Arm 2: Pembrolizumab + neoadjuvant chemotherapy → surgery → nivolumab + adjuvant endocrine therapy	1. pCR 2. EFS
HER2 positive breast cancer				
NCT01996267 (TRAIN-2)	*N* = 437	3	Arm 1: Fluorouracil + epirubicin +cyclophosphamide + trastuzumab + pertuzumab Arm 2: Paclitaxel + trastuzumab + carboplatin + pertuzumab	pCR

(continued)

Table 15.1 (continued)

ClinicalTrials.gov Number identifier	Number of patients	Phase	Treatment arms	Primary endpoint
NCT02003209	$N = 312$	3	Arm 1: Docetaxel + carboplatin + trastuzumab + pertuzumab → surgery + radiation → trastuzumab Arm 2: Docetaxel + carboplatin + trastuzumab + pertuzumab + (premenopausal receive goserelin + AI and postmenopausal receive AI) → surgery + radiation → trastuzumab	pCR
NCT04425018 (MARGOT)	$N = 171$	2	Arm 1: Paclitaxel + pertuzumab + margetuximab Arm 2: Paclitaxel + pertuzumab + trastuzumab	pCR
NCT04553770	$N = 88$	2	Arm 1: Trastuzumab deruxtecan Arm 2: Trastuzumab deruxtecan + anastrazole	pCR
NCT03595592 (APTneo)	$N = 650$	3	Arm 1: Trastuzumab + pertuzumab + carboplatin + paclitaxel → surgery → trastuzumab + pertuzumab Arm 2: Doxorubicin + cyclophosphamide + atezolizumab→ trastuzumab + pertuzumab + carboplatin + paclitaxel → surgery → trastuzumab + pertuzumab + atezolizumab Arm 3: Trastuzumab + pertuzumab + carboplatin + paclitaxel + atezolizumab → surgery → trastuzumab + pertuzumab + atezolizumab	EFS
NCT03726879 (IMpassion050)	$N = 453$	3	Arm 1: Atezolizumab + doxorubicin cyclophosphamide → atezolizumab + paclitaxel + trastuzumab + pertuzumab → surgery → pertuzumab + atezolizumab Arm 2: Placebo + doxorubicin cyclophosphamide →placebo + paclitaxel + trastuzumab + pertuzumab → surgery → placebo + pertuzumab + trastuzumab	pCR

Table 15.1 (continued)

ClinicalTrials.gov Number identifier	Number of patients	Phase	Treatment arms	Primary endpoint
NCT02061423	*N* = 7	1	HER2 pulsed dendritic cell vaccine	1. Compliance 2. Treatment related adverse events
Triple negative				
NCT02425891 (IMpassion130)	*N* = 900	3	Arm 1: Atezolizumab + nab-paclitaxel Arm 2: Placebo + nab-paclitaxel	1. PFS in all randomized participants 2. PFS in participants with detectable PD-L1 3. OS in all randomized participants 4. OS in participants with detectable PD-L1
NCT03036488 (KEYNOTE 522)	*N* = 1174	3	Arm 1: Pembrolizumab + chemotherapy → surgery → pembrolizumab Arm 2: Placebo + chemotherapy → surgery → placebo	1. pCR 2. EFS
NCT03281954 (NSABP B-59/ GBG 96-GeparDouze)	*N* = 1520	3	Arm 1: Placebo → surgery → placebo Arm 2: Atezolizumab → surgery →: Atezolizumab	1. pCR 2. EFS
NCT02620280 (NeoTRIPaPDL1)	*N* = 278	3	Arm 1: Carboplatin + abraxane → surgery → chemotherapy Arm 2: Carboplatin + abraxane + atezolizumab → surgery → chemotherapy	EFS
NCT03150576 (PARTNER)	*N* = 527	2/3	Arm 1: Paclitaxel + carboplatin Arm 2: Paclitaxel + carboplatin + olaparib	1. Treatment-related adverse events 2. pCR 3. Completion rate

(continued)

Table 15.1 (continued)

ClinicalTrials.gov Number identifier	Number of patients	Phase	Treatment arms	Primary endpoint
NCT01057069 (neo-TN)	$N = 310$	2/3	Arm 1: HRD positive tumors: ddAC × 4 cycles + tCTC × 2 cycles Arm 2: HRD positive tumors: ddAC × 3 cycles → carboplatin + paclitaxel × 3 cycles Arm 3: Non-HRD positive tumors: ddAC × 3 cycles →unfavorable response → carboplatin + paclitaxel × 3 cycles Arm 4: Non-HRD positive tumors: ddAC × 3 cycles → favorable response → ddAC × 3 cycles Arm 5: Non-HRD positive tumors: ddAC × 3 cycles → favorable response → carboplatin + paclitaxel × 3 cycles	1. HRD tumors: Average NRI after intensified alkylating therapy in comparison to that after 'standard' neoadjuvant chemotherapy 2. Non-HRD tumor: NRI
NCT04230109 (NeoSTAR)	$N = 100$	2	Arm 1: Sacituzumab govitecan Arm 2: Sacituzumab govitecan + pembrolizumab	pCR
Surgical management and de-escalation				
NCT03820063 (TRAIN-3)	$N = 462$	NA	Paclitaxel + trastuzumab + carboplatin + pertuzumab × 3 or 6 cycles based on rCR → surgery	3-year EFS
NCT04301375 (ELPIS)	$N = 27$	NA	Paclitaxel + trastuzumab + pertuzumab → if achieve pCR, then no surgery; if do not achieve pCR, then surgery	3-year loco-regional DFS
NCT04289935 (VISION-I)	$N = 420$	NA	Neoadjuvant treatment → vacuum assisted biopsy	Sensitivity [proportion of true positive patients (non pCR by both VAB and surgery) given patients with non pCR assessed using surgical specimen]
NCT02800317 (RISAS)	$N = 248$	NA	RISAS → axillary lymph node dissection	1. Sensitivity of RISAS for identifying axillary pCR 2. NPV of RISAS for identifying axillary pCR 3. FNR of RISAS for identifying axillary pCR

Table 15.1 (continued)

ClinicalTrials.gov Number identifier	Number of patients	Phase	Treatment arms	Primary endpoint
NCT04109079 (ATNEC)	$N = 1900$	NA	Arm 1: Axillary treatment (axillary lymph node dissection or axillary radiotherapy) Arm 2: No axillary treatment (axillary lymph node dissection or axillary radiotherapy)	1. DFS 2. Patient reported lymphedema
NCT01901094 (Alliance A01120)	$N = 1660$	3	Arm 1: Axillary lymph node dissection + nodal radiation therapy Arm 2: Axillary radiation + nodal radiation therapy	RFS
NCT01872975 (NSABP B-51)	$N = 1636$	3	Arm 1: Participants with lumpectomy: No regional nodal XRT with WBI Arm 2: Participants with mastectomy: No regional nodal or chest wall XRT Arm 3: Participants with lumpectomy: Regional nodal XRT with WBI Arm 4: Participants with mastectomy: Regional nodal XRT and chest wall XRT	RFS
Novel strategies				
NCT03357120 (ALIENOR)	$N = 180$	NA	Neoadjuvant chemotherapy → surgery → ctDNA mutations analysis post-surgery and then every 6 months for 5 years	Prognostic value of ctDNA mutations on 3-year RFS
I-SPY2	NA	2	Multiple standard or intervention arms used to assess novel agents	1. pCR 2. EFS 3. Distant recurrence-free survival

AI aromatase inhibitor, *ddAC* dose-dense doxorubicin + cyclophosphamide, *DFS* disease-free survival, *EFS* event-free survival, *FNR* false negative rate, *HRD* homologous recombination defect, *IDC* infiltrating ductal carcinoma, *ILC* infiltrating lobular carcinoma, *NPV* negative predictive value, *NRI* neoadjuvant response index, *pCR* pathological complete response, *PEPI* preoperative endocrine prognostic index, *PFS* progression-free survival, *rCR* radiologic complete response, *RFS* recurrence-free survival, *WBI* whole breast irradiation, *XRT* external radiotherapy

IMPACT trial, the risk of relapse is then correlated to scores of 0, 1–3, and ≥4 corresponding to 10, 23, and 48%, respectively [3]. A score of 0 effectively identifies a very low risk population, where NAC can effectively be omitted. The benefit of NET with regard to long term outcomes based on utilization of this index is yet unknown, prompting trial design incorporating PEPI and other biomarkers, namely, Ki-67 to understand this.

ALTERNATE follows suit of assessing tumor response to NET utilizing Ki-67 levels more or less than 10% as a surrogate to identify ER+, HER2- cases more likely to require more aggressive therapies, including chemotherapy, while further evaluating endocrine-sensitive disease rates (ESDR) in cases continuing with NET [4]. ESDR is derived as a proportion of cases with a modified PEPI (mPEPI) of 0 at time of surgery (defined as pT1–2, pN0, and Ki-67 <2.7%, or achieving a pathologic complete response (pCR)). Between groups treated with neoadjuvant anastrozole, fulvestrant, or both, no discernable differences were reported in ESDR or rate of breast-conserving surgeries, although RFS data is lacking at this time [5]. As compared to historical data from similar cohorts not receiving NET, RFS from these studies will clarify whether there is an added benefit to this approach in lieu of current practices employing endocrine therapy in the adjuvant setting alone.

Among pathologic factors appreciated for a heightened response to endocrine therapy, lobular histology tumors are consistently found to be more frequently hormone-receptor-positive (HR+) with a less robust response to neoadjuvant chemotherapy as compared to invasive ductal carcinomas [6]. Collectively, this signals a preferential response to endocrine therapy (ET), which is further being explored in a phase II study (NCT02206984), exclusively investigating the change in Ki-67 levels in invasive lobular carcinomas (ILC) after neoadjuvant therapy with either tamoxifen, anastrozole, or fulvestrant. Meaningful decreases in Ki-67 levels consequent to NET may lead to changes in the clinical approach to ILC, which currently follows standard of care algorithms, utilized irrespective of histology.

The synergistic role of combination CDK4/6 inhibition and ET has cemented this relatively new treatment paradigm in the management of metastatic HR+, HER2- patients. Building on the successes achieved with CDK4/6 inhibitors (CDKIs) in this setting, PALLET [7] and neoMonarch [8] phase II trials independently demonstrated that the addition of a CDK4/6 (ribociclib or abemaciclib, respectively) to ET in the neoadjuvant setting led to enhanced decreases in Ki-67 levels status after a short course of treatment, although in PALLET, no difference in clinical response was observed. A phase III trial (NCT03969121) is currently underway that continues to investigate the benefit of CDK4/6 inhibition (utilizing palbociclib) in combination with ET and will compare PEPI and EndoPredict EPclin scores to assess efficacy. In contrast, the phase III SAFIA trial will include patients on the basis of oncotype dx RS < 31 to investigate the efficacy with regard to pCR upon addition of palbociclib to fulvestrant +/− goserelin (in pre- and peri-menopausal patients; NCT03447132) [9]. Similarly, NSABP FB-13 seeks to expand on PALLET in premenopausal patients with the addition of goserelin to letrozole and palbociclib in an effort to identify patients that achieve Ki-67 <10% as appropriate candidates to continue NET where NAC can safely be omitted [10]. PELOPS is an ongoing phase II trial that specifically enriches for ILC patients and compares fold changes in Ki-67 and pCR in cohorts given neoadjuvant tamoxifen vs. letrozole +/− palbociclib. While cohorts are not stratified by histology (lobular vs. ductal) in PELOPS, emphasis on recruitment of ILC patients ensures more generalizable findings in this sizable subpopulation.

Given advances achieved with immunotherapy (IO) in triple negative breast cancer (TNBC), multiple studies continue to investigate whether IO has a place in the management of HR+ patients. Checkmate 7FL is a phase III study utilizing nivolumab in high-risk ER+, HER2- patients in the neoadjuvant setting vs. placebo in combination with paclitaxel, then an anthracycline plus cyclophosphamide, and continuation of IO vs. placebo with standard ET in the adjuvant setting [11]. Planned primary endpoints include pCR and event-free survival (EFS) rates. Keynote 756 follows a similar design also in high-risk patients, although utilizing pembrolizumab [12]. Interim analysis of these studies has not yet been performed.

HER2-Positive Breast Cancer

Neoadjuvant chemotherapy constitutes the standard of care for stage II-III HER2+ early breast cancer with efficacy largely determined by pCR rates which reliably correlate with patient outcomes [13] as well as influence of adjuvant management. Current guidelines encourage the use of dual HER2 blocking agents, trastuzumab and pertuzumab (HP), with chemotherapy [14, 15]; preferably a taxane and carboplatin [16]. In the adjuvant setting, presence of a single HER2 blocking agent (trastuzumab) combined with carboplatin and taxane regimens have similar efficacy and reduced toxicity as compared to the combination with an anthracycline and taxane [17]. Given significant improvements noted in pCR with dual HER2 blockade [13], TRYPHAENA went on to demonstrate that the combination of trastuzumab and pertuzumab together with an anthracycline was not associated with increased cardiac toxicity when compared to non-anthracycline dual HER2 blockade in the neoadjuvant setting [18]. With the apparent absence of added cardiac toxicity when incorporating anthracyclines to HER2-directed regimens, TRAIN-2 continues to evaluate the combination of epirubicin with trastuzumab and pertuzumab (NCT01996267). TRAIN-2 trial is a phase III, multicenter, open label, randomized study that compares pCR rates between anthracycline- and non-anthracycline-treated cohorts with largely non-significant findings to date. Toxicity has been notably higher in the anthracycline group with higher rates of grade 4 febrile neutropenia (18% vs. 6%, respectively), arguing for the omission of anthracyclines during neoadjuvant therapy, although long-term data is pending [15].

The benefit of chemotherapy and HER2-directed therapy in the neoadjuvant setting is clear with regards to prognosis prediction. In cases of triple positive disease (HR+, HER2+), however, timing of ET is not well defined. The combination of chemotherapy and HER2-directed therapy achieves high pCR rates in HR-, HER2+ patients, although this has consistently been found to be comparatively lower in HR+, HER2+ patients [13, 17, 19–21], suggesting resistant mechanisms more likely to benefit from endocrine therapies and alternative pathways.

The addition of endocrine therapy to HER2-directed therapies in the metastatic and adjuvant settings has been clearly associated with improved outcomes [22, 23,

24]. However, data is lacking in the neoadjuvant setting. In a small study evaluating neoadjuvant HER2-directed targeted therapies without chemotherapy, a 21% pCR rate was seen in ER+ patients in which letrozole was also given, compared to 36% pCR in the ER- group [25].

Similarly, in PerELISA, chemotherapy was omitted in "molecular responder" triple positive cases in which Ki-67 was relatively reduced by at least 20% after a 2-week neoadjuvant treatment of letrozole. pCR was seen in 20.5% after patients continued to receive 5 cycles of HP prior to undergoing definitive surgery [26]. In an ongoing phase III randomized trial, estrogen deprivation therapy (goserlin acetate) and an aromatase inhibitor (AI) will be added in premenopausal patients with AI added alone to postmenopausal HR+ patients receiving standard of care docetaxel, carboplatin, and HP (TCHP). This study will elucidate the added benefit of ET in the neoadjuvant setting for triple positive disease (NCT02003209). Of note, the ADAPT protocol (NCT01745965) previously evaluated the efficacy of T-DM1 with or without standard ET, compared to trastuzumab with ET. While a significantly higher pCR rate was reported for TDM-1 with or without ET compared to the trastuzumab arm, the addition of ET did not appear to have a significant added benefit [27].

Further challenging the standard TCHP regimen is the Neopeaks study, which is a randomized, neoadjuvant phase II study comparing TCHP to T-DM1 and pertuzumab (TDM1 + P), or TCHP followed by T-DM1 and pertuzumab (T-DM1 + P) in both HR+ and HR- patients. Superior pCR rates were achieved with the T-DM1 + P cohort that was notably more prominent among ER+ groups (69% vs. 43.3% pCR rates in TCHP-T-DM1 + P vs. TCHP alone, respectively, $p = 0.047$). Differences were not significant between groups among patients with ER- disease [28]. Altogether, the aforementioned findings indicate that HR+/HER2+ patients may benefit from a modified approach to traditional regimens.

As the role of T-DM1 continues to expand, particularly after KATHERINE [29], Margetuximab is highlighted as another emerging antibody-drug conjugate, which displays enhanced antibody-dependent cell-mediated cytotoxicity (ADCC). Margetuximab is thought to have a higher affinity for both alleles of the Fc receptor CD16A, having shown increased PFS as compared to trastuzumab in advanced HER2-positive BC [30, 31]. In an early phase I study evaluating margetuximab in HER2+ solid tumors where no standard therapy was available, tumor reductions occurred in over half of response-evaluable patients with breast cancer. In addition, analysis of peripheral blood mononuclear cells showed that margetuximab enhanced antibody-dependent cell-mediated cytotoxicity (ADCC), as compared to trastuzumab [32]. The currently recruiting phase II trial (MARGOT, MARGetuximab Or Trastuzumab, NCT04425018) will evaluate pCR rates after treatment with paclitaxel, pertuzumab, and margetuximab (TMP); or paclitaxel, pertuzumab, and trastuzumab (THP), in patients with stage II-III HER2+ breast cancer. Patients will be followed for 10 years after surgery, with some candidates receiving margetuximab for a year post-surgery if response to 12-week treatment is acceptable [33].

On the heels of promising findings reported from another novel HER2-directed agent, trastuzumab-deruxtecan, in DESTINY-Breast 01 in metastatic patients [34], a newly recruiting phase II study (NCT04553770) aims to explore the role of trastuzumab-deruxtecan with or without anastrozole specifically in HER2 low, HR+ patients in the front-line neoadjuvant setting.

The addition of PD-L1 inhibitors to promote adaptive T-cell antitumor activity constitutes a novel approach that has been encouraged by prior experimental and clinical evidence. In HER2+ disease, presence of intratumoral PD-L1 serves as an independent poor prognostic marker of disease-free survival (HR = 1.866, $p = 0.001$), with lower expression of PD-1 among tumor-infiltrating lymphocytes (TILs; $p = 0.011$) [35]. However, recent studies suggest that trastuzumab increases adaptive antitumor immunity, which is further facilitated by anti-CTLA-4 antibodies [36, 37], ultimately leading to the development of the APTneo trial (NCT03595592). This is a phase III, randomized, open-label study that will combine trastuzumab, pertuzumab, carboplatin, and paclitaxel with or without atezolizumab in women with early high-risk and locally advanced HER2+ disease who are suitable for neoadjuvant therapy. The primary outcome will be EFS; whereas, the secondary outcomes will include pCR, clinical objective response (COR), distant event-free survival (DEFS), OS, and adverse events. Of note, the phase II KATE2 trial (NCT02924883) previously evaluated the role of atezolizumab in combination with trastuzumab in the metastatic setting, which did not demonstrate a significant difference in PFS and was stopped due to futility and elevated frequency of adverse events among patients receiving atezolizumab [38]. Despite the discouraging results of KATE2, it remains to be elucidated if the APTneo trial will provide more promise.

Impassion050 (NCT03726879) will similarly evaluate the efficacy and safety of atezolizumab in patients with early HER2+ breast cancer. Patients will be given atezolizumab in combination with dose-dense doxorubicin plus cyclophosphamide, followed by paclitaxel plus trastuzumab plus pertuzumab. The primary outcome is the percentage of pCR among the PD-L1-positive population. Secondary outcomes will include pCR among PD-L1 negative population, pCR based on HR status, and OS.

Dendritic cell vaccines constitute a different avenue to overcome HER2 therapy resistance. HER-2 peptide-pulse dendritic cell type 1 (DC1) specifically promotes T-cell responses against HER2, which is manipulated by a strategy termed *Immune.*

Conditioning via *Activated Innate (autologous) Transfer* (ICAIT). Briefly, ICAIT consists of rapidly activating immature $CD14^{+}$ peripheral blood monocytes into fully functional DCs in vitro. DCs are then pulsed with stimulatory molecules and peptide antigens based on the HER-2/neu sequence, which are then administered back into the patient's lymph nodes [39]. A currently active clinical trial (NCT02061423) is providing a pulse DC1 vaccine to high-risk HER2+ breast cancer patients with residual disease post neoadjuvant therapy. Primary outcomes assessed include participation, compliance, and occurrence of treatment-related adverse events, with immunogenicity and anti-HER2 immunity considered as secondary outcomes.

As HER2-directed therapies seem to be less effective against ER+ than ER- tumors, analysis of Th1-mediated cytokine response has also been studied. Interestingly, no significant differences in Th1 response have been found in blood after DC1 vaccination based on HR status, with or without antiestrogen therapy. Nonetheless, the anti-HER2 Th1 response is higher in ER+ patients treated with anti-HER2 vaccination and antiestrogen therapy, compared to those not treated with antiestrogen therapies. These results were very similar in terms of pCR. Patients with ER+ disease who were vaccinated and treated with antiestrogen therapy had a similar pCR to those with ER- disease (28.6% vs. 31.4%), but significantly higher pCR than those who did not receive anti-estrogen therapy (4%, $p = 0.03$). These results encourage the development of further studies in the neoadjuvant setting [40].

Triple Negative Breast Cancer

Triple negative breast cancer is an active area of research given its comparatively aggressive natural history with no clear biomarkers. Despite the lack of targeted therapies for this patient population, immunotherapy has been found to be uniquely effective. Furthermore, TNBC patients have a higher propensity to harbor BRCA1/2 mutations, which suggests they may exhibit a preferential response to inhibitors targeting the DNA damage repair pathway.

Impassion130 first established a role for immunotherapy in the management of metastatic TNBC. The addition of atezolizumab to paclitaxel in the first-line metastatic setting demonstrated prolonged PFS and a trend for improved OS [41]. NSABP B-59/GBG 96-GeparDouze and NeoTRIPaPDL1 are phase III trials that seek to explore the benefit of atezolizumab in the neoadjuvant setting and notably stratify patients based on PDL1 status. Impassion031 similarly incorporates atezolizumab in the intervention arm with primary analysis demonstrating higher pCR, with the addition of atezolizumab to NAC (57.6% vs. 41.1%; Δ16.5%; 5.9, 27.1; 1-sided $P = 0.0044$) that appears numerically more enhanced in the PDL1-positive cohort (68.8% vs. 49.3%; Δ19.5%; 4.2, 34.8; 1-sided $P = 0.021$, not significant) [42]. The addition of pembrolizumab vs. placebo to NAC, as opposed to atezolizumab, has heralded comparable findings in Keynote-522. At first interim analysis, 64.8% of patients in the pembrolizumab-chemotherapy arm had achieved pCR as compared to 51.2% in the placebo-chemotherapy arm (95% CI, 5.4 to 21.3; $P < 0.001$) [43].

Overlapping molecular features of TNBC and BRCA1/2 mutated tumors have encouraged incorporation of PARP inhibitors in TNBC study designs, which preferentially impact tumors with underlying deficiencies in homologous DNA repair. The addition of veliparib to a platinum containing neoadjuvant regimen did not enhance pCR rates in BrighTNess [44], although multiple trials continue to expand on this central supposition. PARTNER incorporates Olaparib in a platinum containing NAC regimen specifically in basal type TNBC or patients with germline BRCA mutations. Neo-TN (NCT01057069), on the other hand, focuses on whether a more intensified NAC regimen with regard to alkylating agent use will lead to improved responses in tumors with homologous repair-deficient (HRD) tumors.

Finally, sacituzumab govitecan (SG) is a novel antibody-drug conjugate which delivers a topoisomerase 1 inhibitor SN-38 containing the active metabolite of irinotecan, coupled to a humanized monoclonal antibody directed toward tumor antigen Trop-2. SG was recently found to significantly extend OS in the third-line metastatic setting [45] in TNBC and is now being evaluated in the neoadjuvant setting in NeoSTAR (NCT04230109).

Surgical Management and De-Escalation

Early-stage breast cancer patients boast exceptionally high 5-year and 10-year survival and recurrence-free survival rates, which is especially striking compared to most other solid tumors. High success rates status post-multi-modality treatment is largely a function of aggressive therapies that reflect decades of clinical trials. It is becoming increasingly apparent that not all patients benefit equally from the extent of standard of care therapies that are recommended. As a result, multiple trials have been developed to better decipher those patients in whom de-escalation of therapy can be considered.

TRAIN-3 approaches de-escalation in patients with early stage HER2+ disease with the intent of minimizing preoperative chemotherapy. In this single arm, multicenter study, patients that achieve radiologic complete response (rCR) after either cycle 3 or 6 of neoadjuvant therapy, including paclitaxel, trastuzumab, carboplatin, and pertuzumab, may undergo early surgery. The primary endpoint will be 3-year EFS, results of which may encourage further trial design to minimize need for toxic therapies [46].

In the ELPIS study, a prospective, single arm, open-label, unicenter, exploratory study in women with primary operable HER2-enriched breast cancer achieving a complete response following standard anti-HER2-based neoadjuvant therapy with paclitaxel/trastuzumab/pertuzumab, omission of surgery and sentinel lymph node dissection will be evaluated. The primary objective will be to estimate the 3-year locoregional invasive DFS of patients who achieve a pCR based on imaging and stereotactic biopsy, with the intention of omitting loco-regional surgery. The experimental arm will omit surgery, and the no intervention will include surgery. Both arms will be treated with paclitaxel, trastuzumab, and pertuzumab for 5 cycles. If no invasive tumor cells and no in situ disease are identified in the stereotactic biopsy, patients may be able to omit surgery. In addition, trastuzumab and pertuzumab will be continued to complete 1 year of treatment and adjuvant endocrine therapy will be indicated according to hormonal receptor status by immunohistochemistry [47].

While the prospect of forgoing invasive surgery offers great appeal, the risk of encountering a false negative should be acknowledged, which, if present, may deny the patient the opportunity to receive adjuvant T-DM1 as per KATHERINE trial [26]. Thus, accurate interpretation of pCR is paramount. VISION-I (NCT04289935) utilizes a novel technique of vacuum-assisted biopsy (VAB) to more accurately assess for residual tumor status post-neoadjuvant therapy. VAB offers the advantages of a core needle biopsy with the added benefit of using a single insertion line from where multiple samples—including from the tumor center—can be cut and suctioned [48]. The sensitivity of VAB will be compared to regular surgery in assessing pCR status.

Further complicating surgical management in the setting of neoadjuvant therapy is the question of adequate lymph node interrogation and intervention. In this regard, the RISAS study (NCT02800317) investigates the ability of radioactive iodine seeds to predict detection of axillary pCR [49]. The novel procedure contains radioactive iodine seed placement to the axilla prior to initiation of neoadjuvant chemotherapy. The primary outcome of the study is to identify the sensitivity, negative predictive value (NPV), and false negative rate (FNR) of the procedure for detecting axillary pCR. Moving forward, axillary node dissection may be omitted with higher levels of confidence utilizing this technique in the event this procedure is found to predict axillary pCR with high accuracy.

In the phase III British ATNEC study (NCT04109079), axillary radiotherapy in lieu of axillary lymph node dissection is considered for patients with axillary nodal disease present prior to NAC with no evidence of residual axillary disease post NAC. The authors hypothesize that this approach is non-inferior to axillary treatment in terms of DFS and 5-year development of lymphedema, although this remains to be seen. Alliance A011202 (NCT01901094) addresses a similar question, although aims to evaluate whether axillary and regional radiation therapy alone is non-inferior to radiation in addition to axillary lymph node dissection (ALND) in patients with a positive sentinel lymph node biopsy (SLNB) after administration of standard of care neoadjuvant chemotherapy. In contrast, NSABP B-51 (NCT01872975) considers the possibility of radiotherapy omission in breast cancer patients known to be node positive (N1) prior to neoadjuvant chemotherapy that are found to be pathologically node negative (ypN0) at time of surgery. Patients undergoing mastectomy will be randomized to either receive chest wall and regional nodal radiotherapy or no radiation therapy, and patients undergoing breast-conserving surgery will receive whole breast irradiation either with or without regional nodal radiotherapy. Invasive breast cancer recurrence-free interval (IBCR-FI) will be evaluated as the primary outcome of interest and determine to what extent radiotherapy contributes to outcomes in this clinical scenario [50].

Novel Strategies

To provide highly sensitive tools that objectively identify the presence of pCR after neoadjuvant therapy, studies have evaluated the presence of residual circulating tumor DNA (ctDNA). Longitudinal analysis of residual ctDNA during and after neoadjuvant treatment has shown that decrease in patient-specific mutations as measured by ctDNA correlates with response to neoadjuvant therapy, with largest decreases in ctDNA concentration among patients achieving pCR [51]. A prospective, ctDNA collection study of women who received neoadjuvant therapy and surgery, or surgery followed by adjuvant chemotherapy for early breast cancer, irrespective of HER2 or HR status, found that detection of ctDNA during follow-up was associated with relapse (HR 25.2, $p < 0.001$). Furthermore, the presence of ctDNA at diagnosis correlated with RFS (HR 5.8, $p = 0.01$), and distant extracranial metastasis could be detected by ctDNA in 96% of cases [52].

To expand on the value of ctDNA testing, ALIENOR (NCT03357120) is a trial in recruitment stage that aims to assess the prognostic value of mutations in ctDNA. Specifically, samples are to be obtained from patients with invasive breast cancer treated with neoadjuvant chemotherapy who have not achieved a complete pathologic response. The study will perform ctDNA analysis from after surgery every 6 months for 5 years. The primary outcome of the study is to determine the prognostic value of the presence of ctDNA mutations on recurrence-free interval at 3 years. Secondary outcomes include OS and distant metastasis-free interval (DRFI) at 3 and 5 years.

Arguably the most novel strategy with regard to neoadjuvant therapy selection, however, remains to be the I-SPY trial model. In I-SPY 2, patients are classified by their molecular subtype, then randomized to a standard or intervention arm consisting of novel therapies and novel agent combination. The association of pCR with EFS and distant recurrence-free survival (DRFS) is evaluated with information providing real-time randomization of incoming patients to the trial. This multicenter study includes women with operable stage II-III BC who have not had prior surgery or systemic therapy, and whose primary tumor is >2.5 cm. Patients who are not ERBB2 negative/HR positive and have a low 70-gene assay score were excluded. While the rate of pCR varies by subtype, strong associations between achieving pCR and EFS/DRFS (overall HR 0.19, CI 0.12–0.31) have been reported with a median follow-up of 3.8 years, regardless of molecular subtype [53, 54]. I-SPY 2 embodies the goal of personalized medicine to provide patients with the most effective agent individualized in each case in the up-front neoadjuvant setting. Outcomes from individual therapy arms are not yet reported from this highly informative trial.

Future Directions

The management of breast cancer has become increasingly sophisticated and continues to evolve as reported interim and final analyses of the many active clinical trials guide and re-direct the path forward. Advances in patient outcomes with the emergence of multiple novel agents have led to innovative strategies, which challenge standard of care regimens by utilizing these agents in earlier lines and now neoadjuvant settings. Comparatively high survival rates appreciated by breast cancer patients additionally put clinicians in the unique position of considering de-escalation for the appropriate patient. Neoadjuvant endocrine therapy is a particularly attractive avenue in HR+ patients that may spare need for more cytotoxic therapies, although our understanding of predictors to response is still in its infancy. Ultimately, thoughtful trial design will be key in ensuring we can establish parameters for safe de-escalation that does not come at the expense of patient outcomes. The neoadjuvant setting is furthermore distinctly optimal for exploration of the role of molecular and cellular assays, which enhance our ability to provide more personalized care.

References

1. Fisher B, Brown A, Mamounas E, et al. Effect of preoperative chemotherapy on local-regional disease in women with operable breast cancer: findings from National Surgical Adjuvant Breast and Bowel Project B-18. J Clin Oncol. 1997;15(7):2483–93. https://doi.org/10.1200/JCO.1997.15.7.2483.
2. Rastogi P, Anderson SJ, Bear HD, et al. Preoperative chemotherapy: updates of National Surgical Adjuvant Breast and Bowel Project Protocols B-18 and B-27 [published correction appears in J Clin Oncol. 2008 Jun 1;26(16):2793]. J Clin Oncol. 2008;26(5):778–85. https://doi.org/10.1200/JCO.2007.15.0235.
3. Ellis MJ, Tao Y, Luo J, et al. Outcome prediction for estrogen receptor-positive breast cancer based on postneoadjuvant endocrine therapy tumor characteristics. J Natl Cancer Inst. 2008;100(19):1380–8. https://doi.org/10.1093/jnci/djn309.
4. Suman VJ, Ellis MJ, Ma CX. The ALTERNATE trial: assessing a biomarker driven strategy for the treatment of post-menopausal women with ER+/Her2- invasive breast cancer. Chin Clin Oncol. 2015;4(3):34. https://doi.org/10.3978/j.issn.2304-3865.2015.09.01.
5. Ma CX, Suman VJ, Leitch AM, et al. ALTERNATE: neoadjuvant endocrine treatment (NET) approaches for clinical stage II or III estrogen receptor-positive HER2-negative breast cancer (ER+ HER2- BC) in postmenopausal (PM) women: Alliance A011106. J Clin Oncol. 2020;38(15_suppl):504. https://doi.org/10.1200/JCO.2020.38.15_suppl.504.
6. Truin W, Vugts G, Roumen RM, et al. Differences in response and surgical management with neoadjuvant chemotherapy in invasive lobular versus ductal breast cancer. Ann Surg Oncol. 2016;23(1):51–7. https://doi.org/10.1245/s10434-015-4603-3.
7. Johnston S, Puhalla S, Wheatley D, et al. Randomized phase II study evaluating Palbociclib in addition to Letrozole as neoadjuvant therapy in estrogen receptor-positive early breast cancer: PALLET Trial. J Clin Oncol. 2019;37(3):178–89. https://doi.org/10.1200/JCO.18.01624.
8. Hurvitz SA, Martin M, Press MF, et al. Potent cell-cycle inhibition and upregulation of immune response with Abemaciclib and Anastrozole in neoMONARCH, phase II neoadjuvant study in $HR^{+}/HER2^{-}$ breast cancer. Clin Cancer Res. 2020;26(3):566–80. https://doi.org/10.1158/1078-0432.CCR-19-1425.
9. Al-Saleh KA, Bounedjar A, Oukkal M, et al. Prediction of response to neoadjuvant hormonal therapy (NAHT) using upfront oncotype Dx recurrence score (RS): results from the SAFIA phase III trial. J Clin Oncol. 2020;38(15_suppl):594. https://doi.org/10.1200/JCO.2020.38.15_suppl.594.
10. Puhalla S, Yothers G, Sing AP, Julian TB, Wolmark N, Jacobs SA. NSABP FB-13: An assessment of the biological and clinical effects of palbociclib with ovarian suppression and letrozole in the neoadjuvant treatment of pts (pts) with premenopausal (preM) estrogen-receptor positive/HER2-negative primary breast cancer [abstract]. Presented at the 2019 San Antonio Breast Cancer Symposium, San Antonio, TX, December 10–14, 2019. https://doi.org/10.1158/1538-7445.SABCS19-OT2-02-03.
11. Loi S, McArthur HL, Harbeck N, et al. A phase III trial of nivolumab with neoadjuvant chemotherapy and adjuvant endocrine therapy in ER+/HER2- primary breast cancer: CheckMate 7FL. J Clin Oncol. 2020;38(15_suppl):TPS604. https://doi.org/10.1200/JCO.2020.38.15_suppl.TPS604.

12. Cardoso F, Bardia A, Andre F, et al. KEYNOTE-756: randomized, double-blind, phase 3 study of pembrolizumab vs placebo combined with neoadjuvant chemotherapy and adjuvant endocrine therapy for high-risk, early-stage estrogen receptor–positive, human epidermal growth factor receptor 2–negative (ER+/HER2−) breast cancer. J Clin Oncol. 2019;37(15_suppl):TPS601. https://doi.org/10.1200/JCO.2019.37.15_suppl.TPS60.
13. Harbeck N. Emerging strategies in neoadjuvant treatment of patients with HER2-positive early breast cancer. Breast. 2019;48(Suppl 1):S97–S102. https://doi.org/10.1016/S0960-9776(19)31134-8.
14. Gianni L, Pienkowski T, Im YH, et al. 5-year analysis of neoadjuvant pertuzumab and trastuzumab in patients with locally advanced, inflammatory, or early-stage HER2-positive breast cancer (NeoSphere): a multicentre, open-label, phase 2 randomised trial. Lancet Oncol. 2016;17(6):791–800. https://doi.org/10.1016/S1470-2045(16)00163-7.
15. NCCN Clinical Practice Guidelines in Oncology. Breast Cancer. Version 6.2020. Available at: https://www.nccn.org/professionals/physician_gls/pdf/breast_blocks.pdf.
16. van Ramshorst MS, van der Voort A, van Werkhoven ED, et al. Neoadjuvant chemotherapy with or without anthracyclines in the presence of dual HER2 blockade for HER2-positive breast cancer (TRAIN-2): a multicentre, open-label, randomised, phase 3 trial. Lancet Oncol. 2018;19(12):1630–40. https://doi.org/10.1016/S1470-2045(18)30570-9.
17. Slamon DJ, Eiermann W, Robert NJ, et al. Ten year follow-up of BCIRG-006 comparing doxorubicin plus cyclophosphamide followed by docetaxel (AC→T) with doxorubicin plus cyclophosphamide followed by docetaxel and trastuzumab (AC→TH) with docetaxel, carboplatin and trastuzumab (TCH) in HER2+ early breast cancer. [abstract]. Presented at the 2015 San Antonio Breast Cancer Symposium, San Antonio, TX, December 8–12, 2015. https://doi.org/10.1158/1538-7445.SABCS15-S5-04.
18. Schneeweiss A, Chia S, Hickish T, et al. Pertuzumab plus trastuzumab in combination with standard neoadjuvant anthracycline-containing and anthracycline-free chemotherapy regimens in patients with HER2-positive early breast cancer: a randomized phase II cardiac safety study (TRYPHAENA). Ann Oncol. 2013;24(9):2278–84. https://doi.org/10.1093/annonc/mdt182.
19. Salgado R, Denkert C, Campbell C, et al. Tumor-infiltrating lymphocytes and associations with pathological complete response and event-free survival in her2-positive early-stage breast cancer treated with lapatinib and trastuzumab: a secondary analysis of the NeoALTTO Trial [published correction appears in JAMA Oncol. 2015 Jul;1(4):544] [published correction appears in JAMA Oncol. 2015 Nov;1(8):1172. Nucifero, Paolo [corrected to Nuciforo, Paolo]] [published correction appears in JAMA Oncol. 2019 Jan 1;5(1):122]. JAMA Oncol. 2015;1(4):448–54. https://doi.org/10.1001/jamaoncol.2015.0830.
20. Fernandez-Martinez A, Krop IE, Hillman DW, et al. Survival, pathologic response, and genomics in CALGB 40601 (Alliance), a neoadjuvant phase III trial of paclitaxel-trastuzumab with or without lapatinib in HER2-positive breast cancer. J Clin Oncol. 2020;38(35):4184–93. https://doi.org/10.1200/JCO.20.01276.
21. Campbell JI, Yau C, Krass P, et al. Comparison of residual cancer burden, American Joint Committee on Cancer staging and pathologic complete response in breast cancer after neoadjuvant chemotherapy: results from the I-SPY 1 TRIAL (CALGB 150007/150012; ACRIN 6657). Breast Cancer Res Treat. 2017;165(1):181–91. https://doi.org/10.1007/s10549-017-4303-8.
22. Kaufman B, Mackey JR, Clemens MR, et al. Trastuzumab plus anastrozole versus anastrozole alone for the treatment of postmenopausal women with human epidermal growth factor receptor 2-positive, hormone receptor-positive metastatic breast cancer: results from the randomized phase III TAnDEM study. J Clin Oncol. 2009;27(33):5529–37. https://doi.org/10.1200/JCO.2008.20.6847.
23. Montemurro F, Rossi V, Cossu Rocca M, et al. Hormone-receptor expression and activity of trastuzumab with chemotherapy in HER2-positive advanced breast cancer patients. Cancer. 2012;118(1):17–26. https://doi.org/10.1002/cncr.26162.

24. Tripathy D, Kaufman PA, Brufsky AM, et al. First-line treatment patterns and clinical outcomes in patients with HER2-positive and hormone receptor-positive metastatic breast cancer from registHER. Oncologist. 2013;18(5):501–10. https://doi.org/10.1634/theoncologist.2012-0414.
25. Rimawi MF, Mayer IA, Forero A, et al. Multicenter phase II study of neoadjuvant lapatinib and trastuzumab with hormonal therapy and without chemotherapy in patients with human epidermal growth factor receptor 2-overexpressing breast cancer: TBCRC 006. J Clin Oncol. 2013;31(14):1726–31. https://doi.org/10.1200/JCO.2012.44.8027.
26. Guarneri V, Dieci MV, Bisagni G, et al. De-escalated therapy for HR+/HER2+ breast cancer patients with Ki67 response after 2-week letrozole: results of the PerELISA neoadjuvant study. Ann Oncol. 2019;30(6):921–6. https://doi.org/10.1093/annonc/mdz055.
27. Harbeck N, Gluz O, Christgen M, et al. De-escalation strategies in Human Epidermal Growth Factor Receptor 2 (HER2)-positive early Breast Cancer (BC): final analysis of the West German Study Group adjuvant dynamic marker-adjusted personalized therapy trial optimizing risk assessment and therapy response prediction in early BC HER2- and hormone receptor-positive phase II randomized trial-efficacy, safety, and predictive markers for 12 weeks of neoadjuvant trastuzumab emtansine with or without Endocrine Therapy (ET) versus Trastuzumab Plus ET. J Clin Oncol. 2017;35(26):3046–54. https://doi.org/10.1200/JCO.2016.71.9815.
28. Masuda N, Ohtani S, Takano T, et al. A randomized, 3-arm, neoadjuvant, phase 2 study comparing docetaxel + carboplatin + trastuzumab + pertuzumab (TCbHP), TCbHP followed by trastuzumab emtansine and pertuzumab (T-DM1+P), and T-DM1+P in HER2-positive primary breast cancer. Breast Cancer Res Treat. 2020;180(1):135–46. https://doi.org/10.1007/s10549-020-05524-6.
29. von Minckwitz G, Huang CS, Mano MS, et al. Trastuzumab emtansine for residual invasive HER2-positive breast cancer. N Engl J Med. 2019;380(7):617–28. https://doi.org/10.1056/NEJMoa1814017.
30. Marti JLG, Hyder T, Nasrazadani A, Brufsky AM. The evolving landscape of HER2-directed breast cancer therapy. Curr Treat Options Oncol. 2020;21(10):82. Published 2020 Aug 7. https://doi.org/10.1007/s11864-020-00780-6.
31. Rugo HS, Seock-Ah I, Cardoso, et al. Phase 3 SOPHIA study of margetuximab + chemotherapy vs trastuzumab + chemotherapy in patients with HER2+ metastatic breast cancer after prior anti-HER2 therapies: second interim overall survival analysis [abstract]. Presented at the 2019 San Antonio Breast Cancer Symposium, San Antonio, TX, December 10–14, 2019. https://doi.org/10.1158/1538-7445.SABCS19-GS1-02.
32. Bang YJ, Giaccone G, Im SA, et al. First-in-human phase 1 study of margetuximab (MGAH22), an Fc-modified chimeric monoclonal antibody, in patients with HER2-positive advanced solid tumors. Ann Oncol. 2017;28(4):855–61. https://doi.org/10.1093/annonc/mdx002.
33. Krop I. MARGetuximab Or Trastuzumab (MARGOT) (MARGOT). 2020. Available at: https://clinicaltrials.gov/ct2/show/NCT04425018. Accessed January 18, 2021.
34. Modi S, Saura C, Yamashita T, et al. Trastuzumab deruxtecan in previously treated HER2-positive breast cancer. N Engl J Med. 2020;382(7):610–21. https://doi.org/10.1056/NEJMoa1914510.
35. Tsang JY, Au WL, Lo KY, et al. PD-L1 expression and tumor infiltrating PD-1+ lymphocytes associated with outcome in HER2+ breast cancer patients. Breast Cancer Res Treat. 2017;162(1):19–30. https://doi.org/10.1007/s10549-016-4095-2.
36. Müller P, Kreuzaler M, Khan T, et al. Trastuzumab emtansine (T-DM1) renders HER2+ breast cancer highly susceptible to CTLA-4/PD-1 blockade. Sci Transl Med. 2015;7(315):315ra188. https://doi.org/10.1126/scitranslmed.aac4925.
37. Iwata TN, Sugihara K, Wada T, Agatsuma T. [Fam-] trastuzumab deruxtecan (DS-8201a)-induced antitumor immunity is facilitated by the anti-CTLA-4 antibody in a mouse model. PLoS One. 2019;14(10):e0222280. Published 2019 Oct 1. https://doi.org/10.1371/journal.pone.0222280.
38. Emens LA, Esteva FJ, Beresford M, et al. Trastuzumab emtansine plus atezolizumab versus trastuzumab emtansine plus placebo in previously treated, HER2-positive advanced

breast cancer (KATE2): a phase 2, multicentre, randomised, double-blind trial. Lancet Oncol. 2020;21(10):1283–95. https://doi.org/10.1016/S1470-2045(20)30465-4.
39. Koski GK, Koldovsky U, Xu S, et al. A novel dendritic cell-based immunization approach for the induction of durable Th1-polarized anti-HER-2/neu responses in women with early breast cancer. J Immunother. 2012;35(1):54–65. https://doi.org/10.1097/CJI.0b013e318235f512.
40. Lowenfeld L, Zaheer S, Oechsle C, et al. Addition of anti-estrogen therapy to anti-HER2 dendritic cell vaccination improves regional nodal immune response and pathologic complete response rate in patients with ER^{pos}/HER2^{pos} early breast cancer. Oncoimmunology. 2016;6(9):e1207032. Published 2016 Jul 1. https://doi.org/10.1080/2162402X.2016.1207032.
41. Schmid P, Adams S, Rugo HS, et al. Atezolizumab and nab-paclitaxel in advanced triple-negative breast cancer. N Engl J Med. 2018;379(22):2108–21. https://doi.org/10.1056/NEJMoa1809615.
42. Saji S, Mittendorf E, Harbeck N, et al. 3MO IMpassion031: results from a phase III study of neoadjuvant (neoadj) atezolizumab + chemo in early triple-negative breast cancer (TNBC). Ann Oncol. 2020;S1243-7534(20):43197. https://doi.org/10.1016/j.annonc.2020.10.024.
43. Schmid P, Cortes J, Pusztai L, et al. Pembrolizumab for early triple-negative breast cancer. N Engl J Med. 2020;382(9):810–21. https://doi.org/10.1056/NEJMoa1910549.
44. Loibl S, O'Shaughnessy J, Untch M, et al. Addition of the PARP inhibitor veliparib plus carboplatin or carboplatin alone to standard neoadjuvant chemotherapy in triple-negative breast cancer (BrighTNess): a randomised, phase 3 trial. Lancet Oncol. 2018;19(4):497–509. https://doi.org/10.1016/S1470-2045(18)30111-6.
45. Bardia A, Mayer IA, Vahdat LT, et al. Sacituzumab Govitecan-hziy in refractory metastatic triple-negative breast cancer. N Engl J Med. 2019;380(8):741–51. https://doi.org/10.1056/NEJMoa1814213.
46. van der Voort A, Dezentjé VO, van der Steeg WA, et al. Image-guided de-escalation of neoadjuvant chemotherapy in HER2-positive breast cancer: the TRAIN-3 study [abstract]. Presented at the 2018 San Antonio Breast Cancer Symposium, San Antonio, TX, December 4–8, 2018. https://doi.org/10.1158/1538-7445.SABCS18-OT2-07-07.
47. Prat A, Pascual T. Omission of surgery in clinically low-risk HER2positive breast cancer with high HER2 addiction and a complete response following standard anti-HER2-based neoadjuvant therapy (ELPIS). 2020. Available at: https://clinicaltrials.gov/ct2/show/NCT04578106. Accessed on: January 18, 2021.
48. Bennett IC, Saboo A. The evolving role of vacuum assisted biopsy of the breast: a progression from fine-needle aspiration biopsy. World J Surg. 2019;43(4):1054–61. https://doi.org/10.1007/s00268-018-04892-x.
49. van Nijnatten TJA, Simons JM, Smidt ML, et al. A novel less-invasive approach for axillary staging after neoadjuvant chemotherapy in patients with axillary node-positive breast cancer by combining Radioactive Iodine Seed Localization in the Axilla With the Sentinel Node Procedure (RISAS): a Dutch Prospective Multicenter Validation Study. Clin Breast Cancer. 2017;17(5):399–402. https://doi.org/10.1016/j.clbc.2017.04.006.
50. Mamounas EP, Bandos H, White JR. NRG Oncology/NSABP B-51/RTOG 1304: Phase III trial to determine if chest wall and regional nodal radiotherapy (CWRNRT) post mastectomy (Mx) or the addition of RNRT to whole breast RT post breast-conserving surgery (BCS) reduces invasive breast cancer recurrence-free interval (IBCR-FI) in patients (pts) with pathologically positive axillary (PPAx) nodes who are ypN0 after neoadjuvant chemotherapy (NC). J Clin Oncol. 2019;37(15 suppl) https://doi.org/10.1200/JCO.2019.37.15_suppl.TPS600.
51. McDonald BR, Contente-Cuomo T, Sammut SJ, et al. Personalized circulating tumor DNA analysis to detect residual disease after neoadjuvant therapy in breast cancer. Sci Transl Med. 2019;11(504):eaax7392. https://doi.org/10.1126/scitranslmed.aax7392.
52. Garcia-Murillas I, Chopra N, Comino-Méndez I, et al. Assessment of molecular relapse detection in early-stage breast cancer [published correction appears in JAMA Oncol. 2020 Jan 1;6(1):162]. JAMA Oncol. 2019;5(10):1473–8. https://doi.org/10.1001/jamaoncol.2019.1838.

53. Esserman LJ, Berry DA, DeMichele A, et al. Pathologic complete response predicts recurrence-free survival more effectively by cancer subset: results from the I-SPY 1 TRIAL–CALGB 150007/150012, ACRIN 6657. J Clin Oncol. 2012;30(26):3242–9. https://doi.org/10.1200/JCO.2011.39.2779.
54. I-SPY2 Trial Consortium, Yee D, DeMichele AM, et al. Association of event-free and distant recurrence-free survival with individual-level pathologic complete response in neoadjuvant treatment of stages 2 and 3 breast cancer: three-year follow-up analysis for the I-SPY2 adaptively randomized clinical trial. JAMA Oncol. 2020;6(9):1355–62. https://doi.org/10.1001/jamaoncol.2020.2535.

Index

A. Soran, F. Nakhlis (eds.), *Management of the Breast and Axilla in the Neoadjuvant Setting*, https://doi.org/10.1007/978-3-030-88020-0